THE CLINICAL INTERVIEW
USING DSM-III-R

THE
CLINICAL INTERVIEW

USING DSM-III-R

EKKEHARD OTHMER, M.D., PH.D.
SIEGLINDE C. OTHMER, PH.D.

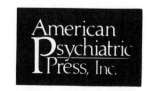

1400 K STREET, N.W.
WASHINGTON, DC 20005

For information about our audio products, write us at:
Newbridge Book Clubs, 3000 Cindel Drive, Delran, NJ 08370

LIBRARY OF CONGRESS
Library of Congress Cataloging-in-Publication Data

Othmer, Ekkehard.
The clinical interview using DSM-III-R / by Ekkehard Othmer,
Sieglinde C. Othmer.
p. cm.
Bibliography: p.
Includes index.
ISBN 0-88048-315-6 (alk. paper)
1. Interviewing in psychiatry.   2. Diagnostic and statistical
manual of mental disorders.   3. Interviewing in psychiatry—Case
studies.   I. Othmer, Sieglinde C.   II. Title.
[DNLM: 1. Interview, Psychological.   WM 141 O87c]
RC480.7.O74 1988
616.89′14—dc19
DNLM/DLC
for Library of Congress   88-16781
CIP

To
Konstantin,
Johann Philipp,
Julia Christie

CONTENTS

CHAPTER 4
FOUR METHODS TO ASSESS MENTAL STATUS 109

LIST OF FIGURES

LIST OF TABLES

ABOUT THE AUTHORS

Ekkehard Othmer, M.D., Ph.D., Professor of Psychiatry at the University of Kansas Medical Center and Medical Director at North Hills Hospital of Kansas City, Missouri, is a member of Psychiatric Institutes of America (PIA). Dr. Othmer is a Diplomate of the American Board of Psychiatry and Neurology and one of its examiners; he is also a fellow of the American Psychiatric Association and a member of the American Medical Association, Society for Neuroscience, American Association for the Psychophysiological Studies of Sleep, Psychiatric Research Society, Society of Biological Psychiatry, and other organizations. Dr. Othmer graduated from the Department of Psychology (Ph.D.) and the Medical School (M.D.) of the University of Hamburg and trained in psychoanalysis at the Psychoanalytic Institute in Hamburg, West Germany. He completed his residency in psychiatry at Renard Hospital, Washington University Medical School, in St. Louis, Missouri.

Sieglinde C. Othmer, Ph.D., is Research Assistant Professor of Psychiatry at the University of Kansas Medical Center, where she is conducting psychotropic investigational drug studies. She is a member of the Society for Clinical Trials and of the Affiliate Staff of Research Psychiatric Center in Kansas City, Missouri. She is the mother of three children. Dr. Othmer studied Romance languages at the Sorbonne in Paris, France, and graduated from the Social Sciences Department of the University of Hamburg, West Germany. She completed a postdoctoral fellowship in genetics at Renard Hospital, Department of Psychiatry at Washington University, in St. Louis, Missouri.

FOREWORD

I read this book with keen interest. Not only because it has DSM-III-R in its title (I had the privilege of being in a leadership role in the development of both DSM-III and DSM-III-R) but also because I have a special interest in teaching clinical interviewing. For almost ten years, I have been teaching a course, on the initial psychiatric interview, to the first-year residents at the New York State Psychiatric Institute. In the course a variety of patients are interviewed, each by both a resident and by me. (The resident and I alternate conducting the first interview, and sometimes one or both interviews are videotaped prior to the class.) In the discussions that follow the interview we attempt to dissect each interview to see what worked, what didn't work, and what alternative strategies either the resident or I could have used that would have made the interview more effective.

The course has always been well received as the students recognize the value of having the opportunity to observe and critically evaluate their own and my interviewing (as well as the interviewing of other senior staff members who help teach the course). However, I have always recognized that with the limited time available (the course is only for about fourteen two-hour sessions), and with the vagaries of patient selection, countless problems encountered in clinical interviewing are never discussed. For that reason I always wished that I could recommend a suitable text that would systematically and comprehensively present the principles of clinical interviewing.

What would be the basic approach of such a text? It would recognize that the clinical interview of a psychiatric patient should have three main goals: to make a tentative psychiatric diagnosis according to DSM-III (and more recently, DSM-III-R), to understand how the patient experiences his difficulties and inner world, and, if possible, to understand what events in the patient's life might have contributed to the current difficulties. Not only are these three goals not incompatible, but they should supplement and complement each other. I am much more confident about a DSM-III-R diagnosis of a major depressive episode if, in addition to information about symptoms included in the diagnostic criteria, I also have information from my interview that the patient experiences his world as empty, his difficulties as overwhelming and his future as bleak, and that the onset of the current difficulties followed an event that was a blow to his self-esteem or reactivated a longstanding inner conflict.

There have been many books (and even more chapters in psychiatric texts) that focus on teaching clinical interviewing. However, none have seemed to me to be successful in the difficult task of integrating these three goals of the clinical interview in a book that is comprehensive, full of examples of clinical interviews (some very good, and some, for illustrative purposes, very, very bad), and fun to read. That is why, as I started to read this book I had two thoughts. The first was that this *is* the kind of book that I have always wished I could recommend to the residents in my interviewing course. The second was that I wished I had written such a book myself!

ROBERT L. SPITZER, M.D.

PREFACE

This book is written for you, the curious person. You have opened this book—mental health professional or layman—because you want to know how to interview, or how to do it better and to compare notes with us.

If you are a medical student on your psychiatric rotation, you are often asked to read books that teach you the nature of psychiatric symptoms and signs. This book will tell you how to assess them.

If you are a psychology student, you learn about abnormal psychology—the psychodynamic, the behavioral, and the descriptive approaches. Here is the book that shows you how to integrate and apply them diagnostically.

If you are a social worker and have seen the impact of stress on your patients and discussed their problems with them, here is the book that can help you to deepen your rapport and to progress to a diagnosis.

If you are a nurse, here is a book that helps you to understand your patients with mental problems better.

If you are a resident and struggle through your psychiatric interviews, because they seem too long, too short, unproductive, or overwhelming, here are some strategies that may improve your interviews.

If you are an old hand at interviewing, and are familiar with psychodynamic methods, and want to catch up with the symptom-oriented approach and with descriptive diagnosis, we have summarized for you what we have learned from some of the masters in the field.

If you are in practice now, you may have expected to learn better interviewing by experience and maybe you did. However, some practitioners have complained to us that interviewing skills were never taught to them and that it is difficult to acquire them in practice. If you share this complaint, here is a book that will help you now.

If you feel that our field is split among the psychodynamic and the descriptive approach, this book attempts to bridge the split. We try to combine the description of symptoms and signs with their interpretation. Therefore, this book reaches beyond descriptive or psychodynamic psychiatry.

If you are one of the born interviewers, then you are the right critic for this book. You will notice our shortcomings; if so, we invite you to write us to tell us how we can improve this text in the future. We extend this invitation to all of you, our interested readers.

Now to the book itself. Some residents have asked us what is the best way to use this book. It is best to start at the beginning and read through to the end because all chapters are designed to complement each other. While you read, use both the DSM-III-R glossary and the glossary in this book which expands on some terms of the DSM-III-R glossary and contains those terms not at all or insufficiently defined in DSM-III-R. You will notice that in the text we have not defined most of the terms because our book focuses not so much on what certain symptoms and signs are, but on how to assess them. Our book does not describe the nature of interviewing, but how to do it.

Before you begin to read please note that this book is about interviewing female as well as male patients. However, the interviewers as well as individual patients are usually referred to in the male gender, since this is the convention in books about both sexes.

EKKEHARD OTHMER
SIEGLINDE C. OTHMER

ACKNOWLEDGMENTS

Our residents sharpened our clinical skills by giving us feedback to our teaching, and our patients gave us understanding of their disorders—we thank them.

Some of our colleagues read sections in various stages of completion and donated significant time and thought to this task. We are indebted to Gerald L. Klerman, M.D.; Arnold M. Ludwig, M.D.; Donald W. Goodwin, M.D.; William V. McKnelly, Jr., M.D.; Elizabeth C. Penick, Ph.D.; Janice Downey, M.D.; Cherilyn M. Desouza, M.D.; William F. Gabrielli, Jr., M.D., Ph.D.; Kevin M. Passer, M.D.; Karen S. Ritchie, M.D.; and Jean Pintar, M.D.

Many thanks to many readers: Elena Gragasin, M.D.; Thomas B. Hall III, M.D.; Eve Hohly, M.D.; Cheryl Holle, M.D.; Linda Keeler, M.D.; Martha Krenn, M.D.; William Levine, M.D.; Barry Liskow, M.D.; Jarek Opechowski, M.D.; Marsha Read, Ph.D.; and John H. Wisner, M.D.

We also thank Marijo Teare, Mary Ellen Vincent, and Christy Stocks for their cheerful criticisms during the many stages of the manuscript.

We thank Donna Simpson for her patience in the countless hours of typing and retyping of the numerous drafts.

We are in debt to our editor at New York University Press, Kitty Moore. She initiated the writing of this book and gave us encouragement. Gently she guided us with constructive ideas concerning organization and design decisions.

Thanks to the initiative of Robert L. Spitzer, M.D., and the support by Allen J. Frances, M.D., this book became a cooperative effort between two publishing houses, New York University Press and American Psychiatric Press.

Dr. Spitzer read the book cover to cover, pointed out weaknesses and suggested how to fix them. He pinpointed flaws, some of which we had tried to overlook. In that sense, he did both a diagnostic and a therapeutic job on us. Also, he drove home the point that the busiest people have the most time when it comes to the important stuff. Thanks, Bob.

Last, but not least, we thank Despina Gimbel, the managing editor of New York University Press and Ann Hirst, the manuscript editor, who scrutinized language and outlay so graciously.

CHAPTER ONE

PROLOGUE: FRAMEWORK

1. Insight- and Symptom-Oriented Interviewing

2. The Four Components

3. The Multiphasic Approach

4. Disorder-Specific Interviewing

SUMMARY

Chapter 1 provides framework and rationale of descriptive psychodiagnostic interviewing. It compares the psychodynamic, insight-oriented interview with the descriptive, symptom-oriented interview and shows their integration.

The interview takes place in four dimensions and therefore has four components: rapport, techniques, mental status, and diagnosing. This interviewing process usually progresses through seven phases. When the patient's pathology interferes with this process, the interviewer has to modify his strategies.

Insanity, even in its mildest forms, involves the greatest suffering that the physicians have to meet.

Emil Kraepelin
Lectures on Clinical Psychiatry, 2d ed., 1906

In 1980, a change in direction took place in American psychiatry. With the publication of the third edition of the *Diagnostic and Statistical Manual of Mental Disorders* (DSM-III), the American Psychiatric Association acknowledged a return to descriptive, atheoretical psychiatry as modeled by Emil Kraepelin. This "neo-Kraepelinian" movement had begun in the 1960s in the Department of Psychiatry at Washington University, under the leadership of Eli Robins, Samuel Guze, and George Winokur.

A look at the definition of depression in DSM-II and DSM-III clarifies this change in concept. DSM-II propagates psychological etiology; it follows a Freudian concept: "Depressive Neurosis . . . is manifested by an excessive reaction of depression due to an internal conflict or to an identifiable event such as the loss of a love object or cherished possession."

DSM-III and DSM-III-R, following Emil Kraepelin, give a menu of signs and symptoms; any assumption of etiology has vanished.

This descriptive approach does not invalidate previous concepts but rather cautions against determining etiology too easily. It restricts itself to classification, prognosis, family history, and epidemiology, all elements empirically verifiable. It is, however, compatible with both a biological and psychological etiology of psychiatric disorders as visualized by Freud.

1. INSIGHT- AND SYMPTOM-ORIENTED INTERVIEWING

The change in concepts of psychiatric illness from DSM-II to DSM-III (and, since 1987, also DSM-III-R) necessitates a change in interviewing styles used by mental health professionals today: from an *insight-oriented (psychodynamic)* to a *symptom-oriented (descriptive)* style. Let us compare in detail both styles, their respective underlying *concept of illness, goal* and *method* of interviewing.

Insight-oriented interviewing originates from the concept that deep-seated, often infantile conflicts become chronic pathogens of the mind which interfere with the patient's actions, distort his perceptions, and lead to symptoms, maladjusted behavior, and suffering.

Insight-oriented interviewing attempts to uncover these unconscious conflicts and bring them to the patient's awareness, with the expectation that he may resolve them. The patient often resists this unraveling by using what have been termed "unconscious defense mechanisms."

The methods used by the insight-oriented interviewer are as follows: he interprets the patient's free associations and dreams; he detects his anxieties, confronts him with his interpersonal behavior toward the therapist and others, identifies defenses and analyzes the patient's resistance to the discussion of his conflicts. He pursues such an interview with the dual purpose of diagnosis and therapy.

Sigmund Freud (1856–1939) developed both the psychodynamic theory of psychiatric illness and the methods of insight-oriented interviewing (Freud 1952–1955). Over the last one hundred years, other investigators have elaborated on this concept and established its place in psychiatry (here are some authors: Adler 1964; Berne 1964; Dubois 1913; Erikson 1969; Horney 1939; Jaspers 1962; Jung 1971; Klein 1952; Masserman 1955; Menninger 1958; Meyer 1957; Rado 1956; Rank 1952; Reich 1949; Rogers 1951; Sullivan 1954; Wolberg 1967).

In contrast, *symptom-oriented interviewing* originates from the concept that psychiatric disorders manifest themselves in a characteristic set of signs, symptoms and behaviors, a predictable course, a somewhat specific treatment response and often a familial occurrence (DSM-III-R 1987). As twin and adoption studies show, heredity as well as learning may contribute to this observed familial occurrence (Goodwin and Guze 1984).

We do not know all etiological factors which contribute to the manifestation of these disorders. Investigators have identified some biological and psychological components but these findings are insufficient to classify these disorders by etiology. Therefore, classification is based on clinical criteria rather than underlying (assumed) pathology (Ludwig and Othmer 1977; Akiskal and Webb 1978).

The goal of symptom-oriented interviewing is to classify the patient's complaints and dysfunctions according to defined diagnostic categories (by criteria in DSM-III/ III-R). Such a diagnosis predicts the future course (prognosis) and helps to select empirically the most effective treatment— but does not allow conclusions about its causes.

The method of the symptom-oriented interviewer is to observe the patient's behavior and to motivate him to describe his problems in detail. The interviewer translates his perception into symptoms and signs for a descriptive diagnosis (DSM-III-R axis I and II). He includes the evaluation of the patient's adjustment and coping skills, his personal way of dealing with his disorder, and an assessment of the patient's medical conditions, social circumstances, and environmental stressors.

Manifestations of the same disorder vary from patient to patient, as do coping mechanisms and treatment responses. Furthermore, comorbidity of major psychiatric and personality disorders and the impact of medical disorders, life stressors, and interpersonal conflicts complicate psychosocial adjustment and prognosis. To acknowledge these factors, the symptom-oriented interviewer incorporates developmental and personality disorders (axis II), physical disorders and conditions (axis III), severity of psychosocial stressors (axis IV), and global assessment of functioning (axis V) in a multiaxial diagnosis.

Goals and methods of this descriptive type of interview have been pursued over the last 3,000 years by physicians of all medical specialties. In psychiatry, this tradition is exemplified in the work of Emil Kraepelin (1856–1926), and of his contemporaries, followers, and critics (Kleist 1928; Leonhard 1979). Since 1980, several books have been published which approach psychiatric interviewing from such a descriptive point of view (Leon 1982; Hersen and Turner 1985; MacKinnon and Yudofsky 1986).

In summary, the insight and symptom-oriented interviews serve different goals in psychiatry and psychology. The insight-oriented interview with an interpretative approach, *explains* signs, symptoms, and behaviors. The symptom-oriented interview with a descriptive approach *classifies* signs and symptoms into disorder categories.

Both approaches are compatible. Mental health professionals seem to agree that they can best understand the patient's personality, conflicts, and problems of living by a psychodynamic approach but that major psychiatric and personality disorders are best assessed by the descriptive method. A synthesis of interpretation and description can bridge the different points of departure.

An interviewer may use both types of interviewing in a two-step fashion. He assumes that a patient may have both major psychiatric and personality disorders and unconscious conflicts. He may diagnose major psychiatric and personality disorders according to DSM-III-R axis I and II by means of a symptom-oriented interview. If, after treatment, interpersonal conflicts persist or surface, he may switch to an insight-oriented interview as a second step, thus complementing his symptom-oriented interview.

Indeed, you can often observe an interaction between both interpersonal conflicts and psychiatric disorders. Psychiatric disorders may revive and magnify existing, or evoke new interpersonal conflicts, while preexisting conflicts may trigger the outbreak or aggravate the course of psychiatric disorders.

E. Bleuler was the first prominent psychiatrist to integrate the two approaches which he did in 1916 (Bleuler 1972). Many psychiatrists followed this integrative approach under the label of eclectic psychiatry. A clearly separated, two-step approach assures appropriately tailoring the interview to the patient's needs.

There Is a Place for Both Methods

The following case report illustrates the two-step method, with description first and interpretation second.

Georgia is a 36-year-old, white single female who has been in treatment for the last six years. Diagnostically, she fulfilled DSM-III-R criteria for major depression, delusional (paranoid) disorder and obsessive compulsive disorder. A worsening of her affective disorder intensified both obsessive compulsive symptoms and persecutory ideas but a remission of the depression was not associated with a remission of either the obsessive compulsive or the delusional (paranoid) disorder. She was functioning professionally but was single and socially isolated. Her symptoms improved with a combination of amitriptyline and thiothixine. Since her persecutory ideas were improved, thiothixine was slowly discontinued to lower the risk of tardive dyskinesia and to respond to the patient's complaint that she felt less alert and lively on thiothixine. Lately, she had lost her job because her company transferred to another city.

She found a new job with a mail order business where she had to correct purchase orders on a computer screen that had the errors highlighted. She loved this type of work and was very proficient and fast in her corrections. Within the first few weeks she managed to make up to 8,000 corrections a day.

Serendipitously, she detected that some of the frames had more than one area highlighted. She realized that she had outperformed her colleagues by working on the false assumption of only one error per frame. She was devastated. She calculated that she literally had messed up thousands of orders, that she possibly had caused irreparable harm to her company—all due to her character flaw of wanting to be the best.

For a few days she concealed the error and continued her routine. Then, she felt she could not take it any more and stayed home from work without notifying her employer. Her supervisor called her, she admitted her mistake, and was grateful that the supervisor did not make a major point out of her failure. Georgia worked for two days, each day looking forward to her job. On the third day, she took some pizzas to work for everybody to express her gratitude.

That afternoon, one of her colleagues walked up to her and said: "Don't you have to cool off your fingers?" and repeated this remark at another occasion. Georgia was shocked. She started to ruminate about this remark. Then she noticed that the number of purchase orders that she had to pick up from a front window was only a tenth of the usual amount—forcing her to interrupt her work frequently, to leave her terminal, walk to the window and pick up a new set of orders. On her way there, she could not help but notice that all other thirty employees in the room typed very slowly, nearly like in a rhythm—tap—tap—tap, and there was no chitchat at all, just tap—tap—tap.

Immediately, she understood what was going on. The small amount of purchase orders were placed there to distract her from her work, so that she had to notice the slow typing, giving her the message:

"You messed up, we have to do your work, slow down so that you don't mess up again."

She realized letting her come back to work was an evil plot to punish her for her failure. Every tap was a condemnation, a revenge for what she had done.

She returned to her work station in tears. They had gotten her good. And she deserved it. It was so mean and cruel, yet so clever. If anybody knew how to torture her, they did.

The next day, she did not report to work and was fired.

Here is how the interviewer uses a two-step approach with this patient.

Step 1: The phenomenological part in Georgia's evaluation is straight-forward. She had persecutory delusions in the past. At times, they were associated with vegetative symptoms of depression and dysphoric mood, never with hallucinations. Since the neuroleptic was discontinued when she became unemployed, she relapsed and the persecutory delusions returned. Georgia's clinical picture again fulfilled criteria for delusional (paranoid) disorder (DSM-III-R 297.10). Treatment with thiothixine was reinstated.

Step 2: We chose an acute psychodynamic, interpretative intervention when Georgia made an appointment and reported the above described problem. Here is a segment of this portion of the interview.

1. I: You went through quite an ordeal.
   P: Isn't it awful? I don't understand how human beings can do that to one another.

2. I: I agree. It is a merciless torture.
   P: I don't understand it. They all seemed so nice, and I really liked my supervisor. He let me come back and he was not down on me at all. I don't understand why he did this to me.

3. I: But it was not him who has done it; it was not them.
   P: (Excited, panicky.) But Dr. O., what do you mean? I just told you what they did to me. How can you say it was not them?

4. I: Because it was you . . . You did it yourself. You thought you deserved that punishment for the big crime you committed. And when the punishment did not come, you brought it on yourself.
   P: (More excited.) But Dr. O. you don't believe me—you were my last hope, you are my only friend—and you don't believe me . . .

5. I: I believe everything you told me. Most of your observations were right. What I have problems with is your interpretations, what you think it all means.
   P: (With slightly lower, less pressed voice.) But how do you explain what the fellow said about my hot fingers, and that they all typed so slowly?

6. I: I don't know. But let me ask you a few questions. Since you worked there, how many new people started in that month?
   P: Six out of thirty.

7. I: You see, in a job like yours there is a high turnover. How do you think a supervisor would get everybody together to type slowly just to punish you? How do you think he'll get that kind of cooperation? They all would think, "if they do it to Georgia, they'll do it to me too." (I. uses Georgia's own persecutory tendencies to break through her delusional beliefs.)
   P: I thought about that on the way home that night, but then I thought no, no—it was all too real.

8. I: Yes, it is real. You have no way of telling that it isn't. And you are right. You made a mistake, and the supervisor made a mistake of not catching your mistake, and I made a mistake of stopping the Navane which would

have helped you to tell apart what is going on on the outside and on your inside. So we all made mistakes. Let's try to correct what we can. I'll give you a new prescription. In a few weeks those things won't happen to you any more.

P: (Shakes her head.) Doctor O., I can't believe that you think I'm that paranoid.

9. I: I know you can't. And I don't expect you to believe what I told you. You may even think I'm in with them too.

P: Yes, that crossed my mind. I thought they had talked to you.

10. I: Yes, that happens. You can't think any differently.

P: (Less intense.) They really did it.

11. I: Do you want to call the supervisor right now?

P: But Dr. O., they would never admit it.

12. I: Would they not just talk to you about your mistake, rather than punishing you like this?

P: Hmm . . . I would think . . .

13. I: Is there anything that would convince you?

P: Yeah . . . if they pay me. Of course, they will not pay me for what I did.

14. I: If they pay you, that will tell you that it might have been you who did the torturing. . . . No matter what, here is a prescription and I want you to start with your medicine now.

Comment: The patient called her company to find out whether there was a check for her which there was. She apologized to the supervisor. At the next visit with me, one week later and back on the neuroleptic:

P: It is terrible how paranoid I am. It still feels real.

I: It will be over soon when the medicine works fully—and we will not stop it again. I apologize for my mistake. It cost you your job.

This case demonstrates the two-step approach. Step 1: Georgia had long-standing symptoms qualifying her for a diagnosis of delusional (paranoid) disorder (DSM-III-R), a diagnosis which may predict return of symptoms when the neuroleptic is stopped.

Step 2: This case also shows that Georgia has a strong punative superego which will punish her when she fails, intentionally or not. A psychodynamic interpretation can explain the content of her delusion to her; however, it cannot remove her tendency to form delusions around stressful or everyday events, when off neuroleptics.

Do not misconstrue this example to mean that the content of every delusion should or can be interpreted, or that the way this case was handled should be considered as a model. The interpretation as presented was intended to give the patient some relief and to motivate her to take medicine again.

Moreover, this type of aggressive interpretation should not be attempted in a first-time interview, with a patient whom the therapist does not know.

This book describes a systematic approach to phenomenological interviewing in psychiatry (step 1). However, our approach is not pure, because it includes a descriptive approach to transference patterns in chapter 2 (Rapport), and defense mechanisms in chapter 3 (Techniques), and chapter 4 (Mental Status) to interface with psychodynamic interviewing (Vaillant 1986).

2. THE FOUR COMPONENTS

The new emphasis on phenomenology requires a fresh look at the interviewing techniques to go along with the new interviewing goal (if one follows DSM-III-R): assessment of signs and symptoms in a psychodiagnostic interview.

A useful comparison to this technique is the way in which twentieth-century artists began to portray the human face and figure. Pablo Picasso's 1957 portrait of Sylvette which hangs in the Chicago Art Institute (Gedo 1980) shows this innovation. Picasso portrayed the woman from all sides: the front, the side and the back, all simultaneously. He gives a "total" picture, a "stereo view" for a comprehensive representation of the persona.

A psychodiagnostic interview requires a similar approach. You see a patient in four dimensions: in his rapport with you; in his response to your interviewing techniques (to get all the data you need and to keep the interview flowing); in his mental status; and in the signs and symptoms of his disorder(s) as they unfold during the interviewing process. You have to keep track of these four components throughout the interview.

Both the insight and the symptom-oriented interview operate in similar dimensions of a four-prong approach.

Rapport: Rapport refers to how the interviewer and his patient relate. Establishing rapport is equally important for the reporter who in an interview chases the four W's—what—where—when—why—as for the businessman who wants to sell his product and has to recognize the customer's needs. Both types of psychodiagnostic interviewing emphasize the importance of establishing, monitoring, and maintaining this rapport. The insight-oriented interview conceptualizes rapport in terms of *transference and countertransference patterns,* thus looking for repetitions of previous infantile relationships in the interview situation. The descriptive approach describes rapport as *patient-interviewer interaction* which progresses from understanding to trust.

Technique: This refers to the methods used by interviewers to establish rapport and to obtain information. Interviewers take pride in theirs. Barbara Walters, the TV host, for instance, wrote a book on "How to talk to anybody about anything." Techniques range from open-ended questions to confrontation, and from interpretation to interrogation.

Both insight and descriptive interviewing emphasize technique, but refer to different methods. The insight-oriented interview uses techniques which uncover unconscious conflicts, such as free association, confrontation, and interpretation, while the descriptive interview stresses techniques that are geared toward the assessment of symptoms, signs, behaviors, and psychological dysfunctions.

Mental Status: This refers to the shape the patient is in while you talk to him. Is he clear or fuzzy in his answers, quick-witted or slow in remembering, pleasant or angry, open or suspicious and concealing, reality-oriented or full of strange and bizarre ideas? This is the same for the insight or symptom-oriented interviewer. He monitors psychological and psychosocial functioning during the interview and recognizes its importance. The descriptive interviewer describes and focuses on dimensions of functions such as psychomotor behavior, speech and thinking, affect, mood, thought content, memory, orientation, insight and judgment, while the insight-oriented interviewer goes beyond the description of these functional disturbances and identifies underlying defense mechanisms.

Diagnosing: The fourth component sounds like something unique to the psychodiagnostic interview. Not quite. It refers to just the special subject matter. Any interview has some central focus. The more the interviewer knows about a subject matter the better he will succeed with his interview. In the psychodiagnostic interview the subject matter is the patient's strengths, weaknesses, and suffering. As in a TV interview, the more the interviewer knows about the subject matter, the more he discovers—the more the health professional knows about the disorder, stressors, and coping skills, the better he can assess them.

Both types of interviews pursue diagnosis but they follow different routes. The insight-oriented interview identifies conflicts and unconsciously directed behavior patterns for a psychodynamic formulation, while the symptom-oriented interview strives to collect a set of symptoms and signs which fit diagnostic criteria of categorical disorders.

Chapters 2 through 5 describe separately the four components of the symptom-oriented, descriptive, psychodiagnostic interview. This dissecting approach to interviewing is similar to the medical school approach to the human body; the same organ system is repeatedly described under the aspects of anatomy, histology, physiology, and biochemistry. Obviously, anatomy, histology, physiology, and biochemistry of the organs do not exist independently from each other. On the contrary, they are one in nature, just different aspects of the same organ system to study, teach, research, and understand the body and its organs and treat its disorders. Similarly interconnected are rapport, assessment techniques, mental status examination, and diagnosing, but for heuristic purposes they will be separately treated.

Interviewing a patient can be compared to two people assembling a puzzle, where the patient has the pieces and the interviewer the image of the completed design.

1. Both must be willing to do it together—rapport.
2. The interviewer must know how to get the right pieces from the patient—he asks him for them, and assembles small sections—which requires assessment techniques.
3. The interviewer has to inspect and move all pieces in front of him continuously—mental status.
4. The interviewer constantly compares with the design what he has put together to see which pieces are still missing—diagnosis.

3. THE MULTIPHASIC APPROACH

All interviewing is a process in time. Most books on interviewing, both psychodynamic and descriptive, divide the interview into three phases: an opening, a middle and an end (MacKinnon and Michels 1971). These phases differ in their respective goals.

In the *opening phase* the interviewer warms up the patient, establishes rapport, and prepares the patient for the main task of the interview.

In the *middle phase* he performs the bulk of the work; therefore it takes the longest time. Some subdivide this phase further to emphasize the shift of interviewing goals. So do we. Obviously, such divisions are arbitrary but of heuristic value.

In the *end phase* the interviewer prepares the patient for the closure. He avoids highly emotional topics, summarizes for the patient what has been learned, and provides an outlook for the future.

We have subdivided the middle phase into four sections and the end phase into two. Thus, counting the opening phase, our standard interview consists of seven phases. The seven phases and their integration with the four components of the interview (see figure 1.1) are described in chapter 6 and illustrated by an edited taped interview in chapter 7.

In your own interviews you will often deviate from such an order of phases because you follow the patient's leads and jump back and forth among phases. Yet, interviewing is easier when you know the order as the default option.

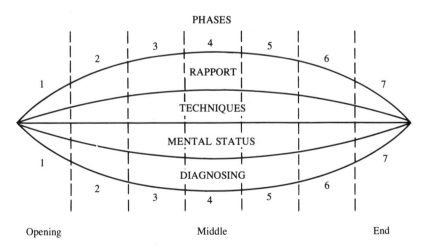

FIGURE 1.1
The seven phases of the standard interview

4. DISORDER-SPECIFIC INTERVIEWING

If a patient is difficult, the skilled interviewer changes his strategies. How else can he get through to the patient or client? What about those who don't understand that you want to help them? Who won't talk? Whether you dig for conflicts or collect symptoms, the patient's shyness, withdrawal, or hostility may get in your way. Thus, the patient's pathology may obstruct a standard approach that you use with the cooperative patient (chapter 7). You have to adjust your interviewing strategies to the patient's behavior typical for his illness. Chapters 8 and 9 describe how to do that for some major psychiatric and personality disorders.

In the chapters that follow, we first show you the general strategies of interviewing, and then their modification for selected disorders. Throughout the book, you can use two measuring sticks to judge the quality of your interviewing technique: short- and long-term outcome.

In the short term, see whether the patient gets involved in the interviewing process and provides useful and spontaneous information. If so, your approach is obviously productive.

In the long term, if your patient returns after the initial interview, cooperates with your treatment, and improves in his functioning, your approach was obviously effective.

CHAPTER TWO

STRATEGIES FOR RAPPORT

1. **Put the Patient and Yourself at Ease**
   Recognize Signs
   Respond to Signs

2. **Find the Suffering—Show Compassion**
   Assess the Suffering
   Respond with Empathy

3. **Assess Insight—Become an Ally**
   Levels of Insight
   Split off the Sick
   Set Therapeutic Goals

4. **Show Expertise**
   Put the Illness into Perspective
   Show Knowledge
   Deal with Distrust

5. **Establish Authority**

6. **Balance the Roles (Transferences)**
   The Empathic Listener
   The Expert
   The Authority
   Carrier of an Illness
   The Sufferer
   The "VIP"

Role Interaction
Dependence on the Interviewer's Authority

SUMMARY

The first component of the interview, rapport, is dissected into six strategies: 1. Putting the patient and yourself at ease, 2. finding the pain and expressing compassion, 3. evaluating the patient's insight and becoming his ally, 4. showing expertise to the patient, 5. establishing authority as a therapist, and 6. balancing the roles in the therapeutic setting.

30 . . . A certain man went down from Jerusalem to Jericho, and fell among thieves, which stripped him of his raiment, and wounded him, and departed, leaving him half dead.

31 And by chance there came down a certain priest that way: and when he saw him, he passed by on the other side.

32 And likewise a Levite, when he was at the place, came and looked on him, and passed by on the other side.

33 But a certain Samaritan, as he journeyed, came where he was: and when he saw him, he had *compassion* on him,

34 And went to him, and bound up his wounds, pouring in oil and wine, and set him on his own beast, and brought him to an inn, and took care of him.

35 And on the morrow when he departed, he took out two pence, and gave them to the host, and said unto him, Take care of him; and whatsoever thou spendest more, when I come again, I will repay thee . . .

37 . . . And then said Jesus . . . , Go, and do thou likewise.

The Holy Bible, King James
Version, Luke 10:30–37

Arleen, a white female in her late twenties, sits tensely on the edge of a chair in the emergency room. She is wearing a light blue dress; her short brown hair is well groomed; she is skillfully made up. She clings to her mother who is standing next to her. Before the interviewer can introduce himself, Arleen shouts with a quivering voice:

P: My mother wants me to talk to a psychiatrist. She thinks I'm getting sick again. Do I have to talk to you? (Patient holds on to her mother's arm.)

I: (With a soft voice.) I need to know more about you before I can answer that.

P: (Shouting.) Oh, you are all alike! You are all in with my husband. I knew it before. (She gets up, ready to run out of the room.)

I: Arleen, don't you think you have suffered enough? (Arleen hesitates and looks back at the interviewer.) I want to help you. (Patient makes one step back towards the interviewer.) I want you to come back . . . As soon as you are ready . . . (Patient proceeds slowly towards the door.) Please think about it . . . (Patient looks back.) I know you want to leave now, but I want you to call me.

P: (Patient hesitates and looks back to her mother.)
I: Your mother will be out in a minute, . . . if you would like to wait outside.

The patient leaves the emergency room; her mother looks puzzled. The interviewer asks her whether Arleen has talked about suicide, or heard voices, or abused street drugs. The mother denies these things but says that Arleen is afraid to be locked up again.

The interviewer explains that he sensed Arleen's panic and that he let her go to put her more at ease. Once her anxiety about being locked up has abated, she may recall his compassion.

The mother agrees to take her home but is surprised, since her daughter had been committed twice before on a similar occasion. "I think Arleen clings to you. You should not have any problems bringing her back," the interviewer explains, "maybe we can get her cooperation; I expect her back on her own."

The interviewer asks the mother whether commitment had worked. "For a while, Arleen did not talk about her husband controlling her mind, but when she was back home, she did not take her medication," the mother replied. "That's my point," the interviewer answered, "sometimes you cannot avoid force, but once you start with it, it's more difficult to regain cooperation. Since your daughter is not suicidal or violent, I like to entice her to return on her own. Her fear of her husband controlling her mind may help." The mother reluctantly agrees to take her daughter home.

What had happened?

The interviewer let the patient go to gain her cooperation; he applied the first strategy for rapport: *Putting the patient at ease.*

Most patients do not come to see us if they do not suffer. The interviewer addressed Arleen's suffering; he applied the second strategy of rapport: *Show compassion.*

By attending to her suffering the interviewer initiated also the split between Arleen's healthy and sick part which will become the object of therapy. Thus, he applied the third strategy of rapport: *Become an ally* (of the healthy part).

He promised help which implies expertise; thus he used the fourth strategy of rapport: *Show expertise.*

He asked her to come back when she was ready; he used the fifth strategy of rapport: *Show authority.*

He allowed her to leave instead of sedating or committing her; he avoided an authoritarian role and allowed her to decide for herself (even though it takes more time in the short but hopefully not in the long run). He responded to her suspiciousness with permissiveness, thus applying the sixth strategy of rapport: *Balance the roles.*

That very afternoon, Arleen called and asked when she could come back. The six strategies had established rapport "on the run." In this chapter we will explore these and other strategies for establishing rapport.

1. PUT THE PATIENT AND YOURSELF AT EASE

The first-time psychiatric patient is often skeptical, apprehensive, and anxious. He overcame the stigma to see a mental health professional, but the taboo about psychiatric or psychological problems lingers in him and troubles him. He is unsure of the people who take care of such matters; he does not know what to expect. He rarely verbalizes what plagues him before the visit:

"Will he listen to me?"
"Will he really understand what I'm telling him?"
"Will he care for me?"
"Will he respect or ridicule me?"
"Will he be able to help me?"
"Can I trust him enough to follow his advice?"

It is your job to convey that you sense these doubts, that you are on his side, respecting him and his concerns and trying to help him—then he will hear an internal all-clear signal and you can carefully initiate rapport with him. But if his fears and hopes are ignored, reservation and frustration will prevail.

When the patient arrives, it is often best to put him at ease by requesting basic information (see also chapter 4.2: Conversation). First, you introduce yourself and ask him for his name and its proper pronunciation. Find out whether he prefers to be addressed by his first or last name. Some authorities recommend to always use the last name to show respect. They argue since the patient usually addresses you with your last name (often with a Dr. in front of it), you should do the same. For many patients this is awkward, creates distance, and raises anxiety.

True, some patients feel compelled to offer you a first name, when they actually prefer a last name. There is no quick way to find that out for sure. Therefore, when you ask, you show that you don't make decisions for him but that you take his wishes into account. One compromise is the southern custom of addressing an older woman as "Miss Edna Joyce" which is less formal yet still respectful.

The numerous interview vignettes that will follow use either first or last names according to the patient's wishes. With patients who seem dependent, very anxious, or psychotic you may skip that ritual (like we did with Arleen).

You may also want to engage the patient in small talk. You might ask how he found out about you, and how he found his way to your office. Hemingway probably put it best—know a man's dialect. Failing that, try to get him to talk of his area of geographical origin, where he was raised, and any common knowledge you might have of places or occupations familiar and comfortable to him.

During this interlude, you can note whether he indeed settles down as you expect him to do, or whether he becomes more tense. Some patients with an anxiety disorder, for instance, may want to get to the point, i.e., their problems; some obsessive patients may figure that they waste time, i.e., money, by beating around the bush.

How do you know what to do when? By reading the patient's signals.

Recognize Signs

The moment you meet a new patient, his mental state may be signaled by a sign. A sign is the nonverbal language of the body often hard to control. It tells you the patient's feelings without words. You can deal with such sign here and now to put the patient at ease and to reassure him that he did the right thing to come and see you. Initiate rapport by reading his signs. They are of different nature:

1. territorial (locomotor)
2. behavioral (psychomotor)
3. emotional (expressive) and
4. verbal.

When he comes in, notice how he moves into the new territory—your office. If he is timid he avoids coming close to you. He shies away from shaking hands. He takes a seat by the door. Your desk becomes a barrier, physical and emotional.

In contrast, the intrusive patient gets too close to you. He may expose you to his breath, spit, loud voice, or the touch of his hands.

His psychomotor fits his locomotor behavior. The timid patient looks down in his lap, avoiding eye contact. The intrusive patient may fiddle with your pencils, rearrange the furniture, turn on your computer, or put his feet on your desk.

Emotional signs surface in the patient's posture, gestures, facial expression, eye contact, and tone of voice. He may walk in with erect posture, chin up, full of energy, or stooped and slowed down. He may smile or look tense, avoiding your eyes. His voice may be quivering or barking. There may be tears.

A patient gives verbal signals about his mental state by the choice of his words.

Pick up his vocabulary, especially his metaphors. He may represent his problems in a visual, kinesthetic, auditory, or more abstract way. Here are examples:

Visual:
"There is no light at the end of the tunnel."
"Everything looks bleak."
"No silver lining."
"Can't see the way out."

Kinesthetic:
"I feel trapped."
"I feel pushed to the wall."
"I'm dead-headed."
"Feels like I'm paralyzed."
"Everything is closing in."
"It's like walking through quicksand."

Auditory:
"There is a constant buzz in my head."
"Everything sounds far away."
"I feel like screaming."

Abstract:
"Feeling depressed."
"Unable to concentrate."

"Confused thinking."
"Less energy than usual."
"No initiative."
"Anxious."
"Getting hypomanic."
"Feeling guilty."

When a patient uses visual, kinesthetic, auditory, or abstract language, pick it up initially. If he says, for instance: "There is no light at the end of the tunnel," ask him, "Since when did things look so dark?" Try to continue his metaphor (Cameron-Bandler 1978). This gives him the feeling you are on the same wave length with him, that you understand and accept him.

To comfort the patient, decode his signals which express his state of mind.

Respond to Signs

The four types of signs—territorial, behavioral, emotional, and verbal—hit you at once. You get an immediate impression. Your patient may be tense, anxious, aggressive, overbearing, elated, depressed, or relaxed. There are different ways of responding to signs.

In the early stages of the interview, you may want to simply observe these signs. You may decide to give the patient space and time—to express himself more—and relax. But you *always* monitor his signs. They are part of his mental status and give you clues for the diagnosis.

In some instances, you may want to alert him to his signs. If you draw his attention to them and discuss their meaning, you may use them as a lead into diagnosing.

In many cases it is best to respond in kind, with or without reflecting on them. This response is often the most effective. For example, you can respond territorially to territorial signals. If your patient avoids you, remain standing, move slowly toward him. Show him you are concerned about his well-being and make inviting gestures. With an anxious patient, who has come accompanied by a family member, you might invite the escort to join. If a patient is intrusive, you can reestablish distance. Your response to intrusion of your personal space can determine whether you stay in control. Make a gesture that stops his advance and follow up verbally.

"Why don't you sit down over there. That way we can talk more comfortably."

While not every interview situation requires strict delineation of boundary lines, their absence can create serious problems, as the following example indicates.

Dr. L. is a 40-year-old, small-framed, oriental psychiatrist who looks younger than his age. He is well trained in his field, but timid. He lets patients stand close to him, and put their hands on his shoulders. He responds by cowering, wincing and backing off. He shows that patients place him in an uncomfortable position. Patients sense his inability to protect his personal space. Disrespect results which is detrimental to rapport with his patients.

With emotional signals you can respond emotionally by shaking your head, or raising your eyebrows; smiling or looking away; raising or lowering your voice.

Hopkinson et al. (1981) found no significant correlation between the rate of a listener's nonverbal response such as head nodding and the amount of emotional expression by interviewed mothers. However, Heller et al. (1966) and Siegman and Pope (1972) contradict this point. No expression or strong emotional expression by the interviewer may inhibit, while a moderate expression may be facilitating for emotional response. Picking up an emotional signal or talking about it, confronting the patient with it, and exploring its origin appears effective for an emotional response. Interviewers who picked up their clients' emotional signals elicited in eight out of nine cases spontaneous self-disclosures—more than three spontaneous self-disclosures in a thirty-minute interview, while interviewers who ignored their patients' emotional signals elicited three spontaneous self-disclosures only in six out of twenty-seven cases.

An example will illustrate how a response to an emotional (and not to a verbal) signal deepened rapport.

Novice: What can I do for you?
    P: I'm so angry and mad, I had two bad years. What these people did to me in North Carolina! (Looks away, bites his lip and clenches his fist.) They stripped me of the right to see my children. I'm angry and depressed about that.

The patient gives two types of signals, an emotional one (looks away, bites his lip, clenches his fist) and a verbal one (I'm angry and depressed). The novice responds to the *word* "depressed."

Novice: You say you are depressed. Did it affect your sleep?
    P: Yeah. (The patient whips his crossed-over leg.)

Novice: What about your appetite?
    P: What about it?

Novice: Was it affected?
    P: Nope. (The patient looks away.)

The supervisor interrupts. He hones in on the suspiciousness and anger which was expressed by body language:

I: (Raises his hand, moves forward on his chair.) Excuse me, you said people have stripped you of the right to see your children.
P: Yes, that's right, they really did me in.

I: (Raises his eyebrows.)
P: The judge and the lawyer down in that little whoretown ... I'm sure you know judges and lawyers in such a place must be crooked. All they deal with is prostitutes, illegal use of drugs, bribery, it is all a big scam.

I: Hmm ... (Shakes his head in disapproval.)
P: At my divorce, these people listened only to my wife. I could not go down there, because I was sick, and my wife paid them off. So they gave me a bad deal.

I: How can we help?
P: I'm so mad, I'm afraid somebody will get hurt if I don't get any help.

The supervisor addressed what the patient had expressed by his body language rather than by words. These signs led him to the patient's persecutory ideas, the core pathology.

As we suggested earlier, you can respond with a metaphor to metaphorical language. Use initially the patient's terms instead of psychological or psychiatric terminology. For instance, when he talks about his "spells," use that word. This gives him the feeling that you understand him. Then ask him to describe what he means by "spell" to help you understand what he is talking about (see chapter 4.3: Exploration).

Later, if indicated, you may introduce technical terms such as seizure, panic attack, cataplectic attack, hypnagogic hallucination, restless leg syndrome, or hyperventilation episode to assure him that you have the expertise to understand his problems.

The following interview section recorded in a rural outpatient mental health center shows how a novice missed picking up his patient's language.

Mr. Huber, a 58-year-old farmer dressed in blue overalls, leans back in his chair with legs spread apart. His face is weather beaten with wrinkles around the eyes from squinting.

> P: I don't know what's going on, I'm not with it anymore!
> Novice: How would you compare your present level of mental functioning with the level you were at prior to the onset of your problems?

> P: What do you mean?
> Novice: I obviously mean how you can concentrate, memorize and think now, in comparison to the time before you got sick.

> P: You mean if I think different now?
> Novice: Yes, that's part of it, but not just thinking, also memorizing and concentrating.

> P: Well, I think a lot about losing my farm and why my son can't take it over.

> Novice: That's not what I mean. I mean, is your thinking slower now, is it more of an effort to get your thoughts out?

> P: You mean if I'm crazy or something?

The novice talks above the patient's head. He interviews him as if the patient were a psychology major. The supervisor continued the interview and it went like this:

> I: You said you are not really with it anymore.
> P: That's right.

> I: Can you give me an example?
> P: Yes, I often stand and stare. Don't know what to do next.

> I: How's that?
> P: Well, I just can't remember what I wanted to do.

> I: You mean it just does not come to you?
> P: Yeah, that's it.

> I: Does that mean that your thoughts just don't pop up in your mind as they used to?
> P: Right. It's just all blank up there. (Patient points to his head.)

In contrast to the novice, the supervisor tunes into his patient's language—therefore, he communicates with him.

To recognize and respond to your patient's signs is difficult if you yourself are tense, anxious, and nervous. This will hinder you to establish rapport. You cannot come up with appropriate questions, you may miss finer points of the mental status, or you may lose contact to the patient, because you focus your attention on yourself. The most powerful technique to help you to overcome self-consciousness and insecurity is to totally shift the focus from yourself to your suffering patient.

2. FIND THE SUFFERING—SHOW COMPASSION

After responding to the patient's signals and putting him at ease, search for the patient's suffering. "Give me a place to stand and I will move the earth," Archimedes allegedly said (c. 287–212 B.C.). This Greek mathematician and scientist illustrated to Hieron II, king of Syracuse in Sicily, that a very great weight could be moved by a very small force provided you have a far out point from which to apply the leverage. In psychiatric interviewing, the point from which you can set the patient's emotions free is his point of suffering.

There are usually two aspects to the patient's problems: the facts and the associated emotions. The facts may be symptoms such as loss of appetite, early morning awakenings, shortness of breath, unexplained abdominal pain; they may be stressors such as the death of a child, marital problems, job loss, and relocation, or recurrent adjustment problems. The emotions are the feelings that these facts stir up in the patient and make him suffer. He may hide this aspect because of fear of being embarrassed. You will intensify rapport if you bring out not only the facts but also his suffering.

Assess the Suffering

To determine the ways in which the patient is suffering, you can try questions such as:

"What is bothering you?"
"What are you going through?"

When the patient describes his problems, often called the *chief complaint*, help him to put his distress into words:

"How did that make you feel?"

indicating that you are interested in his emotions and want to know more about his anguish. In this early phase of the interview it is more important to allow him to ventilate his suffering than to list his symptoms. This approach focuses on him and his pain rather than on you and your need to know the details.

Bringing the patient's affect to his awareness accomplishes two goals: 1. it allows you to judge his affect and mood and to detect the underlying quality, such as depression, anxiety and anger; 2. it shows the patient your interest in his feelings which brings you closer to each other and deepens rapport.

Respond with Empathy

When the patient reveals his suffering, tell him that you understand, show your empathy, and express your compassion. If a patient, for instance,—while telling you that she can hardly make ends meet on her salary since her husband returned to school, and that they may be forced to take out a loan—becomes tense and clenches her fists, avoid focusing on the content of her talk but express empathy for her distress:

"You sounded angry while you said that. You must be fed up with the situation."

Try to be genuine, spontaneous, and accurate in your response to her affect.

"You must feel awful."
"You must feel harassed."
"I can see how that shook you up."
"That must have made you feel deserted."

If you have difficulty in feeling empathy don't try to express it. In that case, attention and appropriate questions convey your interest in the patient better than phony empathy. Patients get annoyed when they are confronted with mannerisms.

I: I heard you say you were apprehensive about coming here.
P: You heard right, damn it, that's what I said.
  or
I: It sounds to me that you were pretty upset when you . . .
P: (Sarcastically) Really? It sounds to you? . . . Doc, you are just playing ther-
  apist—I know that spiel—I have been to too many damn psychologists.

If you express empathy but the patient withdraws from you—check whether you were genuine. Did you really understand his distress? Did you truly feel empathic?

To acquire an empathic, patient-centered, genuine interview style—so that it becomes second nature—recapitulate interviews with difficult patients. Jot down how the patient's attitudes toward you changed, and analyze what caused it. Did you use his vocabulary when you formulated your questions? Were you clearly aware of how the patient's problems affected him? Did you make an effort to explore these feelings? Did you tune into his emotions when you expressed your empathy and your understanding (Rogers 1951)? Were you always aware of and responsive to the patient's attitudinal changes?

It sounds trivial that an interviewer should express empathy if he wants the patient to entrust him with his suffering. Not quite.

Hopkinson et al. (1981) found that the novice uses sympathetic statements in approximately 4% of all his questions and remarks. This figure seems low. However, quality, timing, and context are at least as important as the amount. 51% of sympathetic statements elicited emotional expressions in the patient. This figure rose to 62% when the interviewer expressed his own emotions before he made the sympathetic statement, as compared to 36% when he did not disclose his own emotions. This combined interaction is effective, yet rare. It was used in only 1.5% of all questions and remarks.

If you want to improve on your rapport with your patient, work on your percentages.

3. ASSESS INSIGHT—BECOME AN ALLY

Once you have communicated your empathy, understand your patient's view of his problem, i.e., his insight. This allows you not only to share his emotional but also his cognitive attitude toward his problems.

Why is this assessment necessary? Because you need to use the patient's insight in two ways: 1. When you interview him, you look at his problem from *his* point of view. 2. You use the distance between *his* degree of insight and *full* insight as a measure for his reality testing. It will be part of the therapeutic goal to correct any distortion and help him to gain full insight.

If you misjudge the patient's insight, rapport will deteriorate rapidly. If you treat the patient who feels controlled by a computer as delusional or crazy, he will feel insulted, because he feels his beliefs are true.

Levels of Insight

There are three levels of insight: full, partial, and no insight.

Full Insight

A patient who describes his psychiatric symptoms as a result of a disorder demonstrates full insight. For instance, a patient with panic attacks who recognizes them as "ill" has full insight.

NOTE:

In descriptive psychiatry, insight means that a patient recognizes himself to be ill when he has a psychiatric disease. In psychoanalytical terminology, insight means to understand the conscious and unconscious motives—the *why*—of symptoms and behaviors.

Also, a patient with phobic avoidance or obsessive compulsive worries who considers this behavior as a symptom of a disorder has full insight. Such patients were called "neurotic" in DSM-II.

Rapport comes easily with such a patient. He talks freely about his symptoms because he recognizes them as egodystonic, as part of an illness and not as part of his normal self. He may attempt to withhold embarrassing details such as suicide attempts, or violations of the law, but in general, the patient recognizes his illness and you can interview him for his symptoms. You will find these patients typically in psychiatric outpatient settings, as clients of psychologists, or other mental health professionals.

Partial Insight

In contrast, psychotic patients with schizophrenia, manic depressive illness, or major depression often lack the awareness of being sick; so do drug or alcohol addicts who deny the impact of their illness on themselves and their environment. Since there is such disparity in insight, you have to gauge the patient's ability to understand that he is ill.

Partial insight is also seen in a patient who recognizes that there is something wrong but blames it on external circumstances, as the following example illustrates.

Rose, a 32-year-old, white, single female who lives in an old neighborhood in an industrial city learned to use psychiatric terminology for her problem without accepting it as a disorder. Her mother brought her to the ER.

P: I'm getting paranoid again.
I: What do you mean by that?

P: Well, I think that my neighbors are spying on me again.
I: Why do you call that paranoid?

P: My other doctor told me so.
I: So what do you think we should do about it?

P: I guess I need the prolixin shots again.
I: What does that medication do for you?

P: I'll be less bothered by my paranoia.
I: What do you think the neighbors are really doing to you?

P: One of them comes at night towards my house and listens at my bed-room window. Another one talked to the mailman to tell him to put a bug in my house.
I: Do you really think they are doing this?

P: Of course, what do you think? I'm really paranoid about it.

This patient knows her doctor's view of her condition, that he considers her concerns as sick and in need of pharamacological treatment. But her own beliefs are unshaken in spite of her willingness to cooperate with his treatment—rather than report the neighbors to the police. Symptoms can be elicited from Rose as long as she is not pressed to accept them as indicators of a mental illness. Rose knows that she is suffering and expects that medication will help her even though she does *not* concede that the source of her suffering is an illness.

Your awareness of the patient's level of insight is important for rapport since it determines the phrasing of your questions throughout the interview. For instance, when you ask for family history, it would be a mistake to ask a patient with partial insight:

"Does anybody else in your family suffer from beliefs like you, or show suspicious behavior?"

Rather, ask as if unrelated to the patient's problem; for instance:

"Were there any medical illnesses in your family, or any psychiatric disorders?"

or

"Were some other members of your family also harassed by their neighbors?"

When you discuss treatment, emphasize initially that the medication will make the patient less sensitive to the neighbors' activities; not that it will relieve her delusional suspiciousness.

No Insight

A patient without insight demonstrates complete denial. Characteristic features clue you in right away. He is accompanied by someone who urges him to be treated; his response to your opening question shows passive compliance, angry resistance, or muteness; he does not admit to psychosocial problems, or a psychiatric disorder; and his chief complaint is often noncommital:

"My wife sent me."
"I don't know why I'm here."

If the patient, for instance, is brought in by someone else, find out what leverage this person used to bring him in. Find a motive strong enough to make your patient agree to be interviewed and treated.

Richard is a 37-year-old, white male who works at his father's tobacco farm; he suffers from recurrent delusions and hallucinations:

"Spacemen are coming in at night; they are shooting darts, and I wake up with a splitting headache. Call the FBI, I want to file a complaint!"

The patient recognizes the spacemen as disturbing—but not as a symptom of an illness. To initiate rapport with such a patient you have to consider the spacemen as *his* reality and choose your words accordingly. Do not imitate this psychology student:

Student: Really—have you had these hallucinations for a long time?
    P: What do you mean? I don't know what you are talking about.

Student: I mean your hallucinations about the spacemen?
    P: They aren't imagined, they are real—I get headaches from their shots. Would I get headaches if I imagined that?

Student: Well . . . sometimes our minds play tricks on us.
    P: Maybe your mind plays tricks with you. I better go.

The supervisor interrupts.

I: Wait a minute.
P: (Angry.) Why? I don't want to talk to you either.

I: I see you get annoyed that we don't understand . . .
P: Yeah, you are like my brother. He says I'm crazy.

I: He probably hasn't seen spacemen and has a hard time understanding what's going on. Tell me how long have these spacemen been bothering you?
P: It started again four weeks ago.

I: Is there anything else going on?
P: Well, I have the splitting headache in the morning.

I: Do the spacemen bother you during the day?
P: No, not really.

I: Do they keep track of you in any way?
P: I don't know. They just seem to come at night.

I: Do they have any power over you?
P: No, they just bug me.

I: Can you hear them? Do they talk about you?
P: Well, once in a while at night I hear a whisper that comes from the air conditioner. They say, "See, there he is, see, there he is, and we will get him."

Some patients without insight refuse to be interviewed. Such patients are often accompanied by relatives or friends. Find out from them as much as possible and identify the patient's vantage point of his illness and his suffering. Approach the patient repeatedly from his point of view of the illness and express empathy for what he is going through. He will often open up when he feels you understand him and want to help him.

Split off the Sick

After you have learned what the patient considers as his disturbance, appeal to the healthy observer in him, and offer your help against the trouble. Communicate to him that you are on his side in the battle against his pain. Thus, you create a split between healthy observer and perceived perturbation.

To a patient with *full insight* you can explain the nature of his disorder. Review treatment options and their implementation. Be cautious however and recognize distortions. A depressed patient, for instance, may describe his depressive symptoms in a seemingly distant objective manner, but watch out for depressive distortions! Is his past riddled by guilt feelings? Does he expect a bleak future? Does he underestimate himself? Recognize where the disorder warped his perception.

In a patient with *partial insight* the healthy observer within the patient is harder to define. For instance, Rose truly believes that her neighbors are spying on her. You have to accept her delusions as *her* reality. Therefore, base the phrasing of your questions on *her* perception.

In Richard who has *no insight* the disturbance is the alleged encroachment of the spacemen on him. He feels harassed and is fearful about these persecutors. Express to such a patient how terrible it must feel to be harassed. Offer him the hospital as security against the spacemen, and medication as protection so that the intruders will no longer upset him.

Set Therapeutic Goals

Define two goals, commensurate with the patient's insight: a goal which you discuss with him, and a therapeutic one based on the nature of his illness which you keep to yourself like a trade secret.

In a patient with full insight both goals are one and the same. For instance, you and the depressed patient may view his symptoms as expressions of a treatable illness. State this goal and offer your help.

There are two goals for a patient with partial insight. For Rose, the overt goal is to overcome her neighbors' hostility; your therapeutic goal is to eradicate the delusional thinking—the patient is barred from this insight.

With treatment she will recognize the delusional nature of her beliefs.

Then the treatment of the delusion itself becomes the overt goal. After remission the prevention of a relapse becomes a new overt goal. At this time, the overt and therapeutic goals have merged.

As the delusion melts away, the patient may start to challenge you and ask:

"Do you think my neighbors are really against me, or do you think I'm crazy?"

Ask her what she thinks, and tell her it is more important that you understand her distress rather than worry about how much her neighbors really harassed her. When a patient reaches full insight, she may remark that you probably knew all along that her ideas were nonsense. Counter her statement with a question:

"What would you have said if I told you that six weeks ago?"

For Richard (no insight) the overt goal is to take neuroleptic medication "so that the spacemen bother him less." The therapeutic goal is to abolish his delusions.

Restate the overt goal with the patient's growing insight, often a slow growth. Avoid provocative confrontations and interpretations which may offend him like bad breath. Give him time to see through his problems and have his overt goal merge with your therapeutic one.

Both, overt and therapeutic goals, remain elusive if you do not show the patient that you will help him. The more he distorts reality, i.e., the more the overt and therapeutic goals differ from each other, the more support he needs. Make him feel that you accept him "unconditionally," as Truax and Mitchell (1971) called it. In their research on the effective therapist—the one that initiates change in his client—they isolated three ingredients: empathy for the patient's suffering, genuineness in the patient-interviewer interaction (see above) and unconditionally positive regard for the patient as a person. These ingredients are not restricted to the therapist but also apply to the psychodiagnostic interviewer to create an alliance for both, the immediate interview goal of the patient's self-disclosure and the more remote goal of the patient's improvement.

4. SHOW EXPERTISE

Empathy goes a long way, but empathy is not enough. It tells the patient that you care but it tells nothing about your competence to care.

Convince him that you are an expert. Use three techniques to convince him that you understand his disorder:

a. make him understand that he is not alone with his problem, put his illness into perspective;
b. communicate to him that you are familiar with his illness—show knowledge;
c. deal with his distrust.

This expertise sets you above well-meaning family members or friends. It distinguishes you as a professional.

Put the Illness into Perspective

When the patient describes his problems, you may inject:

"Have you ever known anybody with a problem like yours?"

He may tell you about family members and friends, movies and books concerned with mental illness. Ask him how his own problems fit in. Correct his misconceptions if he has any.

Another patient may claim that he has never heard about a problem like his. Tell him that it is common to hide psychiatric disorders. Then stir up his curiosity for details. Ask him what *he* thinks about his disorder. Discuss with him which features of his illness are common, and which ones are specific to him. Reassure him that many people have similar problems and have gotten well with treatment.

A patient may panic when you mention other patients to him and fear that you file him away as another "case." Put his worries at ease and express that his symptoms may be similar to others but his personality (to deal with them) is unique.

Show Knowledge

Demonstrate expertise to your patient by probing for specific symptoms of his disorder. A patient is sometimes amazed by targeted questions about his condition, wondering: "How did you know that?" Then, he becomes more inclined to trust you and reveal secret concerns such as ruminations, obsessions, or compulsions—since you know anyway.

Another way to establish expertise is to stir up the patient's curiosity about psychology and mental illness which he has read about or seen discussed on TV. Discuss famous examples, such as President Lincoln or Senator Eagleton for depression (also King Saul if the patient has a religious background). Point out how they relate to him. Use phrases such as:

"You got a problem about which we have learned quite a bit recently."
"Your problem is common to middle-aged people."
"Recently, we have made some progress in treating a problem such as yours."

Learn from the patient's response what aspect of his problems interests him. Answer his questions in a concise manner; explain heredity, receptor theories, and psychological formulations, or system theory. Your knowledge is reassuring for the intellectual, obsessive, or educated patient who bases his trust in you more on how much you know than how much you care (for him).

What do you do if you do not know the answer to a question? Admit your ignorance freely. Tell him whether the answer is known, but you don't know it, or whether it is not known at all. Admitting to the limits of your knowledge usually increases the patient's confidence in your honesty. Most patients do not expect you to be omnilegent or omniscient, but if one patient does, discuss his false expectations with him.

Deal with Distrust

Whenever you encounter distrust, when your patient challenges your expertise, decide how to deal with it (see chapter 3: Techniques).

"What caused you to ask this question at this time?"
"Do you have concerns whether I really understand your problems?"

Use counterquestioning, confrontation, or interpretation when you sense a deeper-seated doubt. If you handle him well, he will experience you as an expert. Most patients respect skillful management of their difficulties. We will talk more about this in chapter 3.

5. ESTABLISH AUTHORITY

While empathy roots in your compassion with the patient's suffering, and expertise in your knowledge of his problem, authority originates from your ability to handle him. Establish authority at the moment you meet your patient by taking control of the situation. Take responsibility for his welfare.

The acid test for your authority is his acceptance of your explanations and his willingness to comply with your treatment plan.

Some interviewers overstep their authority. They perceive the patient as a subordinate who should obey. Some patients accept this demanding, or even punative demeanor, and feel strongly guided rather than imposed upon. Obviously, such an interaction fosters dependence. An interviewer who assumes that he knows best, that he does not owe any explanations, and that if the patient does not like it he had better seek help elsewhere—jeopardizes genuine rapport. He patronizes rather than guides the patient.

Most authoritarian interviewers are unaware of their lack of empathy or willingness to explain. They are often insecure and hide their self-doubt behind an authority role. If your patient responds to you with resistance or anxious obedience, examine whether you were too threatening or demanding.

Not only may you get hung up on the authoritarian role, but sometimes the patient pushes you there, even against your will. He may put you on a pedestal and then protest against your authority—or he may be afraid of you, trying to impress or please you, in fear of retaliation—or may admire you as a model or idol to identify with. Make the patient aware of his attempts to push you into the authoritarian role and point out to him his unrealistic expectations, thus counteracting later disappointments.

The grandiose, suspicious, or sociopathic patient may defy your authority, try to disarm you, and demonstrate his disrespect. He may grasp the opportunity to launch remarks such as:

"I have to see about this."
"I usually get a second opinion."
"I don't trust doctors. I've fired them before."
"You either deliver, or else."

Confront him with his behavior:

"You seem to have difficulties in accepting some ideas from me."
"Sure, you should get a second opinion . . . but is it really my opinion or my person (authority) that gives you problems?"

"When you fire doctors it makes you feel as if you are in control. Don't you wish you could also fire your problems?"

"Do you really distrust my delivery or your ability to respond?"

Discuss his difficulties in accepting your authority. For instance, point out the pattern of protest that he repeats with every counselor. But indicate also that you appreciate his concerns which may need further exploration.

6. BALANCE THE ROLES (TRANSFERENCES)

A patient tells Freud that she has the wish to be kissed by him. Freud had just finished a hypnotic session with her. This was the year 1897, the birth of the psychoanalytical term transference (*Übertragung*, Freud, vol. 1, p. 309).

Freud had not consciously evoked any amorous intentions, so he thought. Therefore, he argued, the session must have revived unconscious feelings directed toward somebody else, i.e., the patient's father.

Transference lived on. Not only for the patient, but also for the therapist who has unconscious feelings which were originally directed toward parents but repressed as forbidden. Although repressed, dead they are not. According to Freud, they continue to survive in the unconscious and shape future relationships.

Transference distorts perception, perceives others in roles, or even forces them to adopt roles. The concept of transference has sensitized therapists to the importance of the here and now of the emotional interaction with their patients.

Berne (1961) simplified and popularized this concept. He talks about the parent, the adult, and the child in all of us.

In descriptive interviewing, these concepts are useful. They help to understand patient-interviewer interactions. Berne's "parent" resurfaces in the form of the authoritarian interviewer and the VIP patient (see below). However, both roles may get a tinting of the "child," when interviewer or patient—frustrated in his role assumption—pouts. Berne's "child" surfaces in the patient who presents himself as the sufferer, or in the interviewer who becomes seductive and flirtatious.

The patient who portrays himself as a person with a circumscribed dysfunction but otherwise feels intact, and in control of his skills and faculties assumes Berne's "adult" role. The interviewer role that best corresponds to the "adult" is the flexible professional who assumes roles according to need. A caricature of this role may be the expert who attempts to limit his care to the intellectual dimension.

Long before Freud, the public was aware of different roles that participants in a healing setting play. Hippocrates defined the ethical conduct that physicians should adhere to. Others speak of professional attitude and bedside manners. The French playwright Molière set an early monument to the patient sufferer in his comedy *Le Malade imaginaire* (The Imaginary Invalid).

The psychodiagnostic interviewer learns from these accounts that it is important to be aware of his own and the patient's roles. Only then can he modify and/or discuss the roles and control their interaction to the patient's benefit and the advantage of mutual rapport.

The skillful interviewer balances the roles of empathic listener, expert, and authority throughout the interview. Ideally, he switches these roles according to the patient's needs. However, such flexible interchange—even though ideal—does not always occur. Many interviewers lock into one stereotype and let that dominate their interviewing style. Therefore, it is necessary to monitor the roles that you and your patient slide into and adjust to them if necessary.

The Empathic Listener

The empathic listener puts his patient at ease, is sensitive to his suffering, and expresses his compassion. However, he may become too lenient like a permissive mother with a spoiled child. He may wait for him when he is late, tolerate forgotten appointments, reduce his charges, and even invite him to dinner. In his desire to comfort the patient he may neglect to see limits when indicated, to hospitalize when necessary, or to recommend more intensive treatment measures such as electroshock treatment when all other treatment has failed. As an extreme—he becomes like a compassionate friend or family member developing emotional closeness without professional distance. He falls short as expert and authority.

When you recognize that you overemphasize empathy, start to set limits, take the leadership, and bring your expertise to bear whenever it appears in the best interest of a well-run, economic, yet informative interview.

The Expert

The expert may feel that empathy is a waste of time. What the patient needs is know-how and not compassion. His basic attitude: It is not so important that you want to help—but that you *can*. The expert may ride the high horse of knowledge with an aura of self-proclaimed infallibility. Aloof, he may not care whether the patient follows his recommendations or not, because it is the patient and not him who has to suffer the consequences.

If you are such an "expert," if a warm, friendly tone is missing in your interview, you may try to become sensitive to the patient's suffering. Review the process and determine whether you had empathy. Also, see whether you were supportive and provided guidance where appropriate.

The Authority

From the beginning of an interview, the authoritarian interviewer insists on being in command and expects the patient to follow.

"Compassion?" he may ask with a thin smile of surgical indifference, "What about the patient's respect? Expertise is surely enough—and which patient recognizes it anyway?" Therefore, he expects a patient to put his trust in his hands without having to waste time asking irritating questions.

Patient and interviewer clash if the interviewer insists on his authority and the patient is unwilling to yield. The following took place between a fourth-year psychiatric resident and a 28-year-old patient in the second session of a diagnostic interview. The resident had asked the supervisor for help with this patient whom he had diagnosed as dependent personality. The resident shook hands with the patient and his wife and introduced the interviewer:

Novice: This is the clinic director. He will sit in today. (He neither explained why, nor asked the patient's permission.)

      P: I'm sorry to be late, but we had some car trouble.

Novice: Well, you know the rules of this clinic and have accepted them. We have to charge you for the time that you were late, because I was here and had the time set aside for you.

      P: I understand. By the way, I also brought my wife because she may be able to explain to you better than me what kind of a dilemma we are in.

Novice: I thought we had agreed that you should depend more on yourself and not use others to fight your battles.

    P: But I have such a hard time to get through to you. You told me that most of my problems result from our living with my parents—I was out of a job for six months and we had no reserves. We can stay in my parents' upstairs apartment by paying only for the utilities and repairs. My wife could tell you that my bad feelings don't have much to do with living with them.

Novice: I don't see how I can help you if you don't want to do what we have discussed. You may as well find somebody else.

    P: I guess you are right. I thought I was here to understand myself and my problems better, but I feel bossed around and I don't see how that can help me.

At this point the supervisor stepped in, responded with empathy to the patient's problems, and gave him the opportunity to explain himself.

If you are an authoritarian interviewer you may be unaware of it. Here are some hints that may help you become aware of this problem and therefore help you to correct it.

The patient opposes you and becomes reluctant.
The patient grins and makes undermining remarks.
The patient contradicts you.
The patient becomes very obedient.
The patient becomes uncomfortable and monosyllabic.
The patient becomes anxious and insecure.

If you observe any of these behaviors, examine whether you give the patient enough breathing room, empathy, and support. Obviously, there is more than one reason why the patient may be come obedient, or hostile, but all of us interviewers are well advised to analyze how much we contribute to the patient's maladjusted behavior.

Like interviewers, patients often assume roles. These include: the "carrier of an illness," the "sufferer," and the "VIP."

Carrier of an Illness

As carrier of an illness the patient sees himself only temporarily impaired. He puts distance between himself and his disorder. For instance, he will say it is his sleep not him that is disturbed. Not he has a problem, just his marriage. He puts his problem into quarantine so that it cannot infect the rest of him. Other than the pain in his back he tries to live a "normal life." He does not demand special privileges, or crave sympathy and pity. All he expects is expert medical management. Rapport with him comes easy.

The Sufferer

Such a patient is the opposite from the carrier of an illness. He is consumed by his pain and anguish. His problems flood him with septicemia. He exaggerates his disability. He craves comfort, sympathy, and understanding rather than expert advice. His demands may often become overwhelming, and unbearable. He forces you to set firm limits, yet the expression of your empathy often reestablishes his self-control and containment. Chronic depression and some personality disorders favor the development of this role.

The "VIP"

The "very important patient" sees himself as privileged, entitled to attention at any time of day or night. He is often grossly familiar. He expects preferred treatment. He searches for the very best in the field, the star physician, or best psychologist. Rapport with such a patient may become complex and limit setting unavoidable. The "VIP" attitude can be adopted by anyone from the very successful to the least privileged. Often you will be impressed by the modesty of very successful people. In contrast, the true "VIP" will ring you up at 3 a.m. to tell you he can't sleep.

Role Interaction

Rapport is achieved when interviewer and patient balance their changing roles and act accordingly.

If an adopted role is rejected by either, conflict arises. Monitor the emerging roles and react accordingly. A few patients may resent your expertise as too "brainy" and may long for guidance and leadership: "You are the doctor, don't explain my problems to me; tell me what to do!" In short he may search for the authority whom he can follow, who tells him what to do. Depending on your judgment, you may confront him with that need or you may comply and provide authority.

The following example shows how the interviewer avoided a role conflict, when Bernhard, a 54-year-old, divorced male, openly rejected both the interviewer's authority and expertise.

1. I: What can I do for you?
   P: Before I tell you anything, I want you to know that I'm here to get a second opinion. People have told me that you are pretty knowledgeable. But don't expect that I will believe what you tell me or that I will do what you advise me.

2. I: If you feel like this, why did you come to see me?
   P: I just want to know what you have to say. If I like it, you are on.

3. I: Okay. (Silent.)
   P: What do you have to say?

4. I: Nothing yet. Except that you don't think much about my ability to help you.
   P: That's right.

5. I: You may be right, but I wonder what makes you think that way.
   P: Nobody else could help me before. I lost my job seven years ago.

6. I: Because nobody else could help you, you don't have confidence in me either?
   P: Right.

7. I: I can't promise you anything; I may fail also but I will try!
   P: We'll see.

The interviewer does not defend the role the patient assigns him, nor does he counterattack, but explores the background of the rejection (Q. 2–5). Bernhard's response reveals the reason for his hostility (A. 5). When the interviewer admits that his treatment effort may also fail (Q. 7), the intensity of the patient's rejection abates.

If a patient attacks you, the strategy is *not* to accept the role he has assigned to you—(the target for his aggressions)—but to step aside and to assess the reasons for his aggression. Accept these reasons as the patient's legitimate concerns and communicate this acceptance to him. By not responding to aggression with defense or counterattacks but with analysis of the reason, you may be able to make the patient reflect rather than act out.

Dependence on the Interviewer's Authority

A patient's dependency needs may be as disturbing to rapport as his rejection of the interviewer. The outpatient, Tom, a 27-year-old student of theology, consults the interviewer.

I: What kind of problem brought you here?
P: I don't know whether I should push myself or not.

I: Well, you are bringing up an interesting question. Should you push yourself?
P: Yes, what do you think?

I: I would like to understand why you feel I can give you better advice than you can give yourself.
P: Well, I just want to know if I can hurt myself by pushing too hard.

I: Was that why you asked me?
P: Yes. I think so . . . (pause) but you are right. I just can't make up my mind about anything. I always looked for somebody to tell me what to do.

I: But did you really do what you were told?
P: I don't know. I would have to see whether I agree.

I: That's right, you have to find out for yourself.

The patient attempts to put the interviewer in the role of an advice-giving authority. As in the previous example the interviewer explores the reason. Tom's responses allow the interviewer to direct him to reflection and self-reliance.

You may want to avoid giving advice to the doubting patient who is suffering from depression. Favor empathic listening over authoritarian advice giving. When you listen you allow a patient like Howard to sort out his strengths and weaknesses and come to a decision himself.

P: I hang around the house. I can't stand it. My family avoids me. Should I go back to work?
I: Can you?

P: I don't know, I would just sit there and stare at the desk . . .
I: Yes?

P: . . . and I would be so embarrassed if all the people that work for me see me sitting there not doing a thing.
I: I understand how you must feel. I know you want to work and support your family, but if you try, you fear you may fail.

P: Maybe I should be patient until I feel a little better.
I: It seems to me you don't want to take the risk of failing.

In contrast, it is sometimes therapeutic for a patient if you do accept the authority role. For instance, when the patient is pondering a realistic plan but is still filled with self-doubt because of a depression—your support and encouragement for his plans may make the difference.

Emil, a 45-year-old, white man had suffered from depression for several months without getting relief in spite of intensive therapy.

P: I realize I'm depressed. I don't want to leave the house. I don't feel like hunting for a job. But staying at home and waiting for the kids to come home from school seems to make me more depressed.
I: Hmm . . . and makes you more aware of it?

P: You seem to understand. I think it would be better for me if I pushed myself and took a job!
I: Well, pushing yourself may neither shorten nor lengthen your depression, but I feel it may help you to tolerate your depression better.

P: That's right.
I: I feel that it is a good sign that you want to push yourself and want to go out.

P: I feel I could try it.
I: We will see how it works.

The interviewer accepts the role as authority and supports what he feels is appropriate, without violating the patient's ability to make his own decisions. To invite reflection rather than to support reasonable action may have set the patient back.

In short, assume the role as listener when the patient complains, shows ambivalence, and confusion about his goals. Assume the role as expert when he lacks knowledge about his condition and needs information about his disorder. Assume the role as authority when he has made reasonable decisions, but hesitates with action. Support his decisions and encourage his action.

The skeptic may argue that the professional interviewer will grow into a style and adopt techniques that suit his own personality. Such an argument sounds persuasive but cannot be backed by facts. Michael Rutter et al. (1981) showed that two experienced interviewers in his clinic could change their style at will. They adopted four different styles called the sounding board, the active psychotherapy, the structured, and the systematic exploratory style. Among styles, the number of closed-ended questions, open-ended questions, requests for feelings interpretations, and expressions of sympathy varied vastly and statistically significantly. Rutter et al.'s (1981) results show that interviewing styles are both, teachable and learnable.

Why all this fuss about rapport? Here is one example why rapport is so significant to the success of an interview. A lady in her eighties was sent by a colleague psychiatrist in town for evaluation. I (E.O.) was tired and resentful that I had to see her because I wanted to finish up on this book. Noticing my anger, I thought "What's the use of writing about rapport if you don't use the strategies yourself—every time?" I asked her in. She was skeptical toward the younger fellow with an accent. I put her at ease. I mobilized my empathy for her life story and expressed it. We had a great session. At the end she told me:

"Only after I had seen 20/20 last month I noticed that I'm not alone with my obsessions. And I went to a psychiatrist in town. I dreaded it when he sent me over here. And I dreaded it even more while I was sitting there waiting for you, knowing that I had to talk about my obsessions. But you made it so easy. I told you things that I have not told anybody for 50 years, not even my own children. And I even enjoyed talking about it."

That is one of the reasons to fuss about rapport. What is a better reward than your patient expressing appreciation?

The five minutes you invest at the beginning of the interview to deepen rapport guarantee a high return at the end.

CHECKLIST

Chapter 2: Rapport

The following checklist allows you to rate your skills in establishing and maintaining rapport. It helps you to detect and eliminate weaknesses in interviews that failed in some significant way.

	YES	NO	N/A
1. I put the patient at ease.	___	___	___
2. I recognized his state of mind.	___	___	___
3. I addressed his distress.	___	___	___

4. I helped him to warm up. ___ ___ ___
5. I helped him to overcome suspiciousness. ___ ___ ___
6. I curbed his intrusiveness. ___ ___ ___
7. I stimulated his verbal production. ___ ___ ___
8. I curbed his rambling. ___ ___ ___
9. I understood his suffering. ___ ___ ___
10. I expressed empathy for his suffering. ___ ___ ___
11. I tuned in on his affect. ___ ___ ___
12. I addressed his affect. ___ ___ ___
13. I became aware of his level of insight. ___ ___ ___
14. I assumed the patient's view of his disorder. ___ ___ ___
15. I had a clear perception of the overt and the therapeutic goal of treatment. ___ ___ ___
16. I stated the overt goal of treatment to him. ___ ___ ___
17. I communicated to him that I am familiar with his illness. ___ ___ ___
18. My questions convinced him that I am familiar with the symptoms of his disorder. ___ ___ ___
19. I let him know that he is not alone with his illness. ___ ___ ___
20. I expressed my intent to help him. ___ ___ ___
21. The patient recognized my expertise. ___ ___ ___
22. He respected my authority. ___ ___ ___
23. He appeared fully cooperative. ___ ___ ___
24. I recognized the patient's attitude toward his illness. ___ ___ ___
25. The patient viewed his illness with distance. ___ ___ ___
26. He presented himself as a sympathy-craving sufferer. ___ ___ ___
27. He presented himself as a very important patient (VIP). ___ ___ ___
28. He competed with me for authority. ___ ___ ___
29. He was submissive. ___ ___ ___
30. I adjusted my role to the patient's role. ___ ___ ___
31. The patient thanked me and made another appointment. ___ ___ ___

STRATEGIES TO GET INFORMATION: TECHNIQUES

1. **Complaints**
   Opening Techniques
   Clarification Techniques
   Steering Techniques

2. **Dealing with Resistance**
   Acceptance
   Confrontation
   Looping
   Exaggeration
   Induction to Bragging

3. **Defenses**
   Recognition of Defense Mechanisms
   Handling Defense Mechanisms

SUMMARY

Chapter 3 describes three sets of techniques to get information from the patient. The first set deals with cooperative patients who openly describe most of their problems. The second set is directed toward those patients who consciously conceal part of their problems from the interviewer. The third set of techniques is geared toward patients who—unknowingly (unconsciously)—distort their perception of themselves and others.

I listen. Most people don't. Something interesting comes along—and whoosh!—it goes right past them.

Ted Koppel
Newsweek, JUNE 15, 1987

Examiners for the American Boards of Psychiatry and Neurology are instructed to rate a candidate's interviewing technique by whether he can open up a topic with a broad open-ended question, pursue it by becoming more and more focused, and finally close up the topic by detailed and specific questions. One cannot summarize the general technical approach to psychodiagnostic interviewing any better.

How is this done? Can one learn this interview technique? What are the necessary skills? How do you ask all the right questions? How do you make the patient tell you about his behavior, especially what he sees as his problems?

A patient generally communicates his problems in one of three ways: 1. by pouring it all out (complaints), 2. by revealing some problems but concealing the embarrassing items (resistance), or 3. by obfuscating the most embarrassing part even for himself (defenses).

There are strategies to deal with all three situations.

When the patient communicates by *complaining,* the interviewer only has to help the patient talk, describe his problems in detail, and explore all aspects of them. Three sets of approaches accomplish this: opening, clarification, and steering techniques.

Resistance is more difficult to deal with. Acceptance and confrontation are the most useful techniques in getting a patient to overcome resistance. Indicate that you notice and understand his resistance but, at the same time, try to convince him that it is advantageous for him to give it up.

The use of *defenses* by the patient is the most difficult to handle. In many psychodiagnostic interviews, defenses can be ignored if they don't interfere with your need for information. Occasionally, however, you have to confront or interpret the defense mechanisms in order to maintain rapport or to come to a diagnosis.

1. COMPLAINTS

The patient who comes voluntarily to a mental health professional has a reason for his visit, usually a problem with his functioning, with personal interactions, or with self-conduct and self-satisfaction. When he talks about these problems, the professional listens for the suffering behind the words, and for the patient's complaints (see chapter 2: Rapport). The patient generally expects empathy for his suffering and expertise to identify the source of his malaise. Technically speaking, he expects a diagnosis and a treatment plan (see chapter 5: Diagnosis).

Therefore, the professional needs three sets of techniques to accomplish the following goals: 1. elicit all complaints (opening techniques), 2. translate them into symptoms, long-term behavioral traits, or problems of living (clarification techniques), and 3. cover the territory and move from one set of complaints to another (steering techniques).

Opening Techniques

While interviewing a psychiatric patient you have to find a balance between letting the patient tell his story in his own words and in obtaining information necessary for a diagnosis. If you let him tell his story, he may give an "audition"; if you ask specific questions, your "inquisition" may distort his story. Here are strategies to balance both passive listening and active questioning.

Using a broad, open-ended approach when you begin your dialogue will allow the patient to present his problem in his own words. Useful questions are:

"How can I help you?"
"What can I do for you?"
"What kind of problem brought you here?"
"Where shall we start?"

Such a "patient-centered" approach invites topic selection by him, gives his view of the problem, and should produce his chief complaint. Broad, open-ended questions are the least suggestive and allow the patient to emphasize and elaborate what he sees as important.

Some interviewers only ask open-ended questions throughout the interview. They never follow up on clues or ask for specifics. Such an interviewer may find out, for instance, that the patient was depressed, but will not uncover the length or depth of the depression, unless the patient had volunteered this information. He may also know that the patient had sleep disturbances, but may not have asked him further about the nature of his insomnia. While some advocate this approach, it can work against obtaining information necessary for a proper diagnosis.

Occasionally, you find the opposite type. Once a year, we have a mock examination for our residents in psychiatry. My candidate, Cher, who had to interview a white, middle-aged male, surprised me.

C: I'm Dr. A. You agreed to have this interview.
P: Yes.

C: OK. How old are you?
P: 47.

C: Do you have any siblings?
P: What do you mean?

C: Brothers and sisters.
P: Yes.

C: How many?
P: Three.

C: Are you the youngest?
P: No.

For half an hour this candidate bombarded the patient with closed-ended questions collecting a myriad of small details which she was not able to assemble to a clinical picture, or a diagnostic impression.

These two styles may sound extreme. Yet, the first one is not rare. Milder forms of the second one also occur at the beginning of each batch of students that take up psychodiagnostic interviewing.

There are advantages and disadvantages to both types of questions. Open-ended questions generate genuine, individualized, spontaneous answers. Cox and colleagues (Cox et al. 1981) found that these questions work best in parents who have a vested interest to make the therapist understand their child's difficulty. Probably, we can generalize this finding to all interviewees who are motivated to get their point across. Hopkinson et al. (1981) analyzed naturalistic interviews and found that open-ended questions with few interruptions at follow-up rather than closed-ended questions facilitate emotional expression.

Open-ended questions can also elicit answers that are lengthy, unreliable, vague, and incomplete. As a result, you may discover you lack the details you needed for diagnosis.

Closed-ended questions can generate quick, clear, reliable answers about a circumscribed topic. If a battery of these questions is combined to form a systematic interview, they lead to a fuller coverage of adult patients' mental state than free-style interviews (Saghir 1971). Marquis et al. (1972) support this finding. They show that detailed, structured questions produce a more detailed reproduction of a short movie than free reporting. Cox et al. (1981) also report that a directive style is more effective in obtaining good data about the absence of certain key symptoms. They further found that frequency, severity, context, duration, and qualities of symptoms or problems are better assessed by directive questioning, but did not work better for the assessment of new symptoms or family problems.

Shortcomings of closed-ended questions? In some patients they may force false positive answers, and inhibit the patient's freedom to express himself. In addition, the responses can conform to your preconceptions and thus not yield a truthful picture of the patient's perception of reality.

Table 3.1 shows the pros and cons of open- versus closed-ended questions.

The best approach is to combine questions along the continuum of broad to sharply focused questions. Introduce a new topic with a broad, open-ended question; follow up with targeted ones; and finish with a series of narrow, sometimes closed-ended questions—the yes/no type. This extreme form—the yes/no type—can be used to verify and specify or challenge a response. If you want to avoid closed-ended questions altogether, use sharply focused but open-ended questions. Instead of

"Do you have trouble falling asleep?" (expected answer: yes or no), ask:

"What happens when you try to fall asleep?" (The patient knows that you expect him to talk about sleep onset, but he still has the chance to surprise you with an unexpected answer.)

"I have the weirdest experience. I often see monsters. It is as if I start dreaming when I try to fall asleep." (Hypnagogic hallucinations—a classic symptom of narcolepsy.)

TABLE 3.1
Pros and Cons of Open- and Closed-Ended Questions

Aspect	Broad, Open-Ended Questions	Narrow, Closed-Ended Questions
1. GENUINENESS	High They produce spontaneous formulations.	Low They lead the patient.
2. RELIABILITY	Low They may lead to nonreproducible answers.	High Narrow focus; but they may suggest answers.
3. PRECISION	Low Intent of question is vague.	High Intent of question is clear.
4. TIME EFFICIENCY	Low Circumstantial elaborations.	High May invite yes/no answers.
5. COMPLETENESS OF DIAGNOSTIC COVERAGE	Low Patient selects the topic.	High Interviewer selects the topic.
6. ACCEPTANCE BY PATIENT	Varies Most patients prefer expressing themselves freely; others become guarded and feel insecure.	Varies Some patients enjoy clear-cut checks; others hate to be pressed into a yes/no format.

Thus, the questions change from a predominantly patient-centered to an interviewer-directed format as a topic gets covered. (For more on the different topics of an interview, see chapters 4, 5, and 6.)

Depending on a patient's type of disorder or personality, he may favor one or the other type of question. The obsessive patient prefers closed-ended and circumscribed questions, the hysteric personality broad, open-ended ones. Depending on rapport (see chapter 2) and phase of interview (see chapter 6), choose the appropriate type of questions, their combination and sequence.

After a topic has been initially broached, you then generally need to clarify its boundaries, its specific content, and its connections to other topics. Using clarification techniques will help you with this task.

Clarification Techniques

Some patients answer questions clearly; others are narrow, fuzzy, disjointed, vague, or circumstantial in their response. In such situations, the interviewer needs to get the patient to explain himself more clearly. There are various techniques used to have the patient clarify himself. We call these: specification, generalization, checking symptoms, probing, interrelation, and summarizing.

Specification

The interviewer often needs specific, precise, and explicit information but the patient answers in vague or one-word responses. It is best to switch to a more closed-ended form of questioning as in the following example (Q. 3–6):

1. I: How is your sleep, Mr. Warner?
   P: Lousy.

2. I: What's lousy about it?
   P: Everything.

3. I: Do you have any problems with falling asleep?
   P: Yes.

4. I: How long does it take you to fall asleep lately?
   P: Sometimes an hour, sometimes three hours, sometimes I can't sleep all night.

5. I: Are there nights when you fall asleep all right, but you wake up a few times?
   P: No.

6. I: Do you ever wake up early in the morning and then can't go back to sleep?
   P: No.

Questions 3, 5, and 6 are leading and suggestive, but achieve accurate answers. Their validity has to be judged in the context of the total interview.

For example, if your patient complains:

"I often feel bad."
"My sleep is lousy."

"I'm not eating as I should."
"My sex life is the pits."

feed the vague words "bad, lousy, not eating as I should, is the pits" back to him (Q. 2, 4 below). If feedback fails, tell him how you understand his answer (Q. 5 below). If he responds "That's not it!" let him describe either the most recent or most severe occurence of the event from beginning to end (Q. 6–8 below).

The following interview shows how this technique was used with Lora Carr, a 43-year-old, white, married female with a diagnosis of fibromyositis, a nonspecific illness characterized by pain, tenderness, and stiffness of joints, capsules, and adjacent structures.

1. I: What brought you here, Mrs. Carr?
   P: I feel tired all day.

2. I: Tired?
   P: Because I don't sleep well.

3. I: What's wrong with your sleep?
   P: I have very light and restless sleep.

4. I: (Interviewer focuses on "restless" first and ignores "tiredness.") Well, in what way is your sleep restless?
   P: I guess, I don't know . . .

5. I: You mean you toss and turn?
   P: No, I don't think so.

6. I: When was the last time that your sleep was restless?
   P: That was last night.

7. I: Why don't you describe your sleep starting with the time when you went to bed?
   P: I went to bed at 10:30 and then I was up again a little after 12.

8. I: Yes?
   P: Then at 1 or 1:30 again. It took me a half hour to get back to bed and then I woke up at 4 again, and I don't know when I fell asleep. In the morning I had the hardest time getting up.

9. I: So restless sleep for you means waking up a lot during the night.
   P: That's it.

10. I: (Now, the interviewer shifts to the second part of the problem, the tiredness.) You also said that you feel tired all day.
    P: That's right.

11. I: Does it mostly happen after your restless nights?
    P: No, not necessarily. Some nights I sleep real well and I'm still groggy until 11 o'clock in the morning.

12. I: So then you really seem to have two problems: waking up in the middle of the night and feeling tired during the morning hours.
    P: Yes, that's what's going on.

Restless sleep means having intermittent insomnia (Q. 9). The interviewer examines then the relationship between intermittent insomnia and daytime tiredness, and learns that they are independent.

Generalization

Sometimes a patient will offer specific information when the interviewer needs a sense of his overall recurrent pattern of behavior.

Mr. Allen, a 48-year-old, white, married dairy farmer, had his first depressive episode approximately two years prior to this visit. He experienced a relapse and returned to the clinic.

I: Mr. Allen, tell me, what kind of problems have you had lately?
P: Well, I'm having some problems with my sex life.

I: What about it?
P: Last night I had a terrible problem. We flew in from W. to see you. We checked into the hotel, had a nice meal, but later in bed, I just could not get it up.

I: Do you usually have this problem?
P: My wife is very understanding. She's a good lover.

I: So then you really don't have any sex problems?
P: Last night, as I said.

I: What sex problems do you have regularly, if any?
P: I can't come, no matter how hard I try. It tires my wife out and I get frustrated. But that was not my problem yesterday. I could not get it up yesterday.

I: Were you impotent before you felt depressed again?
P: I did not have any problems then.

The patient has a tendency to bring up a recent, single event which is not representative of his usual symptoms. Therefore, the interviewer repeats his question, but emphasizes the longer time perspective, by using terms like "usually," "regularly," "most of the time," or "often."

If the patient again refers to specific circumstances or situations you may have to explore each situation to appreciate the overall problem.

Checking Symptoms

When a patient's story is vague, the interviewer can present a list of symptoms to help him detect any psychopathology. Depressed patients, for instance, often lack precision and verbal fluency, which prevent them from effectively giving a self-portrait of their thoughts and feelings. In that case you may ask for symptoms. If he still gives vague answers, you may even suggest some symptoms and have him agree or disagree. Cross-check these symptoms to avoid being suggestive. This technique of checking symptoms is used in the following interview.

Joe, a 47-year-old married manager of a small factory, does not provide diagnostic clues in his first seven answers. The interviewer becomes more directive and translates the patient's vague complaint into symptoms:

1. I: Hi Joe. How have things been going lately?
   P: Well, I don't think my wife is really satisfied with me. She says: "Why can't you be your old self again, the way you were when I first met you and when I married you?"

2. I: She thinks you have changed?
   P: Well, we are going to meetings of these Amway people. These are just fabulous people. They try to help you whenever they can. You really have to meet them.

3. I: Your wife thinks you have changed? How does that show in these meetings?
   P: These are fabulous people. They are outgoing and so upbeat. They seem to be so optimistic. I met one of them last Monday morning at 8:30 at the post office. It was one of those gloomy mornings. I asked him how he was doing. He said, "Super, super." He really seemed to glow. There was only one other time that I have seen people act that way. That was in our church.

4. I: So, in what way are you different? What does your wife have in mind?
   P: Well, I don't really know. She is always understanding, but lately she gets impatient with me.

5. I: You mean you cannot tune in with these people?
   P: Right. They stand up, give a long talk and tell you how to motivate others.

6. I: How are you different?
   P: I got up and told them how fabulous they are.

7. I: What's wrong with that?
   P: I don't know! At work they say: "What's wrong with Joe? He was always in a good mood."

8. I: So your mood has changed?
   P: I believe the people at work made funny remarks about me.

9. I: What do you think is wrong with you?
   P: At work, they seem to think that I'm different now.

10. I: It seems that your mood has changed.
    P: Yes, I was always out with the people and joked with everybody and they laughed and said: "There's nothing that can get him down."

11. I: That has changed now?
    P: (Starts crying.)

12. I: Are you down in the dumps?
    P: Yeah, I feel really blue.

13. I: And the people at work, you seem to withdraw from them?
    P: Yeah. I want to be left alone.

14. I: And with the Amway people you just can't get up and give a pep talk?
    P: No, I am just not up to it.

15. I: Are you unable to find the right words?
    P: That's right. I just want to tell them how understanding they are. But I can't even do that. I start crying.

The interviewer first lets the patient tell his story, but the open-ended approach proves ineffective. He attempts to get the patient to be more specific in Q. 2–6, but still does not get a precise description of the problems. Finally, the interviewer checks for symptoms (Q. 8, 10, 12–15). Even though checking for symptoms suggests a complaint and provides words from the interviewer's rather than the patient's vocabulary, this approach is sometimes the only one that allows you to collect diagnostically useful information within a reasonable time frame.

Probing

The interviewer will often find the patient will assign particular significance and meaning to his actions or experiences without explaining why. The interviewer must then try to uncover the reasons for the patient's portrayal of his behavior. This is accomplished by a technique we term "probing."

Probing can best be used in the following instances: when a patient displays an abnormal behavior during the interview; when he assigns significance to an event without indicating why; when he says that someone else sent him to see you; when he seems to be displaying superstitious thinking, clairvoyance, or overvalued ideas. Probing helps to bring out delusional thinking by exposing misinterpretations. Probe at the beginning of the interview when the patient tells you:

"I don't know why I'm here."
"The police brought me."
"My wife made me come."

Ask:

"Why do you think they brought you?"

If he denies knowing anything, continue to probe:

"Why did you go along with them?"

Probe with these "why" questions when the patient tells his story in a bewildered and perplexed way. Ask for his interpretation of his experiences:

"Why do you think these things are happening?"
"What do you think it means?"
"Is it possible that what happened shows us that you are ill?"
"Do you think strange things are going on?"
"Are things not what they appear to be?"

The following case shows how probing was used effectively.

Mr. Stone, a 48-year-old, white, divorced man was brought in by the police because he had been speeding and ignoring the police sirens. When arrested after a brawl, he stated the police prevent fair elections. This and similar utterances got him to the emergency room of the V. A. Hospital in Lexington, Kentucky, where he made the aquaintance of the psychiatrist on call. The interviewer first uses continuation (Q. 1–6, see Steering Techniques below) and then probing (Q. 7).

1. I: What brought you to the emergency room, Mr. Stone?
   P: The police.

2. I: How did you get involved with them?
   P: Oh, it's a long story. I live in (small town in Kentucky) and for the last two years I was thinking of running for mayor.

3. I: Okay.
   P: During the day I work as an accountant. The only time I have to prepare myself for the mayor's job is at night.

4. I: Yes, go on.
   P: In the evening, all of a sudden, my neighbors began coming over. They started to come over nearly every night. They asked if I had time for a beer. I kind of went along with them.

5. I: What happened then?
   P: Two nights ago I thought "This time I'll check up on them." Everything was quiet. My next-door neighbor even had his lights off. But I thought, "They can't trick me." I got my gun out and shot in the air. And when my neighbor opened the window, I told him that I knew that he was watching.

6. I: Alright, what happened then?
   P: He said that I was talking nonsense and that he was going to call the police. I said I wouldn't let him do that. So I jumped in my car and drove off. When I got on the highway, I was stopped by a police car. They said they were stopping me for speeding. I told them I knew why they were really stopping me and I started to get away. But they caught up with me. Finally, they brought me here this morning.

7. I: What do you think this means?
   P: Well, can't you see? Can't you see the plan?

8. I: Well, maybe you can help me along, so I can understand better what's going on.
   P: The neighbors came over, I think because they wanted to steal my time so I couldn't prepare myself for the election. I never told them that I planned to run, but they must have known anyway.

9. I: Why is that?
   P: Because I got some hints.

10. I: What kind of hints?
    P: When I came home I looked through the window, before I entered my house, and I saw a shadow.

11. I: What do you think this shadow was?
    P: I think somebody was in the house looking through my things.

12. I: What do you think the police had to do with this?
    P: My goodness, don't you understand? They don't want me to run for

mayor. They want me locked up. They figure if I get in, I'll clean out that snake pit and reveal all the corruption that's been going on for much too long.

Probing is useful for scanning the patient's thought content for ideas of reference and delusions (Q. 7–12). The interviewer avoids challenging the patient's interpretations because the patient's way of presenting his experience reveals that he has little insight into his reality distortions. Probe also when the patient admits to a significant psychiatric symptom such as a hallucination or delusion. For example, a patient answers a query about having heard voices or seen visions with yes. Get the precise time, place, and frequency of this occurrence. The patient may give a positive answer about hallucinations only to elaborate that such experiences occurred while he was asleep or while drifting into or out of a sleeping state.

Probing is not limited to the patient's interpretation of events. It is a handy tool to pry emotions out of him. In situations where the patient talks about his marriage problem, conflicts at work, or difficulties with his children in a somewhat distant, neutral (objective) way, jump out of the groove of collecting further details of the conflict and ask directly for his emotions.

"How did it make you feel when . . . happened?"

Hopkinson et al. (1981) report that in 55% of such questions and remarks the request for feelings is rewarded. These requests should be made in a nonemotional way. Interviewers who remain neutral have a yield of 61% while those who express their own feelings during such a request harvest only 45%. The direct request for feelings yields an unexpected bonus: nearly 18% of these requests also produce spontaneous self-disclosure by the client which contrasts with 2.5% for all other interventions.

This favorable statistic drives home the point: If you want to know what patients think and feel, ask. Is there any better justification for probing?

Interrelation

To explore overt, illogical relationships is important in a psychodiagnostic interview. As with the technique of probing, it may reveal distorted, disordered, and delusional thinking. If your patient relates two seemingly unconnected elements, tell him:

"Wait! I don't understand what A has to do with B. Please, help me see the connection between them!"

Beatrice, a 39-year-old, white, married woman, mother of five children, is suspicious of her colleagues. When asked about experiences at work, she mentions her son's car accident and relates it to the recent change in her work schedule.

1. I: How are things going at work now?
   P: I don't know. The others seem to avoid me.

2. I: Is there a reason?
   P: I don't know. There might be. Last week when they switched me from the morning to the afternoon shift, my son had a car accident.

3. I: What does that have to do with changing your shift?
   P: They planned the accident.

4. I: What has changing your shift got to do with your son's accident?
   P: The accident was late in the afternoon. That was the first day I had to be at work in the afternoon.

5. I: I still don't understand how you working in the afternoon and your son's accident are related.
   P: Can't you see? They wanted me to be at work when I got the message about the accident, so they could see my reaction. They probably hoped that I would go to pieces. But I didn't give them that satisfaction. I didn't say a word to anyone when I got the telephone message about the accident.

The elements of Beatrice's story are interrelated by her delusional interpretations. The interviewer reveals these delusions by asking the patient how switching her work shift and her son's car accident are interrelated (Q. 3–5).

In the above dialogue, the interviewer asks for logical linkings but does not reflect upon the patient's emotions. If he desired a more emotional discharge, he could have continued the interview by saying:

6. I: You must have felt devastated when you realized that all your colleagues were plotting against you.

Such a remark, if colored by his own empathic feelings, is in 80% of the cases followed by a strong emotional expression by the patient (Hopkinson et al. 1981). What is the value of such an emotional discharge? It allows the interviewer to judge whether the patient's feelings are dominated by guilt, a sentiment of persecution, or hostility. Intellectual interrelating reveals disordered thinking, emotional interrelating brings out disordered affect.

Summarizing

Summaries are useful for clients who are vague, circumstantial, have loose associations, or mild flight of ideas, such as patients with manic-depressive illness or cyclothymia. Summaries focus the patient's attention. Be aware that summaries can lead the patient and you may put words into his mouth. It is helpful to use his vocabulary.

Ron, a 24-year-old, single, male graduate student first contacted the interviewer by telephone with some mild push of speech (see glossary: Speech).

1. I: You told me on the phone that you feel terrible. Just tell me a little bit more about these feelings.
   P: Last Sunday is a good example. It started all of a sudden when I talked to Joan on the phone Saturday night. Then I felt just terrible all of a sudden. On Sunday I did not want to get up. Finally I did, and ran my ten miles. I try to have two ten-mile-days and two fifteen-mile-days a week.

2. I: In what way do you feel terrible?
   P: Just worked up and nervous.

3. I: So how did the rest of Sunday go?
   P: I thought the run would clean up my system, which it usually does, but I still felt all tense and panicky. I could not get anything done. This feeling also affects me when I'm with girls.

4. I: You mean that you have difficulties when you date?
   P: Yes, sexually. I can't relax.

5. I: You have trouble getting an erection?
   P: Yes, it tends to be that way.

6. I: Do you have this problem all the time?
   P: No, it's very bad when I feel tense and rotten. It fluctuates.

7. I: *So you have frequent, short periods where you feel tense and rotten, cannot relax, and have sexual problems?*
   P: That's right. I feel down, can't concentrate on my work, and don't want to do anything.

In his first answer the patient describes "terrible" feelings of short duration. Since he fails to elaborate (A. 2), he is encouraged to go on and to focus on the new topic: the problems with girls (Q. 4). Notice how the interviewer summarizes the patient's statements (Q. 7) and gets his approval.

8. I: For how long have you had those feelings?
    P: As long as I can think back.

9. I: Does it ever get so bad that you think you would harm yourself?
    P: Usually not. I may think about it. Life is precious, but I can understand the tension that some people may have who just go out and take a gun and start shooting people. I would know how to do away with myself. I'm investing in guns. A .45 would take my whole head off.

10. I: Have the terrible feelings ever been so bad that you seem to hear voices?
    P: (Silent, thinks for a while.) No, I don't think so.

The interviewer checks for psychotic symptoms and suicidal ideation. Since hallucinations are absent (A. 10) and suicidal thoughts are presented in a theoretical form and not as a compelling preoccupation (A. 9), the interviewer decides that the patient is presently not psychotically depressed but suffers from moderate depressive mood swings. He therefore explores the presence of normal (Q. 11) and elated mood (Q. 12–16) to check whether the patient is bipolar with rapid mood swings (rapid cycler or cyclothymic disorder), or with long periods of euthymic or normal mood.

11. I: Have you ever felt normal?
    P: Yes, but I really don't know what normal is. I feel very good in between. I can work at a job and go to college, and I'm into investments. I do real well with my money.

12. I: So you have a lot of energy?
    P: Yes, I do. But I'm mainly tense and irritable and high-strung. But I can also feel very good about myself.

13. I: How is your sleep during those times?
    P: Well, for a few days I'm always up and ready to go.

14. I: You mean you stay up all night?
    P: No, I usually sleep 6–8 hours, but I'm wide awake and ready to go in the morning.

15. I: Did you ever do anything foolish during these highs?
    P: What do you mean?

16. I: Well, spending like crazy, getting too involved with girls, or doing things that you really regret later?
    P: Well, no, I never do anything that is really crazy.

17. I: So you have short highs which make you tense and irritable, but also make you feel good at other times. But those feelings never interfere with your sleep or make you do irresponsible things.
    P: That hits it right.

The interviewer *summarizes* his impression of hypomania and gets the patient's approval (Q. 17). He then returns to the assessment of normal mood (Q. 18–21).

18. I: I know I asked you before, but are there any normal times where you are neither down nor high-strung?
    P: You mean, when things just go easy and I don't feel driven or have to kick myself?

19. I: That's right, when things kind of fall in place and seem to run by themselves.
    P: Yes, last year, I had a pretty good semester.

20. I: Do you feel good then for several months?
    P: Usually not that long. Just a couple of months and I start down again.

21. I: Let me summarize. What you describe to me sounds as if you are on a roller coaster, going up and down. The downs seem to be more troublesome than the ups. But the deep downs rarely last longer than a few days. And there don't seem to be many straight stretches or periods when you feel normal.
    P: That's it. That's exactly how I feel.

The interviewer *summarizes* his diagnostic impression of a mild manic-depressive disorder or, possibly cyclothymia (Q. 21).

Another summarizing ploy especially good with patients who might be easily intimidated is to enlist their help as follows:

"I want to see if I have a good idea of what we have discussed; so I'm going to repeat my understanding of our conversation in my own words and I want you to immediately correct any errors I make."

The six clarification techniques carve out the contours of symptoms and assess the interconnections of elements within a topic; they are mostly patient-centered. Steering techniques, which are explained next, help the interviewer to direct the patient's attention from element to element and one topic to another. The interviewer is like the captain of the ship who tells the steerman, the patient, which course to follow. Steering becomes more interviewer-directed than clarification techniques.

Steering Techniques

A vast territory must be covered in order to make a valid diagnosis. How do you get from one topic to the other—cutting the patient off without choking him? Steering techniques offer a way in which to keep the interview on a desired course. The techniques include continuation, echoing, curbing, and transitions.

Continuation

Continuation is the simplest steering technique. It encourages the patient to go on with his story and indicates the course is right. It tells him that he gives diagnostically useful information. This technique includes nonverbal gestures such as nodding, keeping eye contact, inviting hand gestures and statements such as:

"What happened then?"
"Tell me more."
"Okay."
"Anything else?"
"That's interesting."
"I want to hear more."
"I think that's important."
"Go on."
"Keep on talking."
"Hmm."

The advantage of this technique is that you let the patient describe his problems in his own words; no symptoms are suggested.

In the following interview Gary, a 31-year-old, white, single security guard, talks about recent changes in his feelings, which indicate elated mood such as seen in mania, or amphetamine and cocaine abuse. Since this information is diagnostically useful, the interviewer invites continuation whenever the patient stops talking.

1. I: What kind of problem brought you here?
   P: For the last ten days I haven't been able to sleep.

2. I: Hmm.
   P: I just can't fall asleep. I may only doze off for one to two hours toward morning.

3. I: Yes.
   P: And I don't even feel tired during the day at all. (Raises his voice.)

4. I: (Nods.)
   P: Last weekend, I was home with my folks. It seemed that they bugged me a lot. We got into several arguments and I started slamming doors again.

5. I: Any other problems?
   P: Well, I called my friends and tried to arrange something for Saturday evening.

6. I: (Raises eyebrows.)
   P: Both of my friends told me: "You are shouting again on the telephone. Are you getting high?"

7. I: Did anything else happen?
   P: Yes. We went out and I was very attracted to girls. I got so stimulated, I had to go the bathroom twice to masturbate.

8. I: Hmm.
   P: Well, when I came home I had all these fantasies about having sex from behind and I could do it without having to worry about babies.

9. I: What happened then?
   P: Well, I masturbated throughout the night and had wild fantasies. I felt sky-high, but I only had two or three beers.

10. I: Tell me more.
    P: I'm so restless. I try not to talk so much, but it is hard to do. One of these days I feel medication will help me, or I will help myself. But I'm just not there yet.

Directive interventions are avoided, which allows the patient to talk about himself choosing *his* order of importance rather than that of the interviewer.

Echoing

Echoing repeats the part of the patient's answer on which you want him to elaborate. This technique is different from continuation in that *you* selectively emphasize certain elements of the patient's statements, thus enticing him to follow the highlighted parts rather than any other. This technique can be used when the patient offers several leads in his answers but you want him to follow a specific train of thought.

Bernadette, a 36-year-old, white, married housewife, describes her problems in a circumstantial and flighty way. The interviewer echoes reported problems and chooses to ignore her prepared statement.

1. I: How are things going?
   P: They are not going well at all. In fact, I have made a list with all the problems that I have had over the last two weeks. I have written them down every day. My husband agrees with me and he and I think that there may be a problem that I may get sick again.

2. I: You may get sick again?
   P: Yes, I think so.

3. I: What makes you think so?
   P: I don't get my housework done and I'm terrible with my husband and the children. It must be awful to live with me. But let me read from my notes, day by day. Do you want to have them?

4. I: You say you are terrible with your husband.
   P: I'm short and abrupt with him. I have no patience at all. I bite his head off when he hasn't done anything. But I have it all written down here.

5. I: So you are pretty short with him?
   P: Yes, and I'm also terrible with the children. I shout for no reason at all and I'm so tense and irritable. It says here in my notes that I even spanked my little son when he just asked me the same question twice. It seems to be worse when I don't sleep well.

6. I: You can't sleep?
   P: I wake up by 4:30. I can't sleep but I don't want to get out of bed either. I get tense and upset. But I have it written here (points to her diary) much more systematically. Don't you want to hear it?

7. I: I want to hear it from you. You can leave me the notes for later.
   P: Okay, it won't be very organized. I have a terrible time getting my thoughts together. I can't stay on one topic for any length of time. My husband says that if I go on like this I will end up in the hospital again.

8. I: So you are all over the place?
   P: Yes, I am. I start cooking, I start sewing, I call up some people, I start cleaning and I don't seem to finish anything. Nothing gets done.

9. I: So you start many things without finishing them?
   P: Yes. That's typical for my negative highs.

The interviewer selectively echoes some of the patient's formulations to elicit symptoms of her mood disorder: loss of energy, irritability, early morning awakening, distractibility, increase of activity, and experience of a negative high. Without *checking for symptoms,* he obtains a symptom profile typical for an episode with mixed manic and depressive symptoms as seen in roughly 30% of bipolar patients. The echoing technique is useful in patients with some push of speech and who can easily be distracted.

Curbing

The curbing technique tells the patient to stop diverging from the main course and asks him to return after he has strayed from it. Used when patients ramble, get lost in irrelevant details, or discuss other people's problems, curbing is indicated in patients with flight of ideas, tangential speech, push of speech, and circumstantiality.

Stacy, a 25-year-old, white, female graduate student has a hard time staying on one topic. The interviewer curbs her to make her talk about herself which creates a rivalry between his own and the patient's goals.

1. I: What brought you here?
   P: I think I'm having a crisis. I went to the emergency room last night, and this morning and then this afternoon again. They told me to come back to see you.

2. I: What seems to be the problem?
   P: I'm living with Frank. He told me to throw all my medication away. You know he's a mental patient himself. But anybody has to get sick who plays music all night, smokes pot, and takes drugs.

3. I: (Interrupts.) Stacy, why don't we stay with your own problems?
   P: Okay. Well, last night I called home. My mother was not there, just my sister. You know she's dating this black guy and . . .

4. I: Let me interrupt you. Let me ask you why you went to the emergency room yesterday.
   P: Okay. After I talked to my sister I got so upset because I think she's ruining her life. My parents don't like what she is doing at all . . .

5. I: (Interrupts.) So you were upset with her?
   P: Yes, and I started drinking beer, and had pizza. And then I remembered that I should not do these things when I'm on Parnate.

6. I: So you went off your diet?
   P: Yeah, but then I got frightened that my blood pressure might shoot up so I went to the emergency room. My mother will be mad . . .

7. I: Stacy, let's talk about going off your diet. You were upset you said?
   P: Yes, I have not been doing well at all lately. My thoughts seem to race. Last weekend I stayed in bed for two days and I've been up since then. I talked to Frank. You know Frank is . . .

8. I: Stacy, let's go back to your own problems.
   P: Well, I wanted to have sex with Frank. He said: "You are getting sick again. I want you to go back to your own apartment." You know he can be a real stinker. Now he's decided to be straight.

9. I: So Frank tried to kick you out?
   P: He's really worried about me and sees to it that I take good care of myself.

10. I: So this time he wanted you out?
    P: That made me so upset. I called home and just my sister was in, which did not help matters. It reminded me of what she's doing to herself.

11. I: So you were upset? Before you got upset, were you already pretty restless?
    P: That's right. I think it's me and it hasn't really anything to do with Frank or my sister. I'm afraid the voices will come back too. Yesterday it seemed that things were starting to have another meaning again.

The interviewer interrupts Stacy continuously to curb her (Q. 3, 4, 5, 7, 8) and focus her on giving a description of her problems and symptoms. In spite of curbing the yield is often small in comparison to the length of the interview, as the above example shows.

Transitions

During an interview, several topics (see chapters 4–6) have to be covered. You have to entice the patient to change topics. Therefore you need different types of transitions: smooth, accentuated, and abrupt. The choice of transition depends on the patient's mental status. An inattentive patient, for instance, may focus better if a new topic is accentuated, whereas a paranoid patient may become suspicious.

SMOOTH TRANSITIONS:

Smooth transitions lead easily from one topic to the next by giving the impression that both belong together. Here are two types:

Cause and Effect Relationship: You assume that a reported event may affect the patient's functioning. Examples are drug abuse and its effects, life events and their consequences, or a physical ailment and its impact.

Greg, a 16-year-old, black high school student talks about his problem with glue sniffing.

P: Glue has ruined my life. All I can think about is getting a plastic bag over my head and sniffing some airplane glue.
I: Has this sniffing affected your school work?

P: Yes, it's just terrible, I do not even want to go to school and when I go, I'm in a daze.
I: Has it affected your health?

P: I feel dizzy, my heart beats real fast, and I pass out.
I: Has this sniffing influenced your appetite?

P: I have lost several pounds, but I eat ok now.
I: Has the sniffing interfered with your sleep?

P: Yes, sometimes I sleep during the day and can't sleep at night.

The interviewer directs the patient from glue sniffing to symptoms of depression and their severity by causally relating them. Such a transition works if the causal relationship is evident to the patient.

With a delusional patient who is suspicious of anything new, smooth transitions work best. Otherwise, the response will be:

"What does that have to do with it?"
"What a stupid question!"
"I am not going to answer that nonsense."
"Why are you asking me that?"

The smooth cause and effect transition technique worked well with a 27-year-old, white, single assembly line worker with delusional paranoid disorder. The interviewer uses the patient's complaint and connects it with questions that assess the premorbid personality.

I: You told me that people at work have plotted against you. You say this has really changed you. Tell me what kind of a person you were before all this plotting started to mess you up.
P: I was somewhat of a loner, but I always had one or two friends. Now I have nobody.

A cause and effect transition motivates the patient to answer, since his view of his problems is accepted by the interviewer (whereas his usual experience is that his view is rejected).

Temporal Relationship: The transition between symptoms is smoothed by relating symptoms to the same point in time.

I: Kathleen, when you had the panic attacks, did you notice any other changes?
P: Yes, my sleep was real bad. I woke up in the middle of the night and could not get back to sleep.

I: What about your appetite at that time?
P: I forced myself to eat, but I lost several pounds anyway.

I: And how was your social life then?
P: I wanted to hide in the house and not face anybody.

In this example, the smooth transition ties symptoms together that belong to the same syndrome. In other cases you may use time as a reference point to change to an otherwise unrelated topic. For instance, when a patient tells you about his medical problems, but you intend to assess his social history in more detail, you may say:

"When you had all those medical problems, how did you get along with your wife and how were things at work at this time?"

ACCENTUATED TRANSITION:

Accentuated transitions emphasize a shift in topic; they set the previous topic apart from the new one, such as:

"Now let's explore . . ." (medical history for example).
"Let's shift to another area."

An accentuated transition may be introduced by summarizing what you have learned before switching to the new topic.

I: I now know how glue sniffing has affected your life. Let's talk about something different now. Did you have any disciplinary problems when you were in school?

You may use an accentuated transition as partition between the phases—as explained in chapter 6—of the diagnostic interview and as introduction to testing mental status functions (see chapter 4). Here is an illustration for the latter.

"I think we have covered a lot of territory and I feel that I understand most of your problems. Before I give you my recommendations, I would like to cover one more point that does not really seem related to any of your problems. I'd like to get an idea of how well you can respond to some test questions that tell us something about your memory and concentration."

"We have not yet discussed how your memory or thinking may be affected by your problems."

"Would you mind if I asked you a few standardized test questions so I can get a feeling of how well you can concentrate?"

Without explaining such a shift in topic to the patient who, for instance, presents with a marriage problem, he may be surprised if he is subjected to a test of concentration, such as the so-called "serial sevens" backwards (subtracting 7 from 100). However, if you prepare him, he may cooperate.

Accentuated transitions revive the patient's attention and make him aware how many different topics have been covered. Withdrawn depressives, or schizophrenics may liven up. Distractible manics refocus their attention. The circumstantial obsessive compulsive is stimulated by the new topic and cooperates better.

ABRUPT TRANSITIONS:

Abrupt transitions introduce a new topic with little or inadequate warning and can be clumsy and awkward:

"Now, I am going to examine you."
"Let's see, what's the date today?"
"Now I want to ask you a few questions which you may think are really stupid."
"What I wanted to ask you is this . . ."
"Okay, there is something else . . ."

However, abrupt transitions are useful with patients who lie or simulate symptoms in that they catch him off guard.

Mr. Martens, a 43-year-old, white male, was admitted to the Kansas City V.A. Hospital because he claimed severe memory disturbances due to exposure to Agent Orange during the Vietnam War.

1. I: Hi, Mr. Martens, do you remember me? I talked to you last week.
    P: Yes.

2. I: How was your weekend?
    P: I was out on pass.

3. I: How did it go?
    P: I can't remember . . .

4. I: I want you to remember three things: *eyedropper, brown, and justice.* Would you repeat them for me?
   P: Yes . . . eyedropper, brown, and justice.

5. I: Did you watch any television during the weekend?
   P: Oh yes, about the Jews and the Christians in Lebanon. Some mess they have over there.

6. I: Does that concern you specifically?
   P: Yes, I worry about war, especially with Arafat.

7. I: Which leaders on the Jewish side do you fear?
   P: I don't remember their names.

8. I: How is your wife?
   P: She left when I came home.

9. I: Can you remember the three things?
   P: Brown, and . . . and . . . I don't know. But it may come to me if I wait awhile.

10. I: What is the name of the Israeli prime minister?
    P: I don't remember.

11. I: Do you know who Moshe Dayan was?
    P: Wasn't he a Jewish general?

12. I: I am sorry to hear this about your wife. What did you do when she had left?
    P: I wrote her a letter. I told her that I was very disappointed that she left when I came home and I also told this bitch that if she wanted to desert me she should go right ahead. But then I told her that I still love her and that I would like things to work out between us.

13. I: Do you remember the three things?
    P: No, just brown, as I told you before.

14. I: Last week, Dr. X also asked you to remember three things. Do you recall what they were?
    P: No.

15. I: One of the three things was an animal. Do you remember which one?
    P: No.

16. I: I see. You did not remember then either. What did you tell her instead?
    P: I told her *elephant.*

17. I: That's right. But she asked you to remember *lion.*
    P: Yes, it's coming back to me now.

The interviewer jumps back and forth among three topics: television news (Q. 5, 7, 11), marital problems (Q. 8, 12), and recollection of three items (Q. 4, 9, 13–17). The patient claims he does not remember what happened during the weekend but he recalls the TV news. He starts to name the leaders involved in the Middle Eastern conflict, but then claims forgetfulness (A. 10) when he seems to realize that such a recall involves memory. Mr. Martens also recalls the content of the letter that he wrote to his wife. It appears that he was not aware that his memory was tested, because otherwise he would have realized that this recall contradicts his claimed global amnesia.

Regarding the formal memory testing (recall of three items), he claims to have forgotten the items the examiner gave him, but remembers the faulty answer (elephant) he gave the previous week. This inconsistency is not compatible with severe anterograde memory disturbance.

Abrupt transitions have the effect of a cross-examination. They prevent the patient from keeping track of what he wants to portray. They reveal inconsistencies. They are the lie detectors of an interview. Mr. Martens is only cooperative on the surface. He does not address his need for compensation or attention which may underlie his simulations. His behavior is a good lead into the next set of techniques used for patients with resistance.

2. DEALING WITH RESISTANCE

Resistance, in this context, refers to the patient's conscious, voluntary effort to avoid a certain topic. Resistance can surface in several ways. The clearest form is open refusal:

"I prefer not to talk about it right now."
"I don't want to discuss this with you."
"Let's talk about something else."

An indirect form is the patient's attempt to distract you from pursuing a topic: he may answer your questions only briefly, or not at all, or he starts talking intensely about something else, or he is vague, shows reluctance in his facial expression, or pauses before answering. Finally, he may try to dissimulate a problem with expressions such as

"This really doesn't bother me."
"It's not one of my main concerns."
"There are more important things to worry about."

Two reasons for the patient's resistance are common: 1. his wish to keep up an image, 2. his uncertainty about the interviewer's response.

The psychodiagnostic interview often takes place in the first session. Therefore, the patient tries to appear in a good light, and does not want to embarrass himself, or be judged as "crazy." He is uncertain how the interviewer may respond to the disclosure of "senseless" obsessions, "silly" fears, or "strange" hallucinations.

The interviewer has to recognize and deal with the resistance. You have to choose whether you want to tolerate it or persuade the patient to overcome his resistance. If resistance is limited to one particular topic and does not interfere with rapport, you may respect the patient's privacy and move to the next topic. Otherwise, address his resistance.

Use one of six strategies: *Expressing acceptance, confrontation, bypassing* (see below Handling Defenses), *looping, exaggeration,* and *induction to bragging.*

Acceptance

When a patient shows reluctance to talk but not open refusal, it often indicates a concern about ridicule. If the interviewer expresses acceptance of the patient's thoughts and feelings, the patient will feel understood. Free of any moral evaluation, acceptance neither condemns nor praises the patient. To help him to overcome his resistance, encourage him, verbalize what he seems to imply, express that you understand him.

Sharon, a 25-year old, black outpatient law student, has agoraphobia but hesitates to talk about it. The interviewer helps her to overcome her resistance by offering understanding and acceptance.

1. I: What problem brought you here, Sharon?
   P: It's really all so ridiculous that if I tell you, you will just laugh.

2. I: Try me.
   P: I know you will. Why should I try?

3. I: You are afraid I would not understand you and laugh at you?
   P: Yes, that's how I feel.

4. I: It must be a terrible feeling, that you can't talk about what's bothering you. I wish I could help you feel better.
   P: How can you, if it's something so ridiculous?

5. I: It is not ridiculous for you. You are serious, Sharon. And you feel scared.
   P: You really understand?

6. I: Well, you have not told me, but I can feel your fear. It must really torture you.

   P: You are right and it is so ridiculous. Whenever I walk over to the campus all these people stare at me. They sit in front of their houses and they all look at me.

7. I: They look at you? That must make you feel uncomfortable.

   P: I seem to be the only person that walks on the street. All the blacks like to sit in front of their houses in summer. I just feel better when I have reached the campus.

8. I: So you really feel terrible being out there in the street, walking by those houses and having the people stare at you.

   P: Yeah. I hate it. I'm just so scared. I get all these good grades in law school, but I'm so anxious I can't even talk to my relatives when they come over to the house.

9. I: I understand how you feel. It sounds like you are running the gauntlet and I can understand your ordeal. You're doing the right thing by talking to me about it. That's the only way I can understand your feelings and help you.

The phobic patient is often not only fearful about certain objects or situations, but also about the fact that she has to talk about her fear. Acceptance helps the patient overcome such fear and can resolve resistance, but not panic and phobia.

Confrontation

Confrontation focuses the patient's attention on the resistance. It heightens his awareness and invites an explanation. Use this technique when you observe either behavioral clues of resistance such as avoidance of eye contact, blushing, repetitive swallowing, overly controlled affect, tension, restlessness, or if the patient uses monosyllabic and censored speech, distraction tactics, or dissimulates, i.e., minimizes symptoms, or rambles excessively.

The interviewer confronts Mildred, a 34-year-old, white, single secretary, with a behavioral clue. Mildred talks about social isolation and frustration at work. While talking she stares at the interviewer, becomes restless, pauses repeatedly, then resumes talking.

1. I: Mildred, I have noticed that you often look at me without blinking.

   P: What do you mean? (Her posture becomes stiff.)

2. I: I mean you look at me for a long time without blinking.
   P: I guess it's just a habit (patient blushes).

3. I: Are you aware of it?
   P: So you noticed. (Pause.) I was afraid you would. I have had this eye problem since I was 15 years old and had an eye infection. (Patient gives a long-winded history of her eye infection.)

4. I: So what did this infection do to your eyes?
   P: Since the eye infection I think about blinking when I look at people.

5. I: Can you explain?
   P: I always wonder when it would be natural to blink.

6. I: Hmm.
   P: When I look at somebody I always worry about when to blink. If I look too long and don't blink, people think I am staring at them. But when I make myself blink, I think it's unnatural because I did it voluntarily.

7. I: Why didn't you want to talk about it?
   P: It's so embarrassing, you must think I'm crazy.

When confronted with her staring, Mildred minimizes the significance of her behavior (A. 2). Persistent confrontation (Q. 3, 5, 7) yields a full explanation of her symptoms and she gives up her resistance. This confrontation opened up the discussion of obsessions and compulsions.

Mr. Nelson, a 57-year-old, white, married lawyer, was confronted with the irrational reason of his resistance.

1. I: What kind of problems would you like to talk about?
   P: I am thinking over and over whether I would be able to go to sleep tonight. Just tell me if it can hurt me if I take 1 mg of lorazepam when I can't sleep.

2. I: In what way do you think it will hurt you?
   P: My body may be short of enzymes and the drug could accumulate.

3. I: What do you fear could happen?
   P: My breathing may stop and I may not wake up. Tell me if there is a chance this can happen. I worry about these things. But if I don't take the drug I may not be able to sleep. So I'm really in a bind. Damned if I do and damned if I don't.

4. I: Are these the only thoughts that come to your mind time and again?
   P: Yes, these worries.

5. I: Are there ever any other thoughts? Do you have any other repetitive worries?
   P: Like what?

6. I: Some patients wonder how many tiles are on the floor or how many chairs are in the room and they feel they have to count them. Did you ever have any similar experiences?
   P: I don't want to talk about those now.

7. I: So you can only talk about your worries, but not about the other thoughts?
   P: Right.

8. I: What is so different about these other things?
   P: They are so silly and so embarrassing.

9. I: So you don't want to embarrass yourself, but it is very important for me to understand your problems fully.
   P: I can't come back to you if I tell you about them. I feel too embarrassed. As a lawyer I should not have these problems.

10. I: So lawyers are immune to certain illnesses?
    P: Okay . . . I think again and again if I have wiped myself. And I always have to turn my back away from people so that they can't smell it. I know it's nonsense. I wash myself, but it tortures me over and over again.

Initially, Mr. Nelson talked about worries over insomnia (Q. 1–4). A worry is similar to an obsession with respect to its intrusive nature and emotional discomfort, but unlike an obsession, it is ego-syntonic, i.e., the patient identifies with a worry but not with an obsessive thought. Taking the worries as a clue, the interviewer inquires about obsessions but the patient resists this exploration openly (A. 6–7). Confrontation with the resistance (Q. 8–10) achieved the revelation of his obsession and related compulsion.

Mrs. Finch, a 38-year-old, white female, admitted to being nervous at night but denied any other problems. She was confronted with her dissimulation of symptoms:

1. I: What has been troubling you, Mrs. Finch?
   P: At night I'm nervous.

1. I: How do you feel otherwise during the day?
   P: I'm just fine, just nervous at night, that's all.

3. I: Fine?
   P: Yes. Fine. (Patient looks to the ceiling and appears to listen to something, and then looks down.)

4. I: Are you hearing something?
   P: No, they don't bother me anymore.

5. I: Bother you any more? What do you mean?
   P: I'm over them now.

6. I: You mean you don't hear them anymore?
   P: (Patient looks up to the outlet of the air conditioner, shakes her head and mumbles.) Shut up. No, no, no.

7. I: You mean they don't talk to you anymore?
   P: I told you that they don't bother me anymore. (Patient angrily looks up to the ceiling.)

8. I: Since we have been talking together I noticed that they must have been talking to you through the air-conditioning unit.
   P: Why do you say that?

9. I: Well, you just looked up there, made an angry face and talked back to them.
   P: So you heard them too? My sister always says that I am talking nonsense. But my mother and my sister just won't leave me alone. They sneak up on me and say all those mean and awful things.

10. I: So you hear them through the air-conditioning duct even though they are miles away?
    P: Sure, they're sneaky.

11. I: But, you told me that you are not hearing any voices.
    P: That's right. I'm not imagining anything. You know, if I say I hear voices, you will think I'm crazy and imagining things.

Confrontation with her behavior—listening and talking back to the air-conditioning duct—brought out the patient's hallucinations.

Confrontation with Consequences

To use this technique you have to know some of the patient's intentions, because this technique relies on the gratification of the patient's needs. The prospect of satisfaction weakens resistance. This strategy is useful for patients who voluntarily and stubbornly refuse to interact with you.

Mrs. McQueen is a 23-year-old, white, married female who was brought to the ER by her husband because of repeated wrist cutting. Her husband reported that the patient had been a sloppy housekeeper for most of their marriage and had neglected their two children, going to the movies with a girlfriend instead. When he criticized her she threw temper tantrums and lately started to harm herself. Mood, sleep, and appetite were unchanged; according to him she had no hallucinations or delusions. At the ER the patient was shouting and had outbursts of anger; she fell into a state of muteness when committed at her husband's request.

The patient is lying on the bed with her head buried in her hands. She refuses to acknowledge the interviewer but glances briefly through her fingers.

1. I: Hi, Mrs. McQueen. I'm Dr. O. I would like to talk to you.
   P: (No response.)

2. I: Can you tell me why your husband brought you here?
   P: (No response.)

3. I: Do you know that your husband plans to commit you?
   P: (No response.)

4. I: Do you think he is right in doing so?
   P: (No response.)

5. I: Would you like to get out of here?
   P: (No response.)

6. I: I take it that under the circumstances it may be best for you to have some rest. You seem to say: "Leave me alone, until I am ready to talk." Why don't I do that. I'll come back next week and talk to you. Do you want me to let you stay here until next week and then come back?
   P: (Shakes her head.)

7. I: You mean you don't want to take a week of rest?
   P: (Shakes her head.)

8. I: Do you want me to stay and talk to you?
   P: (No answer.)

9. I: Okay. Maybe I should come back later. Is that alright with you?
   P: (No answer.)

10. I: Do you want to stay?
    P: (Shakes her head.)

11. I: Do you want to get out of here?
    P: (Nods.)

12. I: Okay, if you want to get out of here, we have to get a few things straight.
    P: (Talking through her fingers.) You are lying. You won't let me go.

13. I: I have to. I can't hold you if there isn't any reason to hold you. This is not a prison.
    P: (Gets up from her bed and starts to walk toward the elevator, which is in the vicinity.)

14. I: We can't let you go like this. If you want to go, we have to sit down and find out why your husband really wants you here and why you cut yourself. Why don't I give you time to calm down and come back this evening to talk to you?
    P: I don't want to wait that long. I'll talk now.

Because of the patient's immature, even childlike acting out, a personality disorder seems likely. The interviewer feels that the patient's main urge is to go home. He pretends, however, that she may wish to rest before cooperating and arbitrarily suggests one week of that (Q. 7). He assumes that she is not severely depressed and suicidal, but that the self-mutilating behavior is used as a tactic in her marital quarrels. This assumption cannot, however, be confirmed without the patient's cooperation. Since she refuses to stay (A. 7), the interviewer knows that he has tapped a motive strong enough to use for bargaining. He points out that silence will not speed her release. She realizes this, and becomes more cooperative.

When you decide to resolve the patient's resistance rather than to tolerate it, show the patient the advantages of giving it up. Telling her that it is to her advantage may pressure her and increase resistance; breaking down resistance with force is not beneficial for rapport. Therefore, create an atmosphere in which the patient feels supported, can gain insight into her behavior, and experience freedom of choice rather than coercion.

Looping

"You know," Bill McKnelly said when he called us up one Saturday night, after reading chapter 3, "one of the techniques that you should talk about is something one could call looping—it reminds me of that strategy a defensive lineman uses who pulls back from the line and loops around to sack the quarterback. It's a technique lawyers use in court too."

What you do is this: when a patient does not want to talk about something, you let go and get at it from a different angle. It's like coming through the back door.

Mr. Dan Reuben is a 50-year-old, white married schoolteacher, father of three children. As an outpatient he is seeking consultation because of his fading energy, inability to sleep, and worries about the cost of college education for his two oldest sons. During the visit, the interviewer brings up the topic of suicidal thoughts.

1. I: It seems to me that you are carrying quite a burden. Are you able to hold up?
   P: Hmm . . . don't know.

2. I: Have you ever thought of giving in?
   P: How do you mean that?

3. I: I mean has it ever crossed your mind that it is not worth living any more with that much pain?
   P: You mean suicide?

4. I: Yes.
   P: I think that is a terrible sin. It's murder.

5. I: Yes. From a religious point it is . . .
   P: (Interrupts.) It would be an evil deed.

6. I: Have you thought about it?
   P: One should not even think about it—and I don't want to talk about it.

7. I: You are in enough pain as it is. I don't want to burden you more with talking about those thoughts.
   P: (The patient's eyes fill with tears.)

8. I: It seems to me one of your worst worries is your oldest son, whether you can pay those high college costs—and he is such a gifted fellow.
   P: Oh, it's the worst—thinking that I worked all my life so hard as a teacher and can't even give my kid the education he deserves. I feel I let him down . . . and also my other son who is ready to go to college. I let them down, both of them.

9. I: I see. You feel you can't provide what they need.
   P: Right. They would be better off without me. My life insurance would get them through. Isn't it awful?

10. I: That you are worth more to them dead than alive?
    P: Yes. I talked to my agent. If something happened to me, even if it is suicide, they would pay. I always thought the worst way to die would be with a rope around your neck. (Patient starts crying.)

11. I: (Nodding his head.)
    P: Now I feel that's what I deserve. It even feels like peace just hanging there.

In the looping technique, the loop does not have to be wide; just releasing the pressure, shifting the vantage point, often frees the patient and gets him ready to discuss the very topic you were after. In the above example, the thought of committing suicide increases the pathological guilt of the depressed patient to an unbearable degree. Therefore, the thought cannot be pursued. However, the idea of decreasing the guilt through deserved punishment by hanging by his own hand releases the patient's suicidal thoughts at once. For the logical person, not afflicted by depression, the patient's behavior appears contradictory. However, when you understand delusional guilt, you understand why this loop worked.

Exaggeration

An anxious, obsessive, or very conscientious patient is often reluctant to admit to minor wrong doings or failures. He fears the interviewer will reject him if he becomes aware of his character flaws. If you sense such reluctance, decrease the patient's concern by putting it into perspective. If a patient, for instance, slapped her child in anger and is concerned that this was child abuse, you can say:

"You did not bruise or suffocate her?"

Or: A patient is reluctant to elaborate on shoplifting a candy bar when a youngster, you may exaggerate:

"You didn't really rob Fort Knox?"

By comparing the patient's mischief to major harm or crime, the patient usually feels relieved and laughs and experiences clearly that he has not reached your tolerance level where he has to fear rejection. He feels assured instead and can overcome his reluctance.

Induction to Bragging

Patients with sociopathic tendencies often like to make a good impression on the interviewer. They fear that their antisocial acts may tarnish their image, and therefore may attempt to censor the description of such acts. While the exaggeration technique (see above) may also work for these patients, a better technique still is to induce them to brag. For instance, when a patient holds back to talk about his high school troubles, you may challenge him with

"Were you a good fighter?"

Such a statement often seduces him to tell you how he knocked his baseball coach over the head with a bat when he refused to use him in the lineup, or how he tried to beat up on another kid in school who seemed to be interested in his girlfriend.

Or when your patient is lying and cheating but tries to conceal these traits from you, you may encourage him by saying:

"You seem to be sly like a fox—you seem to get away with murder."

Such statements telegraph to the patient that the interviewer is willing to accept the patient's quarrels. Since the patient with an antisocial personality often believes that he was justified in his actions, he feels that your statements indicate your understanding. Your statements tell him that he does not have to fear your criticism.

At a later stage you may have to explain to him that accepting his problems neither means that you encourage him to further antisocial acts nor that you condone and like what he has been doing. It just means that you are willing to give him enough space and attention that he can tell his story with the affect typical for his personality disorder—pride in bragging and interest in impressing others with his deeds (compare chapter 9).

3. DEFENSES

The developmental draft of DSM-III-R (10/5/1985) included a description of defense mechanisms relegated to the glossary in the final DSM-III-R version. This back and forth expresses the ambivalence of the American Psychiatric Association toward psychoanalytical concepts.

Is this inclusion indeed a break with the atheoretical, descriptive approach to psychiatry acclaimed as the basis for DSM-III (1980)? DSM-III conceptualizes disorders as sets of symptoms and signs which satisfy diagnostic criteria. Defenses cannot be fully observed because they postulate specific psychological mechanisms as the underpinnings of observable behavior patterns, signs, and reportable symptoms. The description of defense mechanisms was pursued by the school of psychodynamic interpretative, insight-oriented psychiatry which views psychiatric disorders as results of unconscious conflicts—and symptoms and signs as superficial, changeable manifestations of defense mechanisms, which express the type of unconscious conflict management chosen by the patient.

Some defense mechanisms have intruded into descriptive psychiatry, for instance, denial and rationalization. Empirical studies of ego mechanisms of defense have been conducted (Vaillant 1986). Therefore, their inclusion in descriptive psychodiagnostic interviewing appears defendable.

Being familiar with defense mechanisms helps you understand some of the content and meaning of your patient's psychopathology. Moreover, defense mechanisms may interfere with rapport and history taking. An in-depth assessment and analysis of defense mechanisms is predominantly used in psychodynamic and psychoanalytic interviewing (Vaillant 1986); this book will give only a brief introduction, and will emphasize the descriptive aspect.

The DSM-III-R glossary lists eighteen defense mechanisms:

acting out,
autistic fantasy,
denial,
devaluation,
displacement,
dissociation,
idealization,
intellectualization,
isolation,
passive aggression,
projection,
rationalization,
reaction formation,
repression,
somatization,
splitting,
suppression,
undoing.

This list is not complete; some authors offer others, including introjection, regression, reversal, and turning against the self (A. Freud 1946), affect equivalents, change in the quality of affect, postponement of affect (Fenichel 1945), condensation, symbolization, transference, and transposition (Hinsie 1937).

Recognition of Defense Mechanisms

Defense mechanisms consist of three components: an observable behavior (often a symptom); an unconscious impulse or intent not acceptable to the patient; and a process which links the patient's observable behavior (or symptom) to the unconscious intent. The unconscious intent and the link to the overt behavior or symptom are accessible only by the therapist's inferential interpretation which may or may not be corroborated by the patient.

When you try to decipher the underlying defense mechanisms of overt behaviors or symptoms, you sharpen your skill in recognizing and understanding psychopathology. If you can confirm, by the patient's corroboration, the link between apparently unrealistic behavior and an initially unconscious, embarrassing, aggressive, or libidinous impulse you have identified the defense mechanism.

You will become sensitive to the presence of defense mechanisms if you look for behaviors that indicate unrealistic and unexpected goals, extreme in their intensity, self-incriminating, accusatory, or self-serving in their intent.

Table 3.2 summarizes the triple facet of the eighteen defense mechanisms listed in DSM-III-R plus one which was planned (Draft, DSM-III-R in development 1985) but did not make it into the manual: sublimation.

The defense mechanisms are arranged along a continuum. At one end (top of table) are the defenses which reflect complete repression of painful impulses or events. At the other end (bottom of table) are defenses which allow the appearance of formerly unacceptable impulses after censoring and editing.

To give examples for each of these nineteen defense mechanisms and how they can interfere with the diagnostic interview would exceed the scope of this text. The following will provide only a few examples of how to handle defense mechanisms during a psychodiagnostic interview.

Handling Defense Mechanisms

Defense mechanisms distort the patient's perception of himself and his environment. In an insight-oriented therapeutic interview, the therapist attempts to make the patient aware of his defenses, their underlying mechanism and their unconscious origins, with the expectation that the patient will replace his defensive behavior with a more reality-oriented behavior. In a psychodiagnostic interview the interviewer handles defense mechanisms to the extent that they interfere with rapport and history taking.

TABLE 3.2
Anatomy of Defense Mechanisms According to DSM-III-R

Defense Mechanism	Observable Behavior or Symptom	Unconscious Component	Process
REPRESSION	Amnesia	Painful event, desires, impulses, thoughts, strivings	Unconscious blocking of recall
SUPPRESSION	Avoidance in discussing painful problems, wishes, or feelings, and in exploring sensitive topics	Painful event, sadistic or sexual impulse	Intentional blocking of recall
DENIAL	Stubborn and angry negation of some unpleasant external reality	Painful external reality	Refusal to acknowledge to self or others the awareness of some reality
UNDOING	Compulsive behavior	Sadistic wishes	Symbolic negating of a sadistic impulse
ISOLATION	Obsessions, talking about emotional events without feelings	Painful effect of an event	Splitting of content and affect and suppression of either
DISSOCIATION	Multiple personality, psychogenic fugue, amnesia	Promiscuous, hostile, or irresponsible behavior pattern	Temporary alteration of consciousness and suppression of unacceptable behavior
SPLITTING	Idealization or devaluation of self or others	Negative or positive qualities of self or others	Unacceptable positive or negative qualities of self or others are suppressed
INTELLECTU-ALIZATION	Abstract thinking, doubting, indecisiveness	Disturbing feelings	Avoidance and suppression of the emotional component of an event

Continued on next page

TABLE 3.2—CONTINUED
Anatomy of Defense Mechanisms According to DSM-III-R

IDEALIZA-TION	Unjustified praising of self or others	Negative qualities of self or others	Suppression of negative qualities of self or others
DEVALUA-TION	Derogative statements about others or self, "sour grapes" about a goal	Positive qualities of self, others, or of an unattainable goal	Suppression of positive qualities and exaggeration of negative qualities of self, others, or object
REACTION FORMATION	Devotion, self-sacrificing behavior, correctness, cleanliness	Feelings of hostility, death wish against a close person	Substitution by wishes or feelings opposite of the true feelings
RATIONAL-IZATION	Self-serving explanations and justification of behavior	Socially unacceptable behavior	Give socially acceptable explanations for behavior
DISPLACE-MENT	Phobias	Fear and threat by an object, or love and hate for an object	Transferring a feeling from its actual object to a substitute
PROJECTION	Ideas of reference, persecutory delusions, prejudice, suspiciousness, injustice	Hostility, homosexual feelings, other unacceptable attitudes, wishes, desires	Attributing one's own feelings to others
SOMATIZA-TION	Medically unexplained physical symptoms	Lack of confidence to assert oneself	Production of physical symptoms
ACTING OUT	Violent acts, stealing, lying, rape	Sexual and aggressive impulses	Nonreflective, uncontrolled wish fulfillment
PASSIVE AGGRESSION	Procrastination	Aggressive, hostile impulses	Expression through passivity
AUTISTIC FANTASY	Daydreaming	Unsatisfied impulses and wishes	Fantasized wish fulfillment
SUBLIMA-TION *	Socially acceptable behavior	Unacceptable feelings or impulses	Rechanneling

Note: * not in DSM-III-R

Handling defenses is different from handling resistance. The patient, who shows resistance, is aware of it and voluntarily conceals information. The patient who uses defense mechanisms is often not aware of them and has no voluntary control over them. The pathological behavior takes over and interferes with the interview. Handling defenses means neutralizing their impact but not analyzing and interpreting them.

In the following section, we describe a set of five management techniques that will help you to handle defenses: *bypassing, reassurance, distraction, confrontation, and interpretation.*

Bypassing

Common sense expresses the wisdom of this popular technique in proverbs such as "Let sleeping dogs lie" and "Don't rock the boat."

Every interviewer will meet the patient who clearly distorts his reality perception. A widow may claim that her husband was the best, one wouldn't find a second like him. The record may show that this idolized man was an alcoholic who physically abused her. For the diagnosis of her depression it may not be essential to confront her with her denial, at least not in the first interview, but better bypass or ignore her defense. Her defense mechanism only highlights her mental status.

Reassurance

Reassurance attempts to decrease the patient's anxieties and suspicions and to increase his self-confidence by offering support. Reassurance works by viewing a defense mechanism from the patient's vantage point. This empathic approach will give the patient the feeling of having an ally. It is most effective when the patient appears overwhelmed by his problems.

During a depressive episode, this 45-year-old, widowed father with bipolar illness is ready to give up job hunting and caring for his two children.

1. I: How can I help you, Russ?
   P: (Shakes his head and does not say anything.)

2. I: What's on your mind?
   P: I don't even know why I came!

3. I: What is it, Russ?
   P: (No answer.)

4. I: You seem to be really down.
   P: (Stares at the floor.)

5. I: You look depressed . . . and hopeless.
   P: What's the use. Even if I find a job and I get some money saved and get everything straightened out I get high again and blow it all, and nothing is going to stop me. I went through this before, but it was not as bad as it is this time.

6. I: I think you have learned a lot from the past. This may help you with next time! I believe next time you will come for treatment when you get high.
   P: Do you really think so?

7. I: We both have to work at it. I know you can do it. Things will look better again. You will come out of it, we can talk about it and get you through. Let's talk about your depression now.
   P: If you think so.

Notice that the patient's self-punitive behavior is not addressed and interpreted, but is instead counteracted by the interviewer's support. Rather than assessing special problems, the interviewer feeds him supportive and reassuring statements (Q. 5, 6). The patient livens up when he hears that his therapist does not share the feelings of hopelessness, but sees a better future for him. Reassurance takes advantage of the dependency feelings in the patient. This is most effective if you are perceived as an empathic person.

Distraction

This technique is used for patients who have an abnormal mood state due to a psychiatric disorder such as mania, retarded depression, or intoxication. Such states cannot be changed by addressing underlying defenses. They can be overcome by a stimulus strong enough to get the patient's attention and force him to concentrate at least briefly. Use stimuli such as calling the patient's name, shouting, or using physical contact. The stimulus can be used repeatedly, or can be applied in concert with other stimuli. Ask short and closed-ended questions. You most likely cannot obtain continuous interaction, because the patient will drift off again, but you may get short answers.

Mr. Wilson is an excited 57-year-old, white, divorced male with a history of mania. He reports to the ER smelling of whiskey. He is upset with a nurse who had asked him to stay in one of the examining rooms until the interviewer arrives. He is screaming tirades of protest. The interviewer stands in the doorway and observes the patient for a while. His presence is ignored.

1. I: Mr. Wilson, can I talk to you? (Patient pays no attention and continues to shout in the direction of the nursing station.)
   P: In this damned place everybody thinks they can push you around. But not me. I'll show this bitch.

2. I: (Louder.) Mr. Wilson!
   P: I've never been treated by anybody like this. And I won't take it from this bitch either!

3. I: Hold it! (With an intense pressed voice.)
   P: (Startled, turns around and looks at him, surprised.)

4. I: (Looks him in the eye.) I want to help you. Will you talk to me?
   P: Who are you?

5. I: I'm the doctor on call. My name is Dr. O. I see you have had some problems.
   P: This bitch told me not to leave the room. What do you want? Just stay away from me. I know your kind. First thing you do is give me a shot.

6. I: Mr. Wilson, let's sit down. I want to know what's eating you.
   P: I don't want to sit down.

7. I: Fine with me.
   P: I am just too mad to sit down.

8. I: Can I get you a cup of coffee?
   P: No, you stay here. (Patient gets out his cigarettes.)

9. I: Here is an ashtray for you.
   P: (Lights a cigarette and sits down.)

10. I: Mr. Wilson, can I talk to you? Mr. Wilson, I want to help you. Tell me how I can best help you.
    P: By leaving me alone!

11. I: Fine, but you were alone. All you did was holler. Is this what you came for?
    P: No, I wanted to tell somebody about the problems I'm having in the halfway house.

12. I: Alright, let's sit down, and you tell me about it. (Sits down.) Okay.

To get attention the interviewer addresses the patient with a short command (Q. 3). In response, the patient directs his hostility toward him (A. 5). When the interviewer asks him whether he came to the ER to holler, the patient becomes aware of his self-defeating, acting-out behavior.

Patients who are very excited, who show pronounced push of speech and flight of ideas, or who are intoxicated or delusional may not be distractible. They may need pharmacological intervention before rapport can be established.

Confrontation

Confrontation is used to draw the patient's attention to a particular behavior with the expectation that he will recognize and correct it during the interview.

Carol is a 38-year-old, white, female outpatient. The interviewer had reviewed with her the circumstances that led to her separation.

1. I: How is your relationship with your husband now?
   P: (Looks frightened and hostile.) Why do you ask?

2. I: Well, I just want to know if you are still in touch with him.
   P: (More hostile and angry.) Of course. (The patient gets up and takes her coat.) I better go now!

3. I: Carol, you are getting angry.
   P: Because you know damn well that he is still calling me—goodbye! (Patient is getting up from her chair.)

4. I: Carol, you seem to think that I must be in touch with him. (Superficial interpretation.)
   P: Aren't you?

5. I: You are angry with me and you don't trust me? (Confrontation.)
   P: Nobody is on my side. Not even you. And you are supposed to be my doctor.

6. I: So you feel I am against you too? (Confrontation.)
   P: Aren't you?

7. I: I am on your side, but I notice it is difficult for you to believe me. (Supportive statement and confrontation.)
   P: (Patient turns around, hangs coat over her chair.) I don't know, I try to trust you.

8. I: What is really bothering you about your husband's telephone calls?
   P: I hear the clicking sound in the system. I know he has his tape recorder on and he's recording me again.

9. I: And you think I'm in with him and know about it?
   P: Isn't that why you ask about the calls?

10. I: No, I did not ask you about the calls. I asked you whether you are still in touch with him and that made you very upset and suspicious.
    P: It did. I feel everybody is in with him, even my parents who say that they hate him. Sometimes I don't trust them either.

Reading the patient's delusional suspicion and confronting her with it prevents breakdown of rapport. He combines two techniques: first, he confronts her with her distrust (Q. 3, 5, 6), and second, he shows her support and empathy (Q. 7) by assuring her that he sides with her, which makes her reflect upon her suspicion (A. 7). The combined use of these two techniques works only because the patient has some insight into her suspiciousness (perhaps she is projecting?). Otherwise, she would have refused to discuss the topic any further or left the office.

From a descriptive point of view Carol's beliefs are ideas of reference which border on persecutory delusions, with the exception that *some* insight is preserved. From a dynamic point of view these ideas of reference are conceived as a result of *projection*.

During a diagnostic interview, you have to deal with these reality distortions in order to maintain rapport. You have to decide from case to case whether accepting such ideas of reference as the patient's reality or confronting her with them is more appropriate. When you become included in her delusion, you have to confront the patient with the delusional nature of her thinking. However, if the delusion is fully developed, confrontation will fail to make the patient recognize her reality distortion.

The success of a confrontation is not only dependent upon the patient's insight. According to Pope and Siegman (1965) and Bierman (1969) dissonant and provocative confrontations inhibit the display of emotions, while empathic confrontations according to Anderson (1968) increase self-exploration. Therefore, choose a vantage point for your confrontation that helps the patient understand his inappropriate behavior and at the same time makes him feel your concern. More about this aspect in the section below on interpretation.

Interpretation of Defenses

Interpretation is a statement offering your understanding of the patient's defensive behavior. Whereas confronting can be compared to holding up a mirror,

"Since you have entered the room, you have not looked me in the eye."

interpreting is like using a concave mirror.

"You don't look me in the eye because you fear I can read your thoughts."

Interpretation reflects how you understand the patient; you suggest to him a meaning in his thoughts or an intent behind his behavior. Usually, interpretation follows confrontation, because you have to make a patient aware of his behavior before he can understand your interpretation. Interpretation conveys to the patient that you try to understand his behavior and that you invite him to discuss it with you.

A correct interpretation explains the patient's behavior satisfactorily in the context of all other behaviors. Unfortunately, there is no sure way to be correct. You may feel your interpretation is correct when the patient agrees with it and voluntarily elaborates, when it is in agreement with your clinical experience, and when nothing else in the patient's behavior contradicts it.

The usefulness of a correct interpretation depends on the patient's acceptance. If a patient is unaware of his behavior, an interpretation is usually counterproductive. He will feel criticized and misunderstood, and defend himself against such "accusations." Rapport will deteriorate.

In the patient with persecutory delusions, however, interpretations may lead to a breakup of the interview. He may think that you read his mind and control him. Rather than feeling understood he feels manipulated and walks out. Therefore, it is important to evaluate him for persecutory tendencies before you attempt to use interpretation techniques.

Interpretation is useful with patients who do not initially level with you, or have difficulties expressing their thoughts and feelings. It is used to get the patient more involved and make him realize and understand his attitude.

Hopkinson et al. (1981) found that interpretations offered by the interviewer were followed 44% of the time by the patient's emotional expression. If the patient's emotional response is of value, the interviewer might elect to precede his interpretation by his own expression of feelings; if he does, his client responds in kind in 75% of his interpretations. If he does not, his yield is only 26%.

Interpretation is demonstrated with the defense mechanism of projection. At the same time the three components of a defense mechanism (see above) are illustrated: observable behavior, unconscious impulse or intent, and the patient's behavior that links the two.

Joan, a 28-year-old, black, female law student enters the interviewer's office and, after some introductory small talk, asks:

P: Why are you looking at me like that? It makes me feel as if I'm naked.
I: What do you mean?

P: The way you look at me . . .

The interviewer, who is not aware of having looked at the patient in any particular way, suspects that the patient has a perceptive disturbance which could be described as an idea of reference (the first, i.e., the observable component of a defense mechanism). He decides to probe for the unconscious intent (the second component of a defense mechanism).

I: Do you feel that other men look at you that way, too?
P: Some do. When I walk home from law school.

I: Anyone in particular?
P: Well, one of my teachers. His name is Raoul and he is from South America. He looked at me like that in class.

I: Did he ever say anything personal to you?
P: I'm kind of embarrassed to talk about it.

I: We may both learn something important about you, if we can understand your embarrassment.
P: Well, I kind of thought he was a good teacher. Once, I stayed after class to show him one of my poems. He seemed to enjoy talking to me about it, and took it home with him.

I: Hmm.
P: I asked him if I could come back after the next class to talk about it some more and he agreed.

I: Well?
P: I went back and he analyzed my poem. I was so pleased that I asked him whether I could meet him. He looked at me and I felt all excited and opened my coat. I was naked underneath. He looked at me with a twinkle in his eye

and a smile on his face and said: "Joan, I'm your teacher and I'm also married. Do you understand? I don't want you to feel bad about it. I'm flattered that you feel that way about me."

I: So he understood.
P: I was so embarrassed that I just ran out.

The second component of the defense mechanism, a libidinous intent, emerges. The interviewer infers that the patient may have felt a similar impulse toward him. He attempts to establish the link between the overt behavior and the intent—the third component—namely that the patient projects her intent on to the interviewer, thus sparing her the responsibility for her own erotic wishes.

I: You seem excited when you talk about Raoul.
P: I'm so embarrassed.

I: Do you remember how we got on to this subject?
P: I don't understand your question.

I: Do you remember how we got into the discussion about Raoul?
P: You confuse me. I don't know what you mean.

I: Well, you asked me about the way I look at you.
P: Hmm.

I: And it seemed you felt that I looked at you like Raoul did.
P: Well, that's what I thought.

I: Could it be that you feel toward me as you did toward Raoul?
P: Oh no, that's nonsense. You are jumping to conclusions and that really makes me angry. You are my doctor. I respect you as my doctor. But I don't feel anything else for you. I like you, but not like that.

The patient's resistance to the interpretation is obvious. Without her corroboration, the assumption of projection remains inferential. The interviewer attempts to make the erotic thoughts more acceptable to Joan, thus making her projections less necessary.

I: So you are not really aware of having those thoughts? What would be so bad about them anyway?
P: That you are my doctor. And I also have a boyfriend. He's really something like a fiancé.

I: I don't understand. What do you mean "something like a fiancé"?
P: Well, my mother wants us to stay together.

I: What about you?

P: Well, he's real nice, but he's older and he doesn't have an education and he's awfully jealous.

I: So, if you look at other men, you kind of betray him and also defy your mother's wishes?

P: Now you talk like my psychologist did.

I: Well, I try to understand how you feel and why you were so embarrassed with Raoul. Also why you feel that other men look at you in a certain way.

P: You think it's me?

I: Hmm.

P: You think I'm embarrassed about my wishes?

I: Yes, and that's why you pin them on me.

P: There you go again. (Laughs.) You know, I wondered why you wear such baggy pants. (Laughs.) Maybe, you're right after all. Do you think that's why I have those panic attacks and why I feel uncomfortable when I walk home or when I'm at a restaurant?

I: What do you think? (Pause.) Patients with panic sometimes feel that others look at them in a sexual way, and it is often their own sexual feelings that make them think so. But this is just the content of their panicky feelings, not their cause.

   Even if we talk about these feelings for many hours, and even when you become comfortable with describing these feelings to me, you will still have your panic and still feel uncomfortable in a restaurant. But you may find a different content for your panic.

There are four aspects to interpretation: timing, vantage point, scope, and impact on the patient.

TIMING:

The timeliness of an interpretation is usually easy to judge. When a patient becomes curious about his own behavior, he is ready to explore its meaning.

Bill, a 23-year-old biology student, talks about his relationship with his parents and superiors.

1. I: You are telling me that you still live at home.
   P: Not really. Let's put it this way: I live in the same house as my parents do.

2. I: What does that mean?
   P: It means that I share quarters with them, but I was through with them a long time ago.

3. I: You mean you can't get along with your parents?
   P: They are narrow-minded bourgeois.

4. I: So your social life is not really at home.
   P: Nope.

5. I: How is your life at work?
   P: My supervisor is a real knucklehead. He can't see what isn't in the books— typical product of an American college.

6. I: Did you have better experiences in high school?
   P: I always seem to meet the morons.

7. I: How did you get through college? Did you have a scholarship?
   P: I lost my teaching scholarship. John G. told me I'm not doing what I'm supposed to. The heck with it, it was not worth it anyway. But, so far, I've made some money in computer programming.

8. I: So far?
   P: I don't know if I still have my job. I did some programming of plays for a football coach, but that guy is so authoritarian, he has to have it his way. He can't listen to anybody.

9. I: Do you play football yourself?
   P: No. I was on the swim team.

10. I: You are not swimming anymore?
    P: The coach kicked me off. I was in the locker room when I was supposed to be in the pool. Somebody missed $50 after practice. The coach was mad at me because I didn't follow the rules.

11. I: (Laughs.)
    P: The rules are really stupid. I just needed to get some medication out of my locker and this ass nails me.

12. I: (Laughs again.)
    P: You are laughing. I must come across as a real troublemaker.

13. I: Hmm.
    P: Isn't that what you think? You must think this guy can't get along with his swim team coach, the football coach, or with his teachers.

14. I: And with his bourgeois parents.
    P: I forgot that one. You must think I can't get along with anybody. And that's right. I fly off the handle for any old reason. I wonder what ticks me off?

15. I: Their authority . . . teachers . . . coaches . . . parents . . .
    P: Hmm, it sure looks that way . . . hmm.

16. I: Does it feel that way?
    P: It feels like hitting around a blinder . . . leaching out . . .

The interviewer confronts the patient first with the common thread that runs through different situations (Q. 3, 5, 7, 8, 10). The patient recognizes his problems with others (A. 13). He starts to wonder about it himself by raising questions about his behavior (Q. 14). This is the *time* to attempt an interpretation of the patient's rejection of authority figures (Q. 15). He can then continue to talk of difficulties in following rules, and of possible feelings of revengefulness and vindication (as seen in patients with sociopathic tendencies). The example demonstrates the rule of timing. Make an interpretation when the patient recognizes his behavior as irrational and starts wondering about its meaning.

VANTAGE POINT:

The way you deliver an interpretation is important. Interpretations may be made from your own or the patient's vantage point. With an interpretation from the interviewer's vantage point the patient may feel criticized, annoyed, angered, and compelled to resist. An interpretation made from the patient's vantage point is more likely to be accepted—provided it is correct. Here is an example:

Leslie, a 38-year-old, white female, just divorced from a man her age, reported that she has a tendency to date men in their fifties or older.

Interviewer's Vantage Point: A psychoanalytically inclined interviewer's interpretation was that she was acting on sexual impulses originally directed toward her father. The patient was bewildered:

P: I never had sexual feelings for my father, but I do for these men. They turn me on.

Patient's Vantage Point: An interpretation developed from the patient's vantage point went like this:

I: There must be something about these older men that comforts you, Leslie.
P: (Pause.) I feel more wanted. I feel I don't have to compete all the time with other women.

I: You feel accepted and there is no threat to this acceptance.
P: Right, it relaxes me. I can respond without feeling that I'm taken in. I can believe that the man really means it. I feel I can trust him more than a younger man.

I: What about other women?
P: I feel ahead. I feel first in line.

I: Yes, I see. It must feel like being the darling.

P: (Surprised.) You are right. It just struck me . . . like daddy's darling.

I: Didn't you tell us before that you always had the feeling that your father seemed to like you more than your sisters and brothers?

P: That's right; but I did not mean that that's the reason why I like older men.

I: I know and that is not what I'm really saying. But you felt comfortable with him. You know he meant well. He loved you.

P: He really liked me.

I: And did not just try to have you get into bed with him.

P: That's right.

The patient had wondered about her liking of older men. She was ready to explore the reason for her feelings, which justified the interpretative approach. The interpretation worked because it focused on the elements in her relationship with her father that were closest to her awareness (daddy's darling). This allowed her to recognize her emotional gain in choosing older men after her painful divorce.

SCOPE:

An interpretation can be made regarding a narrow concern, such as an isolated behavior, or larger issues, such as lifestyle and lifelong patterns. Large-scope interpretations can risk to damage the patient's self-esteem and consequently your rapport with him.

Narrowly defined interpretations are used with Karen, a 42-year-old, depressed, white female who talks about her diet. She denies dysphoria, obsessions, and compulsions.

1. I: How do you feel usually?
   P: I'm doing fine. I feel great and I'm proud to be down to 118 pounds from 142.

2. I: So you are on a diet.
   P: Yes, I am watching my calories very carefully.

3. I: How do you do that?
   P: I have coffee in the morning and then at lunch a rare hamburger without bread, but with lettuce. I have a steak for dinner. Once in awhile I get so hungry that I eat a whole quart of ice cream. Afterwards I feel depressed and guilty about it. I also try to be rigid with my smoking.

4. I: What do you mean?
   P: Before I smoke a cigarette I have to wash my hands.

5. I: Can you tell me why you do that?
   P: It's just a habit. I like to have clean hands when I smoke.

6. I: You mean you are afraid of dirt on your hands?
   P: No, but I make breakfast and lunch for the kids.

7. I: And you think some food is still on your hands?
   P: Yes, they may still be greasy. Fat has many calories.

8. I: But why do you wash your hands before every cigarette?
   P: I can never be sure whether I have really washed them completely the time before.

9. I: So you are thinking of still having calories stick to your hands?
   P: (Silent.) . . . I may get them in my body accidently from the cigarettes.

10. I: So these thoughts bother you!
    P: I feel so silly . . .

11. I: It sounds like calories are like bacteria, they can hurt you if they get in your body.
    P: No . . . I guess that's it . . . calories are poison, they make you fat.

In this interview, short interpretations in the form of questions (Q. 6, 7, 9) help reveal obsessive thoughts and compulsions and their unconscious origin. Confrontation (Q. 10) helps her to realize her avoidance of these topics.

Interpretation on a large scope is used to make Janet, a 28-year-old, white, single nurse, aware of how mood swings have affected her choice of partners, and eventually caused the breakup of these relationships. The interviewer points out how she picks fun-loving fellows (often sociopaths, alcoholics, and drug abusers) during her manic episodes and gets disgusted with their irresponsible behavior during her depressive episodes.

1. I: How are things going now, Janet? Are you still with Bob?
   P: Yes, but things are not going as well. Last summer when I asked Bob to move in with me it was just great. We had so much fun together and I really enjoyed having sex with him. And now I don't know what happened. I resent him.

2. I: What is it that you resent?
   P: He's not working. He doesn't even seem to want a job.

3. I: Hmm.
   P: He starts drinking in the morning and it's my money he's using.

4. I: You really sound resentful and angry.
   P: It makes me feel worn out. I oversleep; I don't get my work done, which is unusual for me.

5. I: I remember when you worked two shifts last summer.

   P: I never ran out of energy. Even on my second shift I was faster than every-one else. It didn't bother me then that Bob was that way. It was all fun, and now it's just a drag. I don't think that anybody should hang around like that, live off a woman and be too lazy to do anything.

6. I: Well, something has changed in you.

   P: Yes, I am depressed again.

7. I: That's right. Last summer you had your high. You were much more fun-oriented. Living out that fun was much more important to you than hav-ing a responsible partner.

   P: That's right.

8. I: And you had done the same thing the year before with Frank. You started living with him in August, had a great time, and then got all upset in the spring when he did not want to work, just wanted to party.

   P: Yes, sounds like the same thing.

9. I: When you are high you are like a child, where fun is written in capital letters. And when you are down, you raise your finger like a parent. You see the wrongs in your playmates who still behave like fun-seeking chil-dren.

   P: Yes, that's exactly it.

The interviewer first encourages the patient to tell her story and voice her resentment (Q. 1–5). He then starts to interpret her relationship with Bob (Q. 6). Because of her initial positive responses (A. 6 and 7) the interviewer continues with his interpretations, which the patient readily accepts.

IMPACT ON THE PATIENT:

Interpretations have an emotional impact on the patient. She may gain a new awareness of her situation and feel overwhelmed.

Angela is a 46-year-old, white female. She realized that she took verbal and physical abuse from her alcoholic husband because of feelings of guilt and worthlessness while depressed. The patient had just left her husband and started a job. In spite of past abuse, she still feels a strong sexual attraction to him. The interviewer uses echoing, confrontation, and interpretation to clarify her feelings.

1. I: Where do you stand with your husband, Angela?

   P: When Phil is drunk he gets really mean. Last time he grabbed a lamp and hit me over the head. I had a skull fracture.

2. I: So he is really abusive.

   P: At times he can be so gentle.

3. I: Hmm. So he has another side to him.
   P: Usually he is mean. I cannot stand it anymore. I should have left him two years ago when he hit me with the lamp.

4. I: Would you say you have wasted your time during the last two years?
   P: After a fight he can make up for it—he is really a great lover.

5. I: So physically you are still attracted to him.
   P: Well, that does not make up for the meanness and abuse. If your feelings get hurt it affects everything else.

6. I: Is that why you finally left him, because he is not worth loving anymore?
   P: Yes, but I made a mistake. Before I left him I should have grabbed him and fucked him. Then I should have said: "Now I'm through with you. Now I'll leave you."

7. I: Whenever you tell me something bad about your husband and I agree with you, you turn around and praise him.
   P: (Surprised.) Do I?

8. I: I think you still love him.
   P: (Cries.) But it is a self-destructive love and I know deep inside that I did the right thing, but I feel now terribly lonely.

The interpretation (Q. 8) allowed the interviewer to go beyond the patient's ambivalent vascillations, which hindered the assessment of her feelings about leaving her husband. The patient finally claimed she did the right thing, but that she feels lonely.

This interview shows how an interpretation can overwhelm the patient. The responsible interviewer has to answer the question "Can the patient digest an interpretation at this time?" Enlightening the patient, summarizing his behavior for him, and giving him insight and understanding of it is a goal of the psychodiagnostic interview. But you can only burden him with as much as he can carry through an hour—or he may not return.

CHECKLIST

Chapter 3: Techniques

Indicate which interview technique produced which response listed below; enter the appropriate number on the line provided.

Response:

1 = spontaneous talking
2 = rambling
3 = answering questions adequately
4 = one-word answers
5 = silence
6 = hostility
7 = anger

Interview Technique:

Open-ended, patient-centered questions   _____
Open-ended, symptom-centered questions   _____
Closed-ended questions   _____
Requests to be more specific   _____
Requests to generalize   _____
Requests to give reasons for pathology   _____
Probing   _____
Requests to summarize   _____
Interrelate   _____
Statements to go on and continue   _____
Repeating of patient's statements   _____
Attempts to curb the patient   _____
Questions assessing psychiatric symptoms   _____
Smooth transitions   _____
Accentuated transitions   _____
Abrupt transitions   _____
Confrontations   _____
Expressions of acceptance   _____
Looping   _____
Induction to bragging   _____
Interpretations   _____
Addressing of defense mechanisms   _____
Bypassing defense mechanisms   _____
Penetration of defense mechanisms   _____
Reassurance   _____

FOUR METHODS TO ASSESS MENTAL STATUS

1. **Observation**
   Appearance
   Alertness (Level of Consciousness)
   Psychomotor Behavior

2. **Conversation**
   Attention and Concentration
   Speech and Thinking
   Orientation
   Memory
   Affect

3. **Exploration**
   Mood
   Energy
   Perception
   Content of Thinking
   Multiple Unexplained Somatic Symptoms
   Conversion Symptoms
   Multiple Personality
   Paroxysmal Attacks ("Spells")
   Insight
   Judgment

4. **Testing**
   Level of Consciousness
   Attention, Vigilance, Concentration, and Shifting of Sets

Memory and Orientation
Aphasia, Agnosia, and Apraxia
Affect, Imaging, and Imagining: Suggestibility
Abstract Thinking and Intelligence

SUMMARY

Chapter 4 teaches you how to size up the patient's mental status during the interview. Mental status is a profile of at least twenty psychic functions: Appearance, level of consciousness, psychomotor behavior, affect, speech, formal thinking, attention, concentration, memory, orientation, mood, energy, perception, thought content, insight, judgment, social functioning, abstract thinking, intelligence, and suggestibility. You assess them through OBSERVATION, CONVERSATION, EXPLORATION, and TESTING.

Chapter 4 will tell you what these disturbances mean, not what they are. If you need to know that, consult our glossary for definitions.

Hic Rhodos, hic salta!

According to Aesop, sixth century B.C., athletes gathered on the island of Rhodos, Greece, for competition. When beaten in long jump, one athlete boasted: "At home I did much better." The official's response was: "This is Rhodes; you demonstrate your leaping here."

In the mental status examination it is the here and now that counts.

When you meet your patient, you start to perceive a number of signals. They get condensed into your first impression (Sandifer 1970). Your task as interviewer is to analyze these signals as expressions of the patient's present functioning—his *mental status*. It gives you the cross-sectional view of his strengths, weaknesses, and dysfunctions.

In diagnosing (see chapter 5) you get the historical development of these dysfunctions, the longitudinal view. The integration of both, what you presently witness (including the report on the last twenty-four hours) and what you learn from the patient's history, is the basis for your differential diagnosis.

Keep alert to observe changes in the patient's behavior throughout the interview. With ease you will learn to monitor at least twenty functions: Appearance, level of consciousness, psychomotor behavior, attention, concentration, speech, thinking, orientation, memory, affect, mood, energy, perception, thought content, insight, judgment, social functioning, suggestibility, abstract thinking, and intelligence (Fish 1967; Freedman et al. 1975; Strub and Black 1977; Taylor 1981).

TOOLS

There are four different methods to assess mental status: *observation, conversation, exploration,* and *testing.* The successful use of these methods depends upon the patient's cooperation but there are techniques to best create an environment where they can be used.

Observe all behaviors, such as appearance, consciousness, psychomotor activity, and affect, as they unfold in the first seconds of the interview. Observation is often the only available method in assessing the patient who refuses to speak. Any disturbances that you observe are called signs.

Conversation refers to undirected, casual communication with the patient. You are thus given the chance to appraise his condition when he is somewhat off-guard, unaware the psychiatric examination has begun. As you converse, you can assess the patient's orientation, speech, thinking, attention, concentration, comprehension, remote, recent, and immediate memory. The verbally abusive, hostile, or guarded patient may refuse exploration but not conversation.

Exploration refers to the patient's internal experiences which are not on display, such as mood, motivation, perception, thought content, insight, and judgment. To discern them the patient must be motivated to talk. If he does and tells you about his problems, you are assessing symptoms—and symptoms and signs are what you are after in a psychodiagnostic interview.

Testing helps to determine the patient's memory, orientation, concentration, intelligence, ability to carry on abstract thinking, and suggestibility, if needed. The patient has to be fully cooperative with you to allow testing.

Observation, conversation, and exploration take place throughout the interview but testing, as one might expect, is often reserved for the end.

Sometimes, the interviewer uses them in sequence, as in the following example.

This 35-year-old veteran was brought to the emergency room by the police. He looked disheveled, walked unsteadily, and the smell of alcohol lingered about him. His forearm showed a tatoo.

I: Can I take a look at the American Eagle on your arm? *(Observation)*.
P: Be my guest. (Obviously the patient comprehends what the interviewer is saying and gives a goal-oriented response.)

I: Isn't that what the marines had on their berets? *(Conversation.)*
P: You don't know what you are talking about.

I: Have you had it for a long time?
P: I don't want to talk about it.

I: You mean you are sick of it. (By trying to guess the patient's underlying feelings, the interviewer invites the patient to talk about himself—attempting to start *Exploration.)*
P: The hell—sick of it!? I got it in Nam. We had just survived an ambush and we all got drunk when we did it. Next day I was kicked out. They court-martialed me for stealing and sent me up shitrow.

I: You mean they did you wrong? *(Exploration* with focus on suffering.)
P: Everybody did. I just grabbed a few things to make some bread and get some dope. It was hard to keep going without it.

I: So, in Nam you started to take dope. Are you still doing it?
P: No. It's now mainly booze.

I: Does it get you in trouble?
P: I wouldn't be here, would I?

I: Does it affect your memory? (Interviewer prepares patient for *Testing.)*
P: Bullshit.

I: Then show me. Do you know what place you are at right now?
P: The VA.

I: Do you know what day it is?
P: I haven't paid any attention. Maybe it's Monday or Tuesday (it was Friday). Just get the hell out of here, before I kick your ass.

Conversing about the *observed* tatoo (which may occur more often in patients with antisocial personality), the interviewer learns that the patient is irritable, hostile, and easily provoked by *exploration*. He has a labile affect, but can comprehend and answer questions. He cooperates with *test questions* until his deficiencies become apparent and then resumes his hostile behavior. His answers show that he is oriented to place, but not to time.

1. OBSERVATION

Astute observation of a patient can yield many insights about him. This nurse's report shows how much can be learned through careful observation.

A 22-year-old, white, married woman had just been admitted to the inpatient service:

Rachel was lying in bed on her stomach with her face buried in the pillow. She neither answered questions nor responded to any commands. When I mentioned the doctor would arrive shortly, she did not take any notice. After I left, I peaked through the door window. She got up from her bed, went to the adjacent bathroom, and returned with her hair brushed and makeup on her face, only to resume her position on the bed, face down.

Obviously Rachel is alert, comprehends, and remembers the nurse's remarks. Her motor movements are grossly intact without posturing or stupor, and she can carry out goal-oriented actions.

As this example shows, observation starts before you talk to your patient. Look at appearance, alertness (level of consciousness), psychomotor behavior, and affect. (To appraise affect, you need—besides facial expression—also the patient's thought content, which we will discuss under 2. Conversation.)

Appearance

At the moment you meet the patient, you will note, of course, sex, age, race, nutritional status, body type (see glossary), hygiene, dress, and eye contact. You may notice aspects which are associated with the presence or onset of psychopathology.

Sex and Age

Sex and age are often relevant for the diagnosis, as there are disorders associated more often than not with these factors. For example, in females, anorexia and bulimia nervosa, somatization, and affective disorder are more common; in males, antisocial personality and alcoholism.

In young patients, anorexia nervosa, somatization disorder, antisocial personality, and schizophrenia are seen more often, in older patients degenerative dementia. A patient who appears older than his stated age may have a history of drug or alcohol abuse, organic mental disorder, depression, or physical illness.

Race and Ethnic Background

Race and ethnic background are more than demographic descriptors. They can be one source of stress, of adjustment reactions, and can influence the onset and prevalence of mental disorders. In addition, discrepancy between your background and your patient's can influence your interaction.

If you differ from the patient in race, culture, or nationality, he may react with caution or distrust.

Here is an example.

After a serious suicide attempt (hanging) while on a hospital ward a black, female, lesbian nurse had been resuscitated. Her male resident doctor, an immigrant from Israel, talked with her after the incident and inquired about present suicidal thoughts or plans. The patient denied them emphatically and repeatedly.

He believed her. However, the patient admitted to a black female staff nurse that next time she would not fail and it would be soon. The distance in race, gender, and nationality produced dramatically discrepant assessments.

A racial, national, or cultural difference between you and your patient can also work to your advantage. You may be more objective toward his problems.

Studies have shown that ethnic backgrounds can be associated with psychiatric disorders. For instance, there is more drinking among the Irish, some American Indian tribes, the French, Russians, and Italians, but low rates of alcoholism among Orientals (Goodwin and Guze 1984).

Nutritional Status

Poor nutrition can be the result of a psychiatric or medical illness, for example, anorexia in young females, anorexia due to alcohol and drug abuse, schizophrenia, depression, or medical illness such as cancer, diabetes, or endocrinopathy.

In contrast, obesity may point to an eating disorder, somatization disorder, and affective disorder with hyperphagia, or use of psychotropic drugs such as tricyclics, lithium, and sedating neuroleptics (thorazine and thioridazine).

Hygiene and Dress

Self-neglect can indicate the presence of certain psychiatric disorders such as organic mental disorder, drug and alcohol abuse, depression, or schizophrenia. A three-day-old beard, food stains on clothing, holes in the socks, soiled shoes, body odor, dirty fingernails, or an overdue haircut can point to a disorder. In contrast, extreme neatness and red hands may disclose excessive hand washing as seen in obsessive compulsive disorder.

Dress can reveal many things about a person. It reflects professional status; whether or not someone is engaged in leisure or work activity; adjustment to the season; attitude toward society; or sometimes an extreme mood state such as mania or depression. Some bipolar patients advertise their mood state by their appearance:

When manic, a 65-year-old lady dressed in bright red, wore lots of jewelry, dyed her hair copper, and painted her lips fiery red. When depressed, she let the grey hair grow out, dressed in dark colors, and used no makeup.

In general, a flamboyant outfit, mismatched clothing, and loud makeup can indicate hysteric, organic, or manic symptoms. Highly eccentric, nonconformist, or flagrantly inappropriate attire can be a sign of psychotic behavior. The interviewer must make judgments as to what is inappropriate. The following examples offer some illustrations: the electrician who wears a tuxedo for his appointment; the middle-aged, female lawyer who comes to see you in a bikini top, blue jeans, and barefoot; a patient wearing dark glasses indoors explaining: "I don't want others to see my eyes and read my mind." Such clues should alert but not prejudice you toward a diagnosis.

Eye Contact

Most patients maintain eye contact and track with their eyes the movements and gestures of the interviewer. Aberrant eye movements can be diagnostic: Wandering eyes expose distractibility, visual hallucinations, mania, or organic states. Avoidance of eye contact may express hostility, shyness, or anxiety. Constant tracking may disclose suspiciousness. If appropriate, question the patient about these clues. His answers may lead you right into his pathology.

Alertness (Level of Consciousness)

Level of consciousness is changed by alcohol, drugs, and a number of paroxysmal attacks such as fainting, narcoleptic attacks, petit mal, complex partial, grand mal, and pseudo-seizures. Rarely are the latter observed during an interview with either in- or outpatients. You have to *ask* the patient whether or not he has ever experienced these kinds of attacks (see 3. Exploration).

Lethargy points toward an organic mental disorder (see 4. Testing, Level of Consciousness).

Psychogenic stupor can complicate panic, somatization, and affective disorders, catatonia and organic mental disorder.

Psychomotor Behavior

Psychomotor behavior gives diagnostic clues on alertness, affect, energy level, agitation, and movement disturbance in a wide variety of psychiatric and neurological illnesses. The interviewer should note the patient's posture and four types of movements: expressive, reactive, spontaneous, and goal-directed movements (see 4. Testing).

Erect *posture* may express an increase in energy level, and stooped posture a decrease. Mannerisms, catalepsy, posturing, and waxy flexibility are all signs of either catatonic schizophrenia, atypical affective disorder, or midbrain lesions.

Expressive, reactive, spontaneous, and goal-directed movements are all increased in mania and decreased in depression, parkinsonism, or neuroleptic-induced parkinsonism. In the latter two, the face changes to a mask; expressions freeze and gestures stiffen. (For more about expressive movements, see 2. Conversation, Affect). The patient can be asked to carry out a physical task to allow the interviewer to determine the nature of goal-oriented movements. These can be judged by the latency of initiation, speed, efficiency, ability of completion, and the level and degree of control.

Particular results can indicate pathology. Psychosis may disturb the level of control. A patient may feel that his movements are imposed upon him by an outside force. Anxiety increases reactive and spontaneous movements but often decreases goal-oriented movements. Agitated depression augments spontaneous movements nearly uncontrollably, but impoverishes all other movements. Similar to thought blocking, a catatonic patient shows a blocking of all movements. Such a stupor may be time-limited and without general slowing once the block is overcome. A catatonic patient may refuse to answer but respond hastily after you have turned your back to leave the room. This has been called "reaction at the last moment."

Abnormal Complex Movement Patterns

They include stupor (see above), excitement, and impulsive actions (Fish 1967). You see stages of excitement in agitated depression, mania, paranoid schizophrenia, and catatonia. Catatonic excitement may reduce facial expression but exaggerate, stiffen, and stilt other movements. Senseless violent and indiscriminate destructiveness characterizes postepileptic confusion and pathological drunkenness. Impulsive actions indicate a deficit of insight and/or judgment.

Movements with a neuropathological basis are tremors, akathisia, tardive dyskinesia, choreatic, athetotic movements, and tics. Suspect a tremor to be hysterical if it is limited to one limb, or irregular, and variable over time. Fear and intention increase the tremor, distraction decreases it. Some forms of tardive dyskinesia can also be limited in the same manner. Besides parkinsonian tremor, akathisia and tardive dyskinesia are neuroleptic-induced.

Athetotic movements and choreatic movements indicate neurological disease and differentiate them from catatonia. Both interfere with voluntary actions but disappear during sleep.

Here is an example for tics:

A 19-year-old, white male enters the office accompanied by his mother. While she introduces her son, he throws his head three times to the left side and shouts: "Shit, shit, shit."

This spontaneous movement is a motor tic; it is associated with a vocal tic, the shouting of profanities; these are the essential features of Gilles de la Tourette syndrome.

For abnormally induced movements, see 4. Testing and appendix B.

2. CONVERSATION

While observing your patient, start the verbal part of the psychodiagnostic interview with conversation or "small talk" about any topic other than the patient's problems. With uncooperative patients, you may be restricted to this level of discourse.

Attention and Concentration

When you meet a new patient, ask him about where he has parked or when his appointment was set. This will allow you to determine his level of attention, concentration, orientation, and memory. If his answers are brief, try to follow up and get details. Monitor whether he stays with your questions or drifts off. Is his concentration limited to interesting subjects? Can he concentrate only when he talks, or also when he listens?

Psychiatric disturbances can be revealed during this initial conversation. For example, alcoholic intoxication causes the patient to appear drowsy and inattentive; depression decreases interest and concentration;

patients with a frontal lobe lesion initially are alert and attentive, but soon lose focus.

Speech and Thinking

Speech

To obtain a reading on speech, affect displayed in speech, and on thinking, invite your patient to talk about emotional topics. Then, judge all three dimensions: formal aspects of speech, thinking, and the accompanying affect. For speech disturbances listen to articulation, rhythm, and flow; for thinking monitor word usage, grammar, and sentence structure; for affect notice latency of response, speed, tone, amount, loudness, and inflection.

FORMAL ASPECTS OF SPEECH:

Disturbed *articulation* (dysarthria or slurring of speech) often indicates an organic brain disorder, or intoxication, especially with sedative-hypnotics, and alcohol.

Disturbed *rhythm* of speech is called dysprosody. For example, scanning speech (i.e., pronunciation of words with pauses between the syllables) occurs in multiple sclerosis; staccato speech in psychomotor epilepsy; and mumbling in Huntington's chorea.

Distinguish between *speed* and *flow*. When flow is disturbed, patients talk either in fragments, or contrarily merge their words. If the patient is difficult to interrupt, it can indicate a lack of inhibitory control. Continuous flow of speech, or pressure, is often associated with push of speech, i.e., speech that is difficult to interrupt. Patients with mania, or intoxication with alcohol or stimulant drugs may show both disturbances; patients with anxiety, persecutory delusions, or obsessive compulsive thinking may show pressure only.

Nonfluent speech—with many pauses and without prepositions, conjunctions, and pronouns between the nouns and verbs—is called "telegram style." The patient struggles to find appropriate words and circumscribes what he misses. In these cases, the patient has expressive (motor) aphasia, a destruction of Broca's area in the frontal dominant hemisphere. It may develop suddenly after a head trauma or a stroke, or slowly with brain tumors and beginning senility (Alzheimer's disease).

The circumscriptions help to distinguish between depression and incipient senile dementia. (Older patients frequently forget names. This is senescent forgetfulness, a benign aphasia unrelated to dementia.)

Continuous, senseless word fluency is called "word salad." Pauses are missing, nouns are substituted with incorrect ones (paraphasia). Unable to comprehend what you tell him, this patient has receptive sensory aphasia. Wernicke's area in the temporal lobe of the dominant hemisphere—responsible for decoding speech—is afflicted.

Paraphasic speech (see appendix B) occurs also in some schizophrenic patients or other functional psychosis without known organic disturbance.

Here are pointers for the differential diagnosis. Receptive aphasia shows:

poverty of verbs and nouns
an abundance of conjunctions, prepositions, and interjections
random, nonrepetitive neologisms without fixed meaning
isolated sentences, unintelligible in their grammatical structure (see 4. Testing).

In contrast, a schizophrenic uses the same neologisms over and over again and attaches a private meaning to them. The grammatical structure of sentences remains intact.

Incorrect grammar is used by mentally retarded patients, some schizophrenics, patients with organic disturbance of the speech areas and, of course, by non–English-speaking foreigners. Details of agrammatical sentence construction in speech and writing will be given in Thinking and 4. Testing.

SPEECH AND AFFECT:

The latency of response to your question can indicate various disorders. For example, depressed affect prolongs responses, mania shortens it, and schizophrenia varies it. Distinguish between depressed affect and low intelligence. The patient with mental retardation or organic mental disorder answers quickly to concrete, short, and simple questions but hesitates in his response to more complex questions.

The tone of voice is also an indicator: the manic may be hoarse from talking too much; the alcoholic from cigarette smoking and throat irritation by alcohol. If not due to a hearing problem, shouting indicates lack of inhibition, and could be caused by intoxication or mania. A soft, hesitant, subdued voice may point to depression, anxiety, or suspiciousness.

Inflection of speech should be viewed with respect to content and underlying affect. The depressed or schizophrenic patient may speak in a monotone voice, while patients with mania or somatization disorder modulate excessively. The anxious and excited patient often talks at a higher pitch which drops when he relaxes.

Thinking

Speech and thinking must be separated to effectively assess the patient. Encoding thoughts is speech; their decoding is comprehension. Both are executed by the speech centers in the dominant cortical hemisphere. Their malfunction affects both speech and thinking. Therefore, exclude a disturbance of comprehension and speech before you diagnose a thought disorder. Three criteria help you to judge thinking: Concepts of words, tightness of association, and goal orientedness.

CONCEPT OF WORDS:

Patients with disturbed word concept use words in a concrete or overinclusive manner, or show both simultaneously; their thinking becomes unintelligible. You notice such formal thought disorder often during initial conversation (see appendix A), as the following examples show.

(1) *Concreteness* of thinking:

I: What brought you here?
P: A car. I came in a car.

I: I mean what kind of problem did you have?
P: We did not have any. The car was running smoothly. My brother was driving it.

Notice that the patient cannot grasp the question's abstract meaning about his health but interprets it in a narrow way. Both the mentally retarded and the schizophrenic patient (Goldstein 1964) miss the symbolic meaning of words and limit them to a specific situation. Concrete thinking is therefore not specific for schizophrenia (Payne and Hewlett 1960).

Concrete thinking can be detected by asking the patient to interpret a proverb. (See 4. Testing.)

(2) *Overinclusiveness,* the opposite of concrete thinking, expands the concept of a word (Cameron 1964):

I: What problem brought you here?
P: The west. Everything that comes from the warm to the cold, from the west, drifted in. I live west from here coming with the wind which blows from the west. All problems are more in the east. My problems bring me from the west to the east.

In this case, overinclusiveness of the concept "problem" leads the patient to elaborate on his belief that there is more trouble in world politics in the East than in the West, and then fits himself into this schema. Since he has problems himself he should go to the East. In addition, this patient shows concreteness of thinking by referring to the wind blowing from warm to cold as an analogy to his own problems. Payne and Hewlett (1960) reported that a battery of tests separated schizophrenics from depressed and neurotic patients on a factor called overinclusion, but not on factors retardation and concreteness.

TIGHTNESS OF ASSOCIATIONS AND GOAL ORIENTEDNESS:

How tightly does your patient connect words and sentences? Different forms are: perseveration, verbigeration or palilalia, clang association, blocking and derailment, flight of ideas, non sequitur, fragmentation, rumbling, driveling, and word salad. Logical gaps among sentences are called loosening of association. Tight connections lead to inclusions of very minute details which result in circumstantial speech. Disturbed association frequently leads to a loss of the goal orientedness, to tangential thinking (see appendix A).

Orientation

To check orientation to place, ask the new patient how he found your office. Severely disoriented outpatients are usually brought in by a family member or friend.

Time is a sensitive indicator of orientation. To check orientation to time, ask when the appointment was made. Ask inpatients when they were admitted and how long they have been in the hospital. In a Board Examination ask when the patient was informed about this examination, and by whom.

The demented patient may attempt to minimize deficiencies and claim: "For my daily living I don't need a calendar. What a silly question—I don't need to answer that." Be persistent to learn whether the patient is resistant and unable to perform.

Mentally retarded patients may also be disoriented to time but without using excuses or denial.

Withdrawn or distractible patients appear disoriented, but will answer correctly if you insist.

If the patient is disoriented, focus on the mental status examination rather than on an unreliable history. If you evaluate orientation initially, you avoid the awkward question by novices at the end of their interview:

"Now before we close, do you know what date it is?"

Memory

During the initial conversation you can check your patient's memory in an informal manner. (A formal quantitative approach is described under 4. Testing.) For instance, spell your name when you introduce yourself. When he can repeat it, his immediate recall is probably intact; if he addresses you later by name, his recent memory appears to be working. The same is true if he can describe how he got to the clinic and where he parked. Discussion of past events will reveal his level of intact memory.

Patients with memory disturbances focus on events that they remember. Therefore, introduce topics of *your* choice such as movies, sports events, television series, or political events that you can verify. The patient does not have a vested interest in the subjects, which protects them less from memory extinction.

Conversation can, of course, be used at other times, other than at the beginning of the interview. When you suspect simulation or dissimulation of amnesia, small talk helps you to detect contradictions between facts and intent. Elisa's case demonstrates how *conversation* can aid in the diagnostic assessment.

This 27-year-old, white woman was brought to the hospital emergency room by the highway patrol with the complaint of complete memory loss. She had been found wandering along the highway unable to remember her last name or her address. She claimed she did not know anything about her past. She denied drinking or any king of head injury. There were no signs of trauma. However she was not sure about drug abuse because she just could not remember. During the interview she was guarded and mentioned repetitively that she did not remember. When hypnosis was suggested to recover her memory, she declined.

At the end of the interview the examiner accompanied her from the emergency room to the floor and, while walking with her, mentioned that hyponosis is frightening for many people and that he could understand that she might be scared of it. She replied: "That's right. My father once took me to the carnival in Columbus, Ohio, close to the place where we lived. And they had a show there, and some people from the audience were invited to be hypnotized. I can still see how these volunteers were talking and crying like babies." This unguarded statement contradicted the massive memory disturbance claimed during the "official" interview.

Distortion of Memory

Psychiatric disorders can distort memory. The depressed patient may claim he has been depressed since childhood, or is a born loser, sinner, or criminal. The manic patient may exaggerate his achievements, recalling past hospitalizations as an ordeal of restrictive tortures without recollection of his aggressive behavior that necessitated physical constraints. The schizophrenic may report injustices and persecutions that never happened. The sociopath may invent a life history.

False Memory

Déjà vu and déjà vécu occur predominantly in patients with temporal lobe lesions, but also in people without neurological findings.

Affect

What is affect? Affect is the visible and audible manifestation of the patient's emotional response to outside and inside events, i.e., thoughts, ideas, evoked memories, reflections, and performance. It is expressed in posture, facial and body movements, and in tone of voice, vocalizations, and word selection.

Distinguish affect from mood by four features:

- affect is momentary, lasting as short as one to two seconds; mood lasts longer;
- affect is limited to outside or internal stimuli and changes with them; mood can change spontaneously;

– affect is the foreground, mood is the emotional background.
– disturbed affect is observed by you (sign); disturbed mood is reported by your patient (symptom).

Mood will therefore be discussed in 3. Exploration.

Affect has three functions: (1) self-perception, (2) communication, and (3) motivation.

In the case of self-perception, affect provides us with an emotional value judgment. It tells us whether we like what we experience or hate it. For instance, if you learn unexpectedly that you have been promoted, your heart and breathing rate may increase, you have a warm feeling in your chest, your trunk muscles may firm up, you get a happy expression on your face.

Regarding communication, physical manifestations of affect express our feelings and make them known to others.

In respect to motivation, feelings of anger and rage, for instance, may initiate aggression and destructive behavior; alertness and interest stimulate exploration; fear predisposes to escape. Affect is expressed as a manifestation of emotion; it is a precursor to action.

When we show affect we initiate a goal-oriented action in a rudimentary and incomplete form. For instance, in disgust we curl back our lips so as not to touch any spoiled food with them; we turn up our nose and exhale heavily so as not to smell the stench. In a boring lecture we whip our legs as if ready to escape. Even to an abstract thought we respond with our affect as if it was concrete.

What Is the Origin of Affect?

Recent research has supported Charles Darwin's theory on the innateness and universality of emotional expression, i.e., affect (Izard 1977, 1979). Izard et al. (1983) found nine basic expressive movements to be innate: disgust, surprise, joy, anger, fear, sadness, interest, shame, and content. Their basic expression develops in the first eighteen months of life in a predictable sequence. Thus affect is an inborn mean of interpersonal communication which can be disturbed in psychiatric disorders. The recognition of this disturbance provides diagnostic clues.

All nine affects are disturbed in psychiatric disorders: disgust, perplexity (surprise), elation (joy), anger, anxiety (fear), sadness, interest, shame (guilt), and suspicion (content). In each of the psychiatric disorders one or two of the basic affects dominate at the expense of some others; such as anxiety (anxiety disorders), sadness, disgust and guilt (depression), elation and interest (mania), suspicion (paranoia), and perplexity (organic mental disorder).

How Do You Evaluate Affect?

Watch the flow of gestures and facial expressions. These nonverbal clues emerge before and persist between sentences. The patient expresses it in tone of voice, pitch, modulation, and selection of vocabulary. When you can sense how the patient feels, you have learned to read affect.

The innateness of the basic affects does not preclude their manipulation. We do learn to suppress, exaggerate, distort, pretend, and falsify the expression of our emotions, thus using affect for a purpose. We develop our personal style of display, and can do it on demand.

When Mr. Smith, a successful CPA, became depressed, he still smiled and sought eye contact while talking, but he dropped his smile between sentences. His feet were tapping throughout the interview as if to flee from the situation and his morbid, suicidal thoughts.

Morris (1987) points out that most adults have learned to control their facial expressions but not their legs and feet to convey a desired affect.

To evoke affect, the patient should be asked to talk about sensitive subjects (family situation, personal losses, success or failure at work, frustrations and disappointments, or hobbies). Primary dimensions of affect are quality, intensity, duration, and appropriateness to stimulus; secondary dimensions are range and control.

The expression of specific *qualities* of affect are, for instance, wide-open eyes and frowning forehead which will alert you to anxiety, or a restless and apprehensive look to perplexity. Clenched teeth and fists, and stiff facial muscles portray anger. A head turned sideways and a patient observing you out of the corner of his narrowed eyes demonstrate suspicion. Smiles, rapid changes in expressions, euphoric glimmer in the eyes interrupted by outbursts of anger give away manic excitement. A stiff facial expression with lively moving eyes, as if looking through a mask, and sparse gestures with the mouth in so-called snout spasm indicate catatonia. The omega sign on the forehead, corners of the mouth drawn downward, tearful eyes, and drooping shoulders point toward depression. Some depressed patients smile with their lips, but have "dead eyes." A patient with agitated depression sits in a chair wringing his hands, rocking back and forth, repeating the same phrase: "Please help me, please help me!"

Intensity shows the patient's involvement in a topic. Schizophrenics are often unable to feel involved. Interviewing them is like talking to a computer. Nothing appears to touch them; their affect is flat or shallow. The paranoid schizophrenic however may come alive if you challenge his overvalued ideas or delusions (Leonhard 1979, calls this affect laden paraphrenia).

Duration: Affective response may perk up for a split second or freeze; it may rise and mellow slowly, or be switched on and off.

The affect's relationship to thought content can be *inappropriate,* for example the schizophrenic who giggles about the death of his mother. Another abnormality in the relationship between thought content and affect is the lack of concern that sometimes a patient with conversion reactions (pseudoneurological symptoms) shows. Such a patient may claim he is blind, paralyzed, or has no sensations in his body, yet he shows no concern for his future fate, or for the impact of the symptoms on his life. The French psychiatrist Janet has used the term *la belle indifférence* for this sign (Campbell 1981).

The *range* of affect and its different qualities varies from narrow (as in the withdrawn schizophrenic, the retarded depressive, or the obsessive-compulsive) to wide (as in the intoxicated or brain-damaged patient). Some types of affect may dominate over others, such as suspicion in paranoid disorder, hopelessness and guilt in depression, or irritability and joy in mania.

Judge whether the patient or the stimulus controls the affect. Are the patient's emotions stable and only slightly modulated by the topic of the conversation? Or are they rapidly changing in response to the topic (labile affect), which occurs in the intoxicated or manic patient?

The limbic system of the brain colors speech and actions emotionally (Isaacson 1982), the right (nondominant) parietal lobe recognizes these emotions and the right frontal lobe expresses them (Ross 1982). By evaluation of affect, the interviewer makes a statement about the functioning of subcortical and cortical structures of the brain.

3. EXPLORATION

An interviewer can observe and converse with the patient without his consent. But with the next section of the mental status examination which we call *exploration,* he has to cooperate because *he* becomes its object. You start to explore when you ask: "What brought you here?" When he describes his symptoms you zero in; when you observe signs of disturbed behavior you may confront him and explore their meaning.

When do you question him about symptoms and signs? Immediately if they disrupt rapport, or might be forgotten later, or when they lead into the center of psychopathology.

The following vignette offers an example of how exploration can reveal pathology. John keeps staring at the name plate on your desk, seems distracted, and pays little attention to your questions. Ask him why.

P: I try to figure out how many different words I can make with the letters in your name.

I: Do you often play with letters or words in this way?

P: All the time. I blow three or four hours a day by doing that and other things.

It is best to delay exploration of a sign or symptom if it seems of minor importance, sidetracks you, or is part of a complex psychopathology such as a delusional system that may emerge later.

Mood

Mood, a long-term feeling state through which we filter all experiences, will not be revealed unless the patient is asked directly about it. Sometimes you find an apparent discrepancy between affect and mood; the patient controls his affect by wearing a social mask, but describes depressed mood.

Mr. Brink, a real estate developer in his sixties, slender, tall, wearing coat and tie, entered my office smiling and seemingly in good spirits. He was accompanied by his wife, dressed in designer clothes.

"Why did you come to see me?"

"I heard a friend of mine talk about you and my ears perked up", answered the wife, "because I thought about my husband's problems. He was most active until about fourteen years ago, when he had a bout with depression. He was treated by a local psychiatrist with several antidepressants, but never responded. He finally got better without medication."

"How do you feel now?" I asked Mr. Brink. He smiled and looked at his wife. I continued to look at him.

"Well . . ." he said. "I don't know . . . Bad, I feel bad. I put everything off, don't want to do anything. See . . . I can't even speak up. She does all the talking."

"And it was just the opposite before he got sick", his wife interjected. "It was me who always was nervous."

"What do you feel when you feel bad?"

"I worry. I worried about coming here. I worried all evening and night."

"You worried in the evening. Is that different from the morning?"

"In the morning I'm numb. I don't want to get up. I don't want to do anything. I don't want to talk."

"What feels worse, the morning or evening?"

"I'd have to say the morning . . . like now."

"Is there anything that will make you feel better for a while?"

"No, nothing, nothing at all."

"Yesterday he was feeling good," his wife insisted. "His son was over and took him out. And he always enjoys that a lot."

"Having your son over makes you feel better?" I asked turning back to him. Mr. Brink's face seemed to drop; the lines in his face deepened; he looked ashen.

"Maybe for a while," he said with a doubting, weak voice.

"Talking about your son cheers you up?"

"Not really. Nothing makes a real difference. Talking usually makes me feel worse."

While I spoke with him, he smiled with thin lips, just to look so much older again when I turned toward his wife.

"When I talk to you, you don't seem that depressed," I addressed him again.

"For a short while I can put up a front, but I feel worse behind it."

"He has to do that in his business," his wife said.

"I can't accomplish anything," he said. "I can't do my work. I just sit there. I don't know what to do first."

"How does the future look to you?"

"I will never get better. I wish I wasn't around any more."

Mood has five dimensions: quality, stability, reactivity, intensity, and duration. These can be explored as they emerge in the interview.

Quality

Mood seeks and finds a fitting content, such as themes of guilt and failure in depression. The quality of mood cannot be determined from observed affect—you have to ask. Good questions to uncover mood are:

"How do you feel most of the day?"
"How do you feel now?"

These questions may yield clear answers:

"good"
"energetic"
"high"
"depressed"
"tired"

or ambiguous ones:

"I feel rough."
"I've been sitting on the swing a lot."
"I've been lying around the house lately."
"Okay, I guess."

To explore ambiguous answers, you can offer the patient a range of responses:

"Are you more blue, sad, down in the dumps, low spirited or high, up, on top of the world?"

If a patient cannot describe his mood in his own words, you can ask questions about his everyday activities or vegetative functions:

"Do you enjoy talking to me?"
"Do you get fun from your hobbies?"
"What are you going to do in the future?"
"Do you get satisfaction from your work and the things you do every day?"
"How is your sleep . . . appetite . . . sex drive . . . energy?"

Once you find descriptors of his mood, use them as anchors. Such talk puts the patient in touch with his feelings and can help him assess his own mood.

Stability

A stable patient may remain tranquil and pleasant no matter what adversities he reports: "I feel like the rock of Gibraltar, nothing seems to shake me. That's a real new feeling for me."

Unstable mood changes spontaneously or reactively. Spontaneous mood changes can occur during a single day.

"I feel rotten when I wake up at 4 a.m., unable to fall asleep again. I feel blue most of the morning hours, but my mood picks up after lunch, and evenings are the best for me."

This so-called *diurnal variation* is often associated with an affective disorder. These questions may help you:

"Compare your mood in the morning with your mood in the evening. Are there any differences?"
"When do you feel better—at breakfast or at supper?"
"Do you feel better now or later?"

Reactivity

Lack of reactivity is typical for endogenous depression. For example, nothing could cheer up Mr. Brink, not even his son's visit. In contrast, dysphoric patients with drug and alcohol abuse, somatization disorder, and some personality disorders feel better if their social situation improves.

Intensity

Mood varies between intense and shallow. Patients experience panic, mania, and drug-induced excitement as intense. In contrast, schizophrenics have a flat and shallow mood. Depressed moods can be intense despite a flat affect.

Duration

Duration gives mood its diagnostic value. Dysphoria lasting hours or days is seen in personality disorders, sociopathy, alcoholism, and drug abuse, while depressive mood of affective disorder lasts two weeks or longer. The same is true for elated mood. DSM-III-R proposes, for instance, an arbitrary cutoff of a few days to diagnose mania.

Energy

Energy level can be determined in a number of different ways. Monitor how often a patient brings up a new topic, and how well he elaborates on it. Ask him about how easily he can initiate and carry out actions. Ask him whether he has to push himself and drags through the day. Ask him about his last twenty-four hours. Was it easy to go through daily routines? What about new tasks? Ask whether he plans his day or not.

The depressed patient complains that he cannot plan, decide, initiate, and carry through actions. The obsessive worries about his indecision and repeated checking. The manic initiates lots of things, but oftentimes finishes few. The phobic is restricted by numerous avoidances. The patient with antisocial personality may appear active, but he pursues pleasure rather than accomplishments. The schizophrenic may watch TV all day long.

Perception

Normal perception originates from stimulation of specific sensory receptors. It is disturbed with psychotic patients. Patients with hallucinatory perceptions have images, auditory and olfactory impressions in the absence of verifiable stimulation.

Psychotic patients hear voices without people around, sometimes over enormous distances; these voices come and go capriciously, follow them, and there is no escape. Most hallucinating patients realize the "hallucinatory character" of their perceptions without being able to explain it but they insist that these perceptions are real and not imagined. You can safely ask "Do you hear any voices even when nobody is present?" Or more empathically "Are you bothered or harassed by voices?"

Some patients with schizophrenia are ambivalent whether they should tell you or not:

"What did the voices tell you today?"

may help. If not ask him whether the voices tell him not to talk about them.

Insight into Hallucinations

When you are trying to determine whether a patient has hallucinations, assume that the patient has no insight into their morbid nature. Therefore, ask factual questions:

"Do you hear voices?"

rather than questions that imply morbidity:

"Have you ever been so sick that you heard voices?"

Even though most hallucinating patients realize that others consider their perceptions as "crazy," they themselves do not share that view. They do not have full insight into the morbid character of the hallucinations.

There are five stages of insight:

Stage I: Previously reported hallucinations have now stopped. The patient has full insight into their morbid nature.

"In the past I believed that I heard my mother's and sister's voices calling me names. I must have really been sick. I know they will not do such a thing. And even if they could, they would not do it."

Stage II: Hallucinations were experienced in the past, but are not present now; the patient believes that they were real.

"Some months ago my mother's and sister's voices harassed me. They have stopped now."

Stage III: Hallucinations have been experienced recently but the patient refuses to talk about them. He seems to realize the contradiction between the psychotic perceptions and reality.

"I don't want to talk about my mother's and sister's voices anymore. I just don't care for that nonsense. They don't bother me anymore."

Stage IV: The patient talks about his hallucinations, but does not act upon them.

"I hear my mother's and sister's voices. They are calling me names. I hear them all the time."

Stage V: The patient acts upon his hallucinations. He obeys or responds to the voices:

"My mother and sister scolded me again. I heard their voices, they called me a monkey. I called them up and told them to stop. But they are vicious and lied to me, they denied that they are doing it."

One patient, an Italian immigrant, harassed by voices, had murdered his mother and sister because they denied hearing the same voices he heard and refused to stop them. Obviously, this patient did not comprehend that his hallucinations were unique and limited to him. Usually you can convince a patient that his hallucinations are limited to him. This however does not convince him that they are unreal. With treatment patients become more receptive to this argument. If they insist on the reality of their hallucinations take it as an expression of the severity of their symptoms. Find out whether your patient is aware that the hallucinations are exclusive to him by asking "Can other people hear the voices too? Do you think I can hear them?"

Hallucinations usually appear and disappear by passing through these five stages. They are clinically important for two reasons: First, for discharge, the patient should be at stage I. Clinicians who are unaware of these stages often consider patients at stage III as symptom free and discharge them prematurely. Schizophrenics at this stage are usually not compliant; they often stop their medication and relapse. Second, since nonacute hallucinations reappear in the same order as they disappear, use these stages to titrate medication on an outpatient basis.

Patients talk about their hallucinations in different ways. They may deny them or present them with insight. Here are some techniques to handle this.

1. During stage III: If you suspect that your patient has hallucinations but denies them, ask flatly:

"What did the voices tell you this morning?"

The patient may then describe his hallucinations:

I: Did you hear voices recently?
P: No.

I: When was the last time you heard them?
P: About two or three months ago when I was in the hospital.

I: You have not heard them since?
P: (Hesitates). No, I don't think so.

I: Tell me, what did these voices tell you this morning?
P: They told me everything I should do and they told me not to talk about it.

2. During stages IV and V: If a patient calls his hallucinations "crazy," be reluctant to accept this as an indication of insight. Instead, expect it to be lip service and challenge his statement. He may not have true insight in hallucinations but has learned that others consider them as "crazy." Pursue the topic by asking what he thinks about the nature of his hallucinations; his comments may be quite delusional:

P: I think I'm getting crazy again.
I: Why?

P: I believe some people use waves to transmit their voices into my ears.
I: Is it crazy for you to hear these voices?

P: Not for me, only for others.

A patient may ask you whether you believe that he is crazy. Tell him that you believe that he has these experiences, that they are real for him, and that you want an accurate description from him to understand them better.

3. If a patient resorts to delusional explanations:

"My ears seem to be extremely sensitive."
"A radio station is sending these voices."
"The heating duct works as a loud speaker."

accept his delusional explanations as real and show him empathy for his harassment. Offer him treatment for his suffering. Don't tell him that the medication will give him insight into the morbid character of the voices or make them disappear, because for him they are real.

4. Patients who emphasize the reality of their hallucinations and belittle others who lack the talent to perceive them should not be challenged but be allowed to describe in detail their experiences as if they were reports from another planet.

5. Patients who accuse you of maliciously lying when you deny hearing the voices usually suffer from persecutory delusions and may become dangerous. Let the patient voice his accusations and let him explain why he thinks you are withholding the hallucinatory experience and not leveling with him. Thus, focus on the assessment of the delusion rather than a confrontation with reality.

Content of Thinking

Many psychiatric disorders are characterized by a pathological content of thinking. Here are some suggestions on how to tease it out.

Delusions

Delusions are fixed false beliefs, often about some action that has taken place, such as the neighbors spying and plotting against the patient.

Here are four questions that assess a delusion:

1. What is going on?
   This assesses content. Asking a direct question such as
      "Do you have strange or crazy ideas?"
   does not work when the patient lacks insight. It is much better to ask:
      "Do other people think that you have crazy ideas?"
   This approach works because most patients talk about their delusional ideas to family members and friends and get rebuffed by remarks like "That's crazy!"
      Also, tap key areas known as breeding grounds for delusions: persecution, injustice, discrimination, guilt, grandiosity, love, power, knowledge, jealousy, illness, passivity, nihilism, poverty, ESP, supernatural abilities, or victimization by cosmic waves and x-rays.
2. Why is it going on?
   This gives the patient an opportunity to offer his explanation. He may respond by indicating they punish, harm, control or honor him.
3. Where will it lead?
   This generates the patient's expectations about the delusion. Common responses are they will attack or they want to drive him crazy.
4. What is he going to do about it?
   This will give the patient's reaction. For instance, he will defend himself or surrender.

Bleuler (1972) and Schneider (1959) attempted to correlate the content of a delusion with specific psychiatric disorders, especially schizophrenia. Schneider described eleven so-called first-rank symptoms, seven delusions, one delusion combined with a kinestetic hallucination, and three auditory hallucinations, which he believed to be pathognomonic for schizophrenia. However, recent research has shown that these symptoms are neither sensitive nor specific for schizophrenia. According to Mellor (1970) only 80% of schizophrenics show first-rank symptoms. Especially chronic schizophrenics with negative symptoms and some acute schizophrenics are free of first-rank symptoms. In contrast, approximately 11.5% of patients with an affective disorder studied by Taylor and Abrams (Taylor and Abrams 1973) had Schneiderian first-rank symptoms.

Delusions are not disorder specific. Evaluate them in the context of other psychopathology such as type and age of onset, course, social deterioration, premorbid personality, and association with other affective or organic symptoms.

Delusions with depressive themes (see table 4.1) are seen when a depressed patient suffering from delusions is burdened by guilt feelings. Claiming he has always been wicked but that he has only recently been found out, he expects only one possible outcome: harsh and merciless punishment. He says he will plead for mercy and forgiveness or request to be punished as the only way to rid himself of guilt.

Grandiose delusions (see table 4.2) surface without much probing. Ask the patient what the immediate future holds for him and he will present thoughts flavored with messianic glow, coming wealth, power, and indestructible health.

TABLE 4.1
Delusions with Depressive Themes

Content	Pt's Explanation	Pt's Expectation	Pt's Reaction
GUILT	Wickedness of own character; past sinful, evil intents	Painful suffering, harsh punishment	Plea for mercy, self-accusation, and willful surrender
POVERTY	Unproductivity, worthlessness, moral weakness	Deprivation of all goods and rights, ridicule and expulsion from society	Submission, self-destruction, and suicide
NIHILISM and DEATH	Result of deprivation and punishment	Helpless and powerless victim of others	Self-mutilation
ILLNESS	Weakness and worthlessness of mind and body	Permanent disability and death	Seek help; surrender to the inevitable

TABLE 4.2
Grandiose Delusions

Content	Pt's Explanation	Pt's Expectation	Pt's Reaction
MESSIANIC ABILITIES	Chosen, reborn, special reward for accomplishment	Future admiration, acknowledgment as leader of mankind	Preaching, helping, healing
WEALTH	Deserved reward	Public praise and acknowledgment	Use wealth to abolish poverty on earth
POWER AND GIFTEDNESS	Deserved reward	Admiration	Help and lead mankind; great inventions
INDESTRUC-TIBLE HEALTH, ETERNAL LIFE	Special endowment and gift; chosen	Admiration	Investment in many activities

More difficult to explore are delusions of passivity formerly thought to occur in schizophrenia (see table 4.3). Such a patient often wants to hide them from you. Table 4.3 lists Kurt Schneider's eight delusions which have the following in common:

1. The patient feels under the influence of a strong force such as x-rays, electronic surveillance, magnetic fields, or telepathy.
2. This force is overpowering; it makes him think, feel, want, and act completely out of his own control (feelings of passivity). He experiences other people's feelings and thinks other people's thoughts rather than his own.
3. The reaction to his delusion is submission; he cannot resist; he is the victim.

To induce a patient to describe some of these delusions start with an open-ended question such as

"How do you control your mind, your thoughts, your feelings and your actions?"

If the answer is evasive, become more specific and ask if anybody ever tried to tamper with his thoughts, his feelings, or control him or force

TABLE 4.3
Delusions of Passivity

Content	Pt's Explanation	Example	Pt's Reaction
INSERTION of SENSATIONS (SOMATIC PASSIVITY)	Experience of feeling the controlling force	"My boss gives me evil looks which run down my body and give me tingling sensations in my genitals."	Passive submission
THOUGHT BROADCASTING	Radio waves, magnetic waves, telepathy	"My head is a radio; it transmits all my thoughts so everybody can hear them."	Lack of control; no action taken
THOUGHT WITHDRAWAL	Magnets, a black hole, vacuum suction or evil people steal thoughts	"In the evening they turn on the big wind pump and suck all my thoughts out of my head."	Complaints and submission
THOUGHT INSERTION	Feeling of a foreign thought's being forced into mind by micro- or radio waves	"Mr. X on TV uses my head to think with."	Passive compliance
INSERTION of FEELINGS ("MADE" FEELINGS)	Outside agent projects feelings onto patient	"My dead sister transmits her anger into me. She shouts and cries, and uses my body to do that."	Patient displays feelings, knowing that they originate on the outside, or he is forced to feel that way.
INSERTION of IMPULSES ("MADE" IMPULSES)	Impulse manufactured by outside agent and imposed on patient	"The devil turns my head and makes me look at all men's crotches."	Submission to imposed impulse
INSERTION of an OUTSIDE WILL	Outside force pulls the strings and controls patient's actions	"The university computer sends impulses to all my muscles, makes	Patient complies like a marionette

Continued on next page

TABLE 4.3—CONTINUED

Content	Pt's Explanation	Example	Pt's Reaction
		them move, and detects my actions."	
DELUSIONAL PERCEPTION	Patient has a real perception and suddenly recognizes its true meaning	"The doctor crossed his legs. Then I knew he wanted me to go home and masturbate."	Patient follows and complies with message perceived through observation

him to do things against his will. For instance, when you check for thought insertion:

"Is it really somebody else's thought?"

Assure that the patient is delusional and not just describing anxious feelings of derealization, where "things appear as if they are not real." The patient with a delusion of alienation does not have the "as if" experience, but is convinced of living in an unreal world without being frightened by it.

Manic patients may report that other people can read their mind, a claim also often voiced by patients with schizophrenia. To make a distinction you can ask for the total delusional profile.

I: Danielle, what kind of thoughts did you have when you were hospitalized last?
P: I thought other people can read my mind.

I: What was the reason for that ability?
P: My thoughts were so fast, so intense, and so loud that I believed other people must hear them. I wasn't aware of the difference between saying something or just thinking it.

I: So what did you do when you had this experience?
P: I got so frustrated about other people because they did not respond to my thoughts, so I started to throw things at them.

I: How did you get back in control?
P: When I calmed down, I noticed that I had to talk in order to get a response. My thoughts became slower, I could sort them out and put them into words.

Danielle was not a passive victim of outside forces like a patient with schizophrenia would describe herself, but experienced the fast and intense thoughts typical for mania. Throwing objects was not due to hostility, as a patient with schizophrenia would report, but to her frustration as a manic patient, to sense that her physical limitations constrain her self-expression.

Persecutory and grandiose delusions (see table 4.4) are seen in the affective disorders, paranoid disorders, schizophrenia, organic mental disorders, and drug abuse. If you assess the complete profile of these delusions, the flavor of the underlying disorder will emerge.

Besides persecution and grandiosity, another delusional theme deserves attention: jealousy. Premorbidly, such a patient may have been suspicious, jealous, and preoccupied with marital infidelity. At the outbreak of the delusion he may start to interrogate his spouse for hours, during most of the night, claiming that her vagina is moister than usual and that she looks exhausted with bags under her eyes. In the case of a female delusional patient, she may be inspecting her husband's underwear for stains of semen. Even though this delusion is disorder-nonspecific, it seems to be more common in alcohol addicts.

Overvalued Ideas

Similar to delusions, overvalued ideas cannot be corrected by logical arguments, yet sometimes they are not obviously false. They can be persistent; their importance is exaggerated. The patient realizes his emotional engagement but justifies it.

Similar to delusions, overvalued ideas center around injustice, discrimination, disappointment, betrayal, jealousy, or grandiose plans, but they are less intense. The following types of questions may elicit them:

"Is there anything going on that concerns you a great deal?"
"Have you been a victim of injustice, discrimination or unfair treatment?"
"Do you have any important plans or goals?"
"Are you working on an invention?"
"Will you become famous one day?"

Occurring in patients with schizophrenia, affective disorder, organic brain syndrome, phobias, obsessions, and personality disorders, overvalued ideas have no specific diagnostic value, but can be harbingers of a delusion.

TABLE 4.4
Profile of Persecutory and Grandiose Delusions and Their Diagnostic Correlates

Content	Patient's Explanation	Patient's Expectation
PERSECUTION	Jealousy of persecutors	Battle and friction, but final victory by the patient
PERSECUTION	Moral failure, sin	Punishment
PERSECUTION	Misunderstanding of good intentions by persecutors	Final recognition of good intentions
PERSECUTION	Bewilderment, inability to figure out the reason for persecution	Unclear; hope for cessation of persecution
GRANDIOSITY (DELUSION OF ENTITLEMENT)	Superiority, elevation above others	Spectacular victory and annihilation of opponents
GRANDIOSITY	Enlightenment, self-improvement, giftedness	Effective as healer and helper
GRANDIOSITY (MARTYRDOM)	Chosen to suffer for the evil of all mankind	Punishment as a symbolic victim
GRANDIOSITY (PER SE)	Past accomplishments, evidence, no need for explanation	Acceptance by everybody without questions

Phobias

Phobias consist of a specific phobic stimulus, an unreasonable, unexplained anxiety of being exposed to it, and the avoidance behavior. In the interview it is best to focus on one aspect at a time. Phobic objects or situations can be assessed by questions such as

Patient's Reaction	*Probable Diagnostic Correlation*
Careful guardedness, outbreak of verbal or physical attacks	Schizophrenia, Delusional (paranoid) disorder
Self-accusation, surrender to punishing authorities, plea for mercy	Depression
Demonstration of good intentions, and values	Mania
Fearful or hostile self-protection, complaints, accusations	Organic mental disorder
Hostile and arrogant depreciation of others	Schizophrenia, irritable mania
Messianic-like and forceful preaching	Mania
Self-sacrifice	Manic depressive, depression
Grandiose mannerisms and claims	Organic mental disorder (general paresis)

"Is there anything like animals, sharp objects, or heights that you dread?" (to assess simple phobias).

"Do you feel comfortable talking to a crowd? Does it bother you to be watched by a group of people?" (to assess social phobias).

"Does it bother you to eat in crowded restaurants, visit a movie theater on Friday night when they are filled to the rim? Does it bother you to wait in line with a huge crowd of people?" (to assess agoraphobia).

Since phobias are classified by the type of the dreaded and avoided object, be specific about this aspect. Ask for unreasonable fears:

"Do you experience any excessive unreasonable fears?"
"Do you have any anxiety that is ridiculous?"

Finally, ask for avoidance behavior:

"Is there anything you have to avoid under all circumstances?"

Explore whether panic attacks preceded the development of a phobia, often the case in agorahobia. You can choose the order which fits best in the flow of the interview. Find out what impact the phobias have on the patient's life. Do they choke his social activities, prevent his advancement, or take an unusual toll on his time?

Obsessions

Obsessions should be differentiated from repetitive, enjoyable thoughts such as sexual fantasies, and from overvalued ideas and delusions that beset the patient's mind but are acceptable to him (egosyntonic); and from depressive worries which also are unwanted, but not resisted, because the patient identifies with them.

To elicit obsessions is difficult because the patient feels embarrassed. Ask directly whether he attempts to resist any embarrassing, silly, or time-consuming thoughts, or focus on the common content of obsessions:

"Do you have thoughts of hurting somebody? Do you have dirty thoughts or thoughts of getting contaminated or doubts about having forgotten something?"

If he concurs, go on to confirm that the thoughts are useless, unacceptable, and resisted by the patient.

I: Mr. Neil, do you often have embarrassing thoughts that pop into your mind—against your will—again and again?
P: (Hesitating.) No, not really.

I: Or thoughts that torture you, that you can't resist—that you spend a lot of time on?
P: How do you know?

I: I'm asking you because some of my patients are bothered by intrusive thoughts.
P: Well, I'm embarrassed to tell you, even though the thoughts are not embarrassing; just that I have them, they drive me crazy.

I: Tell me about them.

P: Well, I had to quit my job last month, because I was so slow. Whenever I picked up a tool, a thought came up: Does God want me to pick up the tool? Does he want me to pick it up now? Do I do the right thing? Should I do something else instead? I know it's silly, but I have no control over these thoughts.

Compulsions

Compulsions, by definition, are recognized by the patient as meaningless acts that he feels compelled to perform. Because of this insight you can ask directly:

"Do you have to perform some acts against your will?"

If he is reluctant, embarrassed, and afraid you will consider him "crazy," express empathy, as the interviewer did with Mr. Solinsky:

I: Have you ever felt compelled to carry out an activity, even though you knew it was nonsense?
P: (Hesitates.) What do you mean?

I: Some patients have the feeling they have to do things, like counting, unnecessary cleaning, or checking . . .
P: Yes, I do that sort of thing. I have to light my cigarette over and over again.

I: Can you tell me why?
P: There is no real reason. Just a nonsense, stupid thought.

I: Tell me about it.
P: It's really stupid. You must think I'm crazy.

I: Well, I understand your embarrassment. What is that stupid thought about?
P: I think about my father's death. I am afraid he is going to die. If I light the cigarette I think it brings his life back. And then I think it's nonsense. I shouldn't do it and I put the cigarette out; and then the thought comes back and I have to light the cigarette again.

I: You know it is nonsense?
P: Absolutely, there is no connection. It is ludicrous.

I: Why do you do it?
P: I couldn't live should anything happen to him and I didn't try anything to help him. It's not a big deal just to light a cigarette. So I just do it.

Sometimes obsessions and compulsions gain a delusional quality, when patients start to defend their obsessive thoughts as meaningful.

For instance, Benjamin, a 32-year-old freelance artist, at first was obsessively concerned that his heart would stop beating when he fell asleep. He considered this repetitive thought as nonsense but felt compelled to call the therapist for reassurance. After two years he made it a habit to call his sister, a nurse, for reassurance every night. At this stage he identified fully with his concern and defended his calling as necessary and therapeutic. The thought could not be considered egodystonic any longer—it approached a delusion.

Multiple Unexplained Somatic Symptoms

Multiple, medically unexplained somatic symptoms typify somatization disorder. A recently developed test (Othmer and Desouza 1985) helps to screen them economically. Ask female patients for target symptoms: *S*hortness of breath, *D*ysmenorrhea, *B*urning sensation in sex organs, *L*ump in throat, *A*mnesia, *V*omiting, and *P*aralysis. Remember these symptoms by a mnemonic: "*S*omatization *D*isorder *B*esets *L*adies *A*nd *V*exes *P*hysicians." Women with two or more of these symptoms are suspected to have somatization disorder if the symptoms have interfered with their life, are medically unexplained, and occurred prior to age 30.

Conversion Symptoms

Conversion symptoms are medically unexplained neurological symptoms such as paralysis, blindness, or deafness. Spot conversion symptoms by open-ended questions such as:

"Did you ever experience any nerve problems, for instance, with your vision—such as being blind—or with walking—such as being paralyzed?"

Go through a laundry list (DSM-III-R) of common conversion symptoms. They occur under stress alone or together with multiple somatic symptoms and often result in secondary gain. They can be seen in any psychiatric disorder.

Multiple Personality

Multiple personality is relatively rare but it is not difficult to assess. Direct questions often yield the answer:

"Do you switch into any other personality?"

or

"Do you have periods of memory loss?"

In addition, family or friends have often witnessed such a blackout and told the patient that he had assumed a different name, dressed differently, spoke with a different voice, and claimed to be unaware of his identity. By hypnosis you can often restore lost memory or induce personality switching in such a patient.

Paroxysmal Attacks ("Spells")

Frequently overlooked are paroxysmal phenomena. Patients do not consider them as psychiatric but as neurological, or medical symptoms. Assess paroxysmal phenomena directly.

"Do you have any kind of spells, such as losing consciousness, falling asleep during the day, feeling weak, or dizzy, feeling your heart pound real hard, or feeling as if you were having a heart attack, a seizure, or a memory blackout?"

If the answer is yes, let the patient describe the spells, their symptom profile, duration, when and how often they occur, what triggers them, and their different types. Here is an account of the most common attacks:

Fainting (Syncope): "Things start to turn and I feel dizzy and black out when I get up, or have to stand for a long time, or when I get very hot. I may have to lie down. The atttack lasts from a few seconds to minutes and subsides as soon as I am in a horizontal position with legs and arms up and head down."

Narcoleptic Attacks: These are sudden, irresistible sleep attacks. Patients sleep enough during the night but have several sleep attacks during the daytime. The naps last 15 to 30 minutes and the patient can be awakened. Emotional excitement, anger, or jokes can trigger the attacks.

The attacks are often spaced 90 minutes or multiples of 90 minutes apart. They may be associated with three auxiliary symptoms: 1. Cataplectic attacks. Patients report sudden muscle weakness of the whole or of parts of the body such as in arm and jaw. 2. Sleep paralysis. Patients wake up during the night and are paralyzed for a few minutes but are able to breathe. 3. Hypnagogic and hypnopompic hallucinations. Patients report visual and auditory hallucinations while falling asleep at night (hypnagogic hallucinations) and/or when waking up in the middle of the night or in the morning (hypnopompic hallucinations).

Grand Mal Seizures: The patient passes out and wakes up confused, weak, with headaches and often generalized muscle aches; sometimes he has injured himself, bitten his tongue, or became incontinent. Others have told him that his arms and legs contracted and relaxed rhythmically when he was passed out.

Pseudo-Seizures: Patients may report epileptic "seizures," but they admit that they can still hear and see what is going on around them, that they cannot talk, that their body is shaking, and their arms and legs are contracting. They rarely injure themselves, bite their tongue, become incontinent, or confused afterwards. Most of these patients are suggestible—they can be induced to pseudo-seizures under hypnosis.

Complex Partial or Temporal Lobe Seizures: The patient reports that he has amnestic attacks during which he carries out certain automatic stereotyped activities such as unintelligible, inappropriate, or irrelevant verbalizations, lip smacking, chewing, swallowing, patting, rubbing a part of the body, or fumbling with parts of his clothing. At the end the patient feels confused, has partial amnesia, and is fatigued. Recovery may last up to 20 minutes before the patient can resume his usual activities.

Panic: The patient reports that he often has attacks that feel like a heart attack. Reported symptoms include trouble breathing, palpitations, chest pain, choking feelings, dizziness, vertigo, feelings of unreality, paresthesias, hot and cold flashes, sweating, faintness, trembling or shaking, and fear of dying. The atttacks often start in young adulthood. Individual attacks may last from 15 to 30 minutes, are most intense after onset for five minutes. Sometimes physical exertion may bring them on, but mostly they occur spontaneously without being triggered by outside events.

Amnestic Attacks (Alcoholic Blackout): See 2. Conversation, Memory.

Psychogenic Amnesia: See 2. Conversation, Memory.

Fugue State: The patient travels unexpectedly away from home or work, assumes a new identity, and is unable to recall his previous identity. Perplexity and disorientation may occur even though usually there is no evidence of an organic mental disorder. After recovery the patient does not remember what took place during the fugue.

Hypoglycemic Attack: A patient reports that he often feels sweaty, tremulous, and hungry one to two hours after a meal.

Transient Global Amnesia: The patient reports that he lost memory for close to a whole day. He had no preceding conflicts; hypnotic sessions could not recover the lost memory. These attacks occur sporadically in patients over the age of 60 and may be due to circulatory insufficiency of brain structures involved in memory recall, such as the hippocampus.

Transient ischiemic attacks (TIAs): The patient reports a focal neurological deficit which lasts less than fifteen minutes such as blindness in one eye, paresis

paresis in one arm or leg. These attacks occur in patients with cerebral vascular disease.

Insight

Get a feeling for your patient's insight into his symptoms right from the outset of the interview, as discussed in chapter 2. Monitor insight whenever new symptoms or problems surface by probing:

"What do you think about . . . ?"
"Do you consider this normal for you?"
"Do you need help for it?"

If he responds with

"That's what I'm here for!"

he demonstrates at least some insight. Then counterprobe:

"What are your strengths?"

This double-barreled approach helps the patient to recognize the border between intact and disordered functions. If he defends his symptoms as reality-based, he has limited insight.

Patients rarely have insight into persisting current, nondrug-induced hallucinations and delusions. The reason is simple: insight is based on a cognitive awareness of consensual reality and this process is disturbed in the delusional hallucinatory state. If a patient hallucinates or displays delusional thinking, the pathological process affects the very function necessary to recognize disordered perception and thinking as sick.

Patients can identify disordered emotions more easily than disturbed cognition. This is true for depressed and schizophrenic patients. The manic patient is more capable of recognizing his behaviors as disturbed—such as his spending sprees, overtalkativeness, or indiscriminate sexual affairs—than his persistent feelings of euphoria or irritability. He experiences anxious and depressive moods earlier as disordered than elated moods.

Compulsions, phobic avoidances, and substance abuse rarely occur without the patient's insight into their pathological nature. With the exception of some substance abusers, a patient has little problem in identifying them as disturbances. He has however a problem in controlling or changing them.

Judgment

Judgment is the ability to choose appropriate goals, and to select socially acceptable and appropriate means to reach them. It reflects reality testing, intelligence, and experience. Since judgment requires an integration of outside reality, internal needs, and living skills, it is a sensitive indicator of disturbed mental functions.

Interviewers often explore judgment by probing general knowledge and problem-solving abilities. Clinicians ask, for instance, why rivers flow into oceans, why the stars come out at night, why the government collects taxes. The answers demonstrate some aspects of social intelligence but fail to address the gist of judgment.

Questions which require the patient to verbalize about his view of his own potential and limits in a social context will help to elicit his sense of judgment. You might ask about his future plans:

"How does the future look to you?"
"What are your chances of making a new start in life?"
"Do you think you can make a major invention?"
"Is there any chance that you may become famous?"
"What is the likelihood that you will become a leader of some kind?"

These questions invite the patient to make connections between his present state and his future. They explore the self-perception of his own abilities and assess his estimate of the risks involved in certain actions and how much risk he is willing to take. Here are typical answers from various types of patients to these questions:

A patient with an *organic mental disorder* describes highly unrealistic plans for his future, selects inappropriate and illogical means to achieve them, and shows disregard for his lack of ability, experience, or track record to reach them.
A patient with *schizophrenia* often answers a judgment question completely inappropriately. He may say:

"I will stop the battles of colors."
"I will insulate my bedroom so that the x-rays from the big machine can't penetrate my body."

A patient with an *affective disorder* gives divergent answers depending whether he is depressed or manic: When depressed, he underestimates his abilities, is pessimistic about the outcome of his actions, overestimates risks, and abhors taking them. Therefore his future looks bleak, there is no perspective of growth or success. When manic, no goal is too high to achieve; he perceives his abilities as unlimited, risks are negligible, and his willingness to take them is high. His future glows in bright colors. Mishaps are quickly forgotten, and even without completion of the tasks, happiness is assured.

An *anxious* patient recognizes his abilities but overestimates the risks and shies away from taking them. He views his future with guardedness; he expects obstacles and controversies everywhere and does not expect satisfaction.

You can gauge your patient's judgment by comparing it to his past accomplishments. If his future plans are in line with his track record, lie within his capabilities and control, and are independent of others, the better is his judgment; the greater the discrepancy, the poorer the judgment.

Since symptoms of most psychiatric disorders affect judgment, it is best to systematically and intensively assess your patient's judgment in each case. It will improve your psychodiagnostic evaluation. Even mild symptoms can have a great impact on judgment. When a patient changes his job, location, spouse, career goals, business partners, or investment strategies, evaluate whether such a change reflects an impairment in judgment triggered by a mood, anxiety, or substance-abuse disorder.

4. TESTING

A test *measures* mental functions. Most readers are aware of many available tests and how to use them. Here we will explore how to quantify them. As testing requires the patient's full cooperation, he must expose his deficits. Except for the hostile, or paranoid patient, most patients will cooperate. But a refusal can be as diagnostic as a test result.

Tests are used in neurology, psychology, and psychiatry. Neurological testing identifies deficits of higher functions due to brain lesions by showing failure in a circumscribed task. Psychiatric and psychological testing often measures functional disturbances quantitatively by comparing test scores with age-adjusted standards, for example the Wechsler Adult Intelligence Scale (Wechsler 1981).

Whom Do You Test?

Tests should be used selectively; not every patient has to be tested for everything. If a patient presents a reliable history, answers questions appropriately and in a detailed manner, and behaves adequately, assume that attention, comprehension and expression of language, psychomotor behavior, memory and intelligence, and abstraction are grossly intact.

Testing is appropriate when *exploration* fails to establish the level of functioning, such as in a patient who conceals his mild intellectual impairment, or deterioration (Alzheimer type dementia), or his lack of concentration, or who shows pseudo-neurological symptoms.

When Do You Test?

There are two basic times when testing can be done. 1. When a dysfunction first emerges in the interview, as the following example illustrates:

"You just told me that you have difficulties with your memory. That's very important. I would like to examine it further. Would you mind if we conduct a little test, so I can get a better feeling for your problems?"

2. At the end of the interview when it does not interrupt the flow of interviewing. When you delay testing, tell your patient about it.

How Do You Test?

Before you start, explain to your patient what and why you test. Test higher functions—for economical reasons—in a reversed hierarchy from complex to simple (Strub and Black 1977; Ludwig 1985). Complex functions are impaired first; disturbance of lower functions indicates severity; in other words, you examine, for instance, problem solving and abstraction, and when you detect gross difficulties you trace them back to memory and orientation, and when you find difficulties there, you may want to check attention, vigilance, concentration, and shifting of sets.

In the following layout, we will start with the more basic functions first and progress to the more complex ones.

Here is the hierarchy from simple to complex:

Level of consciousness
attention, vigilance, concentration, shifting of sets
memory, orientation
knowing, performing, communicating

imaging and imagining
problem solving and abstraction
insight and judgment

Focal disturbances do not affect whole hierarchical layers, but a segment of them. For instance, a brain tumor of the right motor strip may lead to a paresis of the left arm and hand and eradicate its most rudimentary movements, yet abstraction, thinking, language, and memory may all be preserved.

Level of Consciousness

If consciousness is impaired, as in the intoxicated, sedated, or sleep-deprived person, all other higher functions will be affected proportionately. Testing of consciousness is simple and has been mentioned under 1. Observation (see above). Even when you address the patient with a loud voice, the lethargic, in contrast to the somnolent patient, does not pay attention. His thinking is not goal-oriented, his movements are decreased, and his awareness limited. Lethargy may be due to drug intoxication, alcohol, or metabolic disturbances.

Stuporous or semicomatose patients respond even to persistent and vigorous stimulation only with groaning or restlessness. Special forms are akinetic mutism (see glossary) and Gjessing's periodic catatonia (see glossary).

The comatose patient is unresponsive even if you pinch him.

Attention, Vigilance, Concentration, and Shifting of Sets

Attention is the ability to focus one's perception on an outside or inside stimulus. Test *attention* by having the patient repeat up to seven digits, forward and backward, presented to him at one-second intervals. The lower level of normal performance is five digits forward and four backward.

Vigilance refers to sustained attention to outside stimuli. Ask the patient to tap on the table whenever he hears an *A* among a series of spoken random letters such as *K, D, A, M, X, T, A, F, O, K, L, E, N, A* . . . The number of errors will show his ability to sustain his attention. If he taps after each letter he shows perseveration.

Concentration is sustained attention to an internal thought process. Ask the patient to subtract seven from one hundred and repeat the subtraction from each remainder $(100-7=93-7=86-7=79$, etc.). Have patients with an IQ below 80 subtract three serially from thirty. Record time and number of errors.

Concentration, Attention, and Vigilance (CAV) can be assessed in combination by asking the patient to name all the months in reverse order, or to spell words backward.

The ability to switch from one thought content to another, called *set shifting,* is measured by visual, auditory, and tactile stimuli. Failure to shift is called perseveration. Examples:

Visual: The patient is asked to copy a given pattern, as shown in figure 4.1.

The patient with visual perseveration cannot continuously shift back and forth between a rounded and a pointed design. He starts the perseveration on the rounded design (upper portion of figure). The same patient is also unable to juxtapose loops; he breaks off the pattern after two loops. Instead, after his first acceptable try he continues the loops in one direction only and also increases the number of loops.

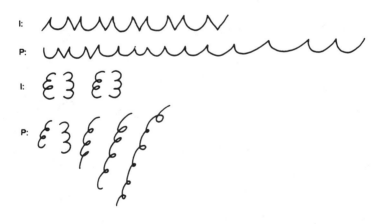

FIGURE 4.1
Perseveration

Auditory: The patient is asked to count the letters of the alphabet A1, B2, etc. Educated and intelligent patients count by 3: A3, B6, C9, etc.

I: A1 B2 C3 D4 . . .
P: A1 B2 C3 D4 E4 F4 G4

The patient with auditory perseveration manages initially to pair consecutive letters of the alphabet with consecutive numbers but after D4, he perseverates on 4.

Patients with impairment in the reticular activating system or the limbic lobe fail tests of attention, vigilance, and concentration, as in severe mania, depression, and intoxication with sedatives. Patients with frontal lobe deficiencies may fail tests for set shifting since they perseverate. For more extensive testing use the Halstead-Reitan Battery (Reitan and Wolfson 1985), or Luria's Neuropsychological Investigation (1966).

Memory and Orientation

Memory

Differentiate immediate, short-term, long-term, recent, and remote memory:

Test immediate memory (recall after 5–10 seconds) by repetition of letters, numbers (see Attention), or four unrelated words *(grey, watch, daisy,* and *justice).* Immediate memory requires registration and reproduction involving the reticular activating system, frontal lobe, limbic system, and central speech area (see 2: Conversation, Speech).

You can test visual immediate memory, which is regulated mostly by the nondominant temporal lobe, by having the patient copy abstract drawings (figure 4.2). The following instructions (Strub and Black 1977) are useful in testing memory:

I am now going to show you a simple drawing. I want you to look at the drawing carefully so that you can draw what you have seen from memory. Do not draw the design until I have told you to begin. You will copy a total of four drawings.

After you have said this, hold the first design for 5 seconds in front of him. After withdrawing the design wait five seconds, then tell him to draw the picture (see figure 4.2).

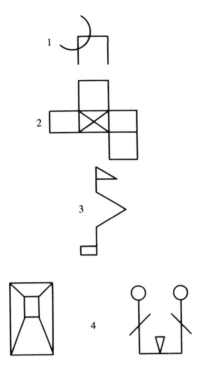

FIGURE 4.2

Test items for visual design reproduction test, Strub and Black (1977)
(Permission to reproduce granted by the F. A. Davis Co.)

SCORING: Score each design on a four point scale with values from 0 to 3:

0—Poor: Given for a failure to recall and reproduce the design.

1—Fair: Recognizable, but distorted, rotated, partially omitted, or confabulated designs.

2—Good: Easily recognizable with minor errors of integration, omission, or addition.

3—Excellent: Perfect (or near perfect) reproductions.

The average patient reproduces all designs with a score of 2 or 3. Low scores indicate a deficit in visual memory (Strub and Black 1977).

Short-term memory is the ability to recall information after 5–10 minutes. Test visual short-term memory by having the patient repeat the figure drawings (figure 4.2) 5 to 10 minutes after exposure. Test short-term auditory memory by asking the patient to repeat four words: *grey, watch, daisy,* and *justice,* and recall them after 10 minutes.

You can test complex auditory memory by testing the recall of a story. There are many such stories; we like the butcher story (source unknown). Instruct the patient to pay attention to the following short story, because he will have to repeat it in detail and discuss it. Then slowly read the following:

$$\overset{1}{\text{On December 18/}} \overset{2}{\text{one week/}} \overset{3}{\text{before Christmas/}}$$

$$\overset{4}{\text{Giovanni Scapini/}} \overset{5}{\text{a 51 year-old/}} \overset{6}{\text{married/}}$$

$$\overset{7}{\text{butcher/}} \overset{8}{\text{of Italian descent/}} \overset{9}{\text{from Columbia/}}$$

$$\overset{10}{\text{Missouri/}} \overset{11}{\text{was cutting meat/}} \overset{12}{\text{in back/}} \overset{13}{\text{of his/}}$$

$$\overset{14}{\text{shop./}} \overset{15}{\text{While working he/}} \overset{16}{\text{accidentally/}}$$

$$\overset{17}{\text{cut off his/}} \overset{18}{\text{left/}} \overset{19}{\text{hand./}} \overset{20}{\text{He got so mad/}}$$

$$\overset{21}{\text{that he picked up/}} \overset{22}{\text{the cleaver/}} \overset{23}{\text{and cut off/}}$$

$$\overset{24}{\text{his right hand too./}}$$

By clinical judgment, the patient should recall at least twelve of the twenty-four elements and grasp the story's illogical nature (compare the campaign trail story by Strub and Black 1977 p. 69). It is desirable that story and scores become standardized and validated which is, however, not the case.

To test *long-term memory* (recall after 30 minutes to days) have the patient reconstruct the interview with him, or have him recall the four words, after 30 minutes. Patients who fail on short-term memory tests usually fail the same test again when asked at a later interval as shown for the alcoholic blackout (Goodwin et al. 1970).

Clinicians often combine short-term and long-term memory as *recent memory* and distinguish it from remote memory. Recent memory assures everyday functioning and learning. Test it, for instance, by having an inpatient describe his last breakfast, lunch, and dinner and verify it with the staff.

Table 4.5 summarizes the memory tests which have been described.

Recent memory depends upon registration (cortex), consolidation (hippocampus), storage (convexity of cortical temporal lobe) and retrieval system (hippocampus, and both dorsal medial nuclei and pulvinar of the thalamus, but not the fornix, amygdala, and mammillary bodies

TABLE 4.5
Dimensions of Memory

	Immediate	*Recent*	*Remote*
TIME SPAN	*Seconds*	*Minutes–Months*	*Years*
MEMORY PROCESS	Registration	Consolidation	Storage
LOCALIZATION	Central cortical language center	Hippocampus Pulvinar Medial dorsal nuclei of thalamus	Association cortex
TESTS	Repeat: 4–7 numbers forward 4 backward 4 objects Abstract pictures Story Word association	Immediate memory tests Repeat after 10 minutes Describe last meals	Facts about verifiable past
TYPES OF AMNESIA	Inattention Central aphasias	Anterograde: Impaired new learning, amnestic state	Retrograde
DISORDERS:			
FUGUE	Intact	Intact	Intact
KORSAKOFF	Intact	Impaired	Intact
EARLY ALZHEIMER	Impaired	Impaired	Intact
LATE ALZHEIMER	Impaired	Impaired	Impaired

as previously thought (Baker and Joynt 1985). The dominant temporal lobe regulates verbal, the nondominant temporal lobe visual learning.

The symptoms of recent memory disturbance are anterograde amnesia (inability to learn new material) and confabulation (willingness to fill gaps with made-up stories).

The following disorders interfere with recent memory:

1. Alcohol amnestic syndrome DSM-III (Korsakoff syndrome); alcohol depletes vitamin B_1 (thiamine) which lesions the mammillary bodies and the dorsal medial nuclei of the thalamus.

2. Assess with which hand he writes, holds a knife, throws a ball, or stirs his coffee.
3. Head injury with concussion interrupts temporarily hippocampal functions. The anterograde amnestic disturbed storage period persists but the associated retrograde amnesia disturbed retrieval shrinks with recovery.
4. Transient global amnesia occurs when the posterior cerebral arteries obstruct the supply to the memory center of the medial temporal lobes.

Isolated disturbances occur in which memory retrieval, but not storage, is affected. Impairment of retrieval can be tested by examining recognition:

If a patient cannot recall any of the four words after 10 minutes, give him a multiple choice which includes one of the words in question. For instance, if he misses WATCH, DAISY and JUSTICE and remembers only GREY, ask him: "Was one of the words flower, stone, DAISY, or pencil?" If he can identify DAISY he can store but not retrieve.

Retrieval is impaired in normal forgetfulness, and in retrograde amnesia.

Patients who show disturbances in recent memory may be examined further with Strub and Black's (1977) Paired Associates Test (see appendix B).

Test *remote memory* (recall after months or years) by having the patient talk about historical events, such as World War II, the Korean or Vietnam War, the last six U.S. presidents, or verifiable personal events, such as date of birth, marriage, or military discharge. Remote memory is regulated by the appropriate association cortex, but not the hippocampus, mammillary bodies, and the dorsal medial nuclei of the thalamus. Therefore, patients with Korsakoff's or early Alzheimer's disease still have intact remote memory, whereas in advanced Alzheimer's and Pick's disease remote memory becomes impaired due to cortical atrophy.

Functional psychiatric disorders—such as severe anxiety, depression with psychomotor retardation or agitation, or mania with severe distractibility—can interfere with memory functions due to a lack of attention.

In dissociative disorders, such as fugue state and multiple personality, retrograde amnesia occurs as a result of suppression or repression. This functional retrieval amnesia is not associated with anterograde (storage) amnesia. Therefore, new learning occurs. These conditions are reversible through hypnosis.

Patients with Ganser syndrome, as often seen in prison populations, also claim memory disturbances. They consistently give answers that come close to being correct:

I: How many legs does a horse have?
P: Five.

I: In which month is Christmas?
P: January.

Psychogenic amnesia, a functional retrograde amnesia, may wipe out remote memory completely. Such patients may claim that they do not remember anything but their own first name and they appear to believe this claim themselves. Hypnotize these patients and recover the lost material.

Orientation

Ask the patient to state his name, time of day, date, year, present location, and situation. Disorientation in time and space are less severe indicators of cognitive impairment than disorientation to person.

Aphasia, Agnosia, and Apraxia

Whenever you notice that the patient is perplexed, has difficulties communicating with you, or is indecisive in his goal-oriented actions, such as walking to his chair, or lighting a cigarette, test him for deficiencies of comprehension and expression of language (aphasia), of recognition of complex sensations (agnosia), and of execution of routine acts (apraxia). Testing will prevent you misinterpreting aphasia as schizophrenic thought disorder, agnosia as psychomotor retardation, and apraxia as catatonia (see appendix B). More detailed testing of the frontal, parietal (Critchley 1953), temporal, and occipital lobes is described elsewhere (Taylor 1981).

Handedness

Before you test for aphasia, the patient's handedness should be determined. Handedness and cerebral dominance are closely allied:

1. Ask whether he is right- or left-landed.
2. Assess with which hand he writes, holds a knife, throws a ball, or stirs his coffee.

3. Ask whether first-degree relatives are right- or left-handed (handedness is hereditarily influenced).
4. Observe the patient while writing. The natural right-hander keeps his hand below, the forced right-hander above the line of writing.

Right-handers have a left dominant hemisphere, left-handers have sometimes a right dominant hemisphere. Footedness coincides 98% with hemispheric dominance while handedness coincides only 80–85%. (Note: Evaluate handedness prior to the administration of unilateral ECT which should be given to the nondominant hemisphere).

Frontal Lobe Reflexes

Complement the testing of apraxias by testing the frontal lobe reflexes which are abnormal when inhibitory pathways in the frontal lobe are interrupted.

Snout Reflex: Snout appears when the upper lip is tapped.

Sucking Reflex: Sucking movement appears when the upper lip is lightly stroked.

Palmomental Reflex: Downward movement of the ipsilateral angle of the mouth appears when the inner surface of the hand is firmly scratched from the thenar to the hypothenar eminence.

Grasp (Forced Grasping) Reflex: The patient grasps the examiner's index finger when his palmar surface between thumb and index finger is stroked.

Glabella Reflex: Tap the forehead above the bridge of the nose. The eyes blink after the first few taps; if no extinction occurs (perseverative glabella reflex) the test is positive, which is an extrapyramidal sign observed in Parkinson's disease and neuroleptic-induced parkinsonism.

Motor Functions

The patient carries out *abnormal induced movements* by demand, often regardless of the consequences. For instance, if the patient is asked to stick out his tongue he will repetitively obey, even if he receives a pin prick each time. *Waxy flexibility* occurs where the patient remains in the position the examiner puts him in. For other tests of abnormal induced movements, see appendix B. Most, if not all, of these movements occur in catatonia.

Affect, Imaging, and Imagining: Suggestibility

To differentiate disturbed affect due to right hemispheric cortical lesions from that of functional psychoses, see appendix B.

Suggestibility is the patient's willingness 1. to imagine a feeling or picture such as:

"Let your head hang down so that it starts to feel heavy and pulls on your neck muscles."

and 2. to comply voluntarily with a request such as

"You start to breathe slower and slower."

High suggestibility (autosuggestion) may be associated with conversion, dissociative, or somatization disorder in some of these patients. Even if true, not suggestibility as such, but uncontrolled uncritical autosuggestion would be necessary to explain the symptoms in these disorders. To test suggestibility, consult appendix B (DeBetz and Sunnen 1985).

Abstract Thinking and Intelligence

Abstract Thinking

To test abstract thinking, ask for the meaning of proverbs, for example:

"Don't cry over spilled milk."
"A stitch in time saves nine."

If the patient responds that one should not worry over past mishaps, or one is better off to fix a small problem before it becomes a big problem, he can abstract. But if he answers:

"If you cry over spilled milk you have not only lost milk, but also tears."
"If you make one stitch you don't have to make another one."

he shows concrete thinking.

Patents with schizophrenia sometimes give awkward interpretations of proverbs:

"Milk is white and tears are clear. They don't mix."

Abstract thinking is regulated by the language area of the dominant hemisphere. One of the drawbacks of the proverb test is that the patient who has experienced many psychiatric evaluations has learned the correct answer. Proverb interpretation is not standardized and normative data are lacking. Some investigators have reported that only 25% of non–brain-damaged adults can interpret proverbs correctly (MacKinnon and Yudofsky 1986). Proverbs are culture-dependent and have therefore little diagnostic value (Taylor 1981). Concrete thinking appears to be a function of low intelligence rather than of schizophrenia (Payne and Hewlett 1960).

COMPLETION TEST:

Ask the patient to complete several conceptual series (e.g., 1, 3, 5, ?, or A, 2, B 4, C, ?).

SIMILARITY TEST:

Ask the patient to find similarities:

"What do an apple and a banana have in common?"
"A car and a submarine?"
"A wheel and a chair?"
"Peace and justice?"

PROBLEM SOLVING:

Test problem-solving ability by asking patients to perform hidden calculations, for instance:

"If you have a total of 27 beer bottles, with twice as many in one refrigerator than another, how many bottles are in each refrigerator?" or
"If you can get to work by bike in 45 minutes but drive there three times as fast by car, how long would it take you to drive?"

Intelligence

Intelligence functions can be crudely assessed with the Rapid Approximation Intelligence Test which consists of a multiplication task: 2×3; 2×6; 2×12; 2×24; 2×48, etc. The nonretarded patient should be able to multiply 2×24. Patients who cannot multiply 2×24 have an 85% probability of having a WAIS IQ score of less than 84 (Wilson 1967).

A test that assesses more verbal abilities and thinking than calculation is the intelligence test by Grace H. Kent (see appendix B, table B.4). A more refined and age-controlled test is the Wechsler Adult Intelligence

Scale (1981). Intelligence tests should be used by a qualified psychometrist or psychologist.

For the diagnosis of dementia, the Mini-Mental State Examination is reproduced in appendix B (table B.5, Kent 1946).

MENTAL STATUS FINDINGS AS SUPPORT FOR DIAGNOSIS: CAVEAT

We have described the mental status examination as a source for clues, since major psychiatric disorders have their typical mental status. The patient's behavior has an immediate diagnostic impact to the point that some interviewers claim they can "guestimate" a diagnosis in the first 20 seconds. However, such reliance on the mental status may herald misdiagnosis, since the mental status can change dramatically within 24 hours.

Mental status assessment is only one of three essential elements of diagnosis, the other two being psychiatric history and family history (see chapter 5). Mental status assessment complements the longitudinal aspect of the patient's psychopathology with cross-sectional data. Gauron and Dickinson (1966) found that the experienced clinician "depended less on the presence . . . paid more attention to the clinical picture in relation to past history. . . ."

Let us focus on this point in the next chapter.

CHECKLIST

Chapter 4: Mental Status Examination

This checklist is designed to give even the perfectionistic interviewer guilt feelings about the completeness of his mental status examination. What have you forgotten? To receive the full benefit of the guilt trip, answer each question for those patients that you interviewed without being able to make a diagnosis. Mark the nonassessed items in red. Look up in the glossary any unfamiliar terms.

Which one of the listed mental status characteristics did you observe? Fill in the appropriate numbers.

1. The patient's willingness to cooperate allowed me to use the following assessment methods (list up to four):
   1 = observation
   2 = conversation
   3 = exploration
   4 = testing   ____ ____ ____ ____

OBSERVATION

Appearance
2. The following characteristics of the patient's appearance were of diagnostic interest (list up to three):
   1 = none
   2 = race
   3 = difference in appearance of age vs. stated age
   4 = nutrition
   5 = body type
   6 = hygiene
   7 = dress
   8 = eye contact   ____ ____ ____

Level of consciousness
3. The patient's level of consciousness indicated:
   1 = alertness
   2 = lethargy
   3 = sleepiness
   4 = stupor
   5 = coma   ____

Psychomotor behavior
4. The following functions were disturbed (list up to three):
   1 = none
   2 = posture
   3 = expressive movements
   4 = reactive movements
   5 = spontaneous movements
   6 = complex movements   ____ ____ ____

5. The following abnormal movements were observable:
   1 = none
   2 = tremors
   3 = athetotic movements
   4 = choreatic movements   ⎯⎯ ⎯⎯ ⎯⎯

CONVERSATION

Attention and concentration
   6. During the interview the patient appeared:
      1 = attentive
      2 = distractible
      3 = apathic   ⎯⎯

Speech
   7. The patient had the following problems with speech (list up to three):
      1 = none
      2 = disturbed articulation
      3 = dysprosody
      4 = nonfluency
      5 = pressure of speech
      6 = circumscriptions
      7 = paraphasic language
      8 = neologistic language
      9 = faulty grammar   ⎯⎯ ⎯⎯ ⎯⎯

Thinking
   8. The patient had the following thought disturbances (list up to three):
      1 = none
      2 = concrete word use
      3 = overinclusive word use
      4 = circumstantiality
      5 = tangentiality
      6 = perseveration
      7 = palilalia
      8 = clang association
      9 = blocking and derailment

10 = flight of ideas
11 = nonsequitur
12 = fragmentation
13 = rambling
14 = driveling
15 = word salad   ____ ____ ____

Orientation
9. The patient showed the following types of disorientation (list all if present):
   1 = none
   2 = to person
   3 = to day of the week
   4 = to day of the month
   5 = to time of the day
   6 = to month
   7 = to year
   8 = to season   ____ ____ ____

Memory during conversation
10. The patient gave the following evidence of immediate recall, short-term, long-term, and remote memory:
    1 = repeat your name (or *grey, watch, daisy, justice*)
    2 = immediately recall the spelling of your name (or four words)
    3 = recall your name (or four words) during the course of the interview
    4 = recall events of last 24 hours
    5 = discuss verifiable remote events
    Which ones were tested?   ____ ____ ____ ____ ____
    Which ones was he able to perform?   ____ ____ ____ ____ ____

Affect
11. Which of the following affects predominated in your patient during the interview?
    1 = sadness
    2 = elation

3 = disgust
4 = anxiety
5 = anger
6 = perplexity
7 = guilt
8 = suspicion
9 = content   ____

12. Which ones of the nine affects were missing? Use the key from question 11.   ____ ____ ____ ____ ____ ____ ____
13. The patient's affect was mostly expressed in:
    1 = gestures prior to talking
    2 = facial expressions prior to talking
    3 = posture prior to talking
    4 = gestures during talking
    5 = facial expressions during talking
    6 = posture during talking
    7 = tone of voice
    8 = pitch of voice
    9 = selection of vocabulary
(Limit of three ranked by importance)   ____ ____ ____
14. The patient regulated his affect predominantly by:
    1 = suppression
    2 = appropriate control
    3 = acting out
    4 = faking
    5 = none of the above   ____
15. How did you judge the intensity of your patient's affect:
    1 = high
    2 = medium
    3 = low   ____
16. The duration of his affective display was usually:
    1 = less than two seconds
    2 = two to seven seconds
    3 = more than seven seconds   ____
17. The range of the patient's affective display was:
    1 = narrow
    2 = medium
    3 = wide   ____

EXPLORATION

Mood

18. Name the terms which the patient used to describe the quality of his mood.

19. How stable was the patient's mood over the past 24 hours? If there were changes in mood, list the type and how they occurred.

20. How reactive is your patient to good news? Describe at least one good event and the patient's reaction to it.

21. Give examples that demonstrate the intensity of the patient's mood.

22. Describe if the patient's predominant mood changed in the past four weeks and how long it lasted.

Energy

23. Describe how energetic your patient is.

24. Is he organized in his planning?   YES NO
25. Is it easy for him to get started   EASY PROCRASTINATES
    or does he procrastinate?

26. Is he persistent in pursuit of his goals?   YES NO
27. Does he complete the tasks?   YES NO

Perception

28. In case the patient ever had hallucinations, describe their content.

29. Determine the patient's stage of insight (I–V) into the hallucination (compare 3. Exploration—Perception).

Content of thinking

30. In case the patient ever had delusions, describe their content.

31. Determine the patient's stage of insight (I–V) for the delusion (compare 3. Exploration—Perception).

32. Classify the patient's delusion according to its content as predominantly:
    1 = manic
    2 = depressive
    3 = schizophrenic
    4 = nonspecific   ____

33. Describe the patient's overvalued ideas, if any.

    _____

34. Describe the content of the patient's phobias.

    _____

35. List the patient's obsessive ideas, if any.

    _____

36. List his compulsions, if any.

    _____

Multiple somatic symptoms
37. In female patients, indicate which of the seven symptoms of the rapid screening test for somatization disorder are present:
    1 = shortness of breath
    2 = dysmenorrhea
    3 = burning sensation in sex organs
    4 = lump in throat
    5 = amnesia
    6 = vomiting
    7 = pain in extremities
                                    ____ ____ ____ ____ ____ ____ ____

38. In the answer to question 37, circle those symptoms that fulfill both onset before age 30 and lack of medical explanation.

Conversion symptoms
39. List the pseudo-neurological symptoms (conversion symptoms) that your patient reported, if any.

    _____

Multiple personality
40. Describe whether your patient ever had amnestic periods in which he assumed another personality.

    _____

Paroxysmal attacks
41. List your patient's paroxysmal attacks, if any:
    1 = fainting
    2 = narcoleptic attacks
    3 = grand mal seizures
    4 = pseudo-seizures
    5 = complex partial seizures
    6 = panic attacks
    7 = alcoholic blackouts
    8 = psychogenic amnesia
    9 = fugue state
    10 = hypoglycemic attacks
    11 = transient global amnesia
    12 = transient ischiemic attacks
    13 = Tourette's tics

                                         ___ ___ ___ ___ ___

Insight
42. Classify the patient's insight into his disorder:
    1 = he recognizes symptoms as part of a disorder
    2 = he recognizes symptoms but provides a rational explanation
    3 = he denies that his symptoms are expressions of a disorder

                                         ___

43. Describe your patient's future plans. Are they realistic?

TESTING	YES	NO	N/A
44. I selected appropriate tests to complete my diagnostic assessment.	___	___	___
45. The patient had problems with attention and concentration.	___	___	___
If yes, I assessed attention and concentration by:			
digit span	___	___	___
serial sevens (threes) backward	___	___	___
naming the months backward	___	___	___
spelling words backward	___	___	___
46. The patient showed signs of perseveration.	___	___	___
If yes, I assessed perseveration by:			
copying of changing patterns	___	___	___
repeating number-letter combinations	___	___	___
tapping at certain letters	___	___	___

47. The patient had impaired memory.   ____ ____ ____
    If yes, I assessed immediate memory by:
      word repetition   ____ ____ ____
      figure drawing   ____ ____ ____
      story repetition   ____ ____ ____
48. I assessed short-term memory by:
      recall of four words after 10 minutes   ____ ____ ____
      description of last meal   ____ ____ ____
49. I assessed long-term memory by:
      recall of the beginning of the interview   ____ ____ ____
      paired associates test   ____ ____ ____
50. I assessed remote memory by:
      recall of historic events   ____ ____ ____
      personal, verifiable dates (birthday, marriage etc.)   ____ ____ ____
51. The patient was disoriented.   ____ ____ ____
    If yes, orientation was assessed by asking for:
      his name   ____
      place of the interview   ____
      day of the week   ____
      day of the month   ____
      time of day   ____
52. I assessed handedness/footedness by:
      asking for it   ____
      asking with which hand the patient writes,   ____
      holds a knife,   ____
      throws a ball,   ____
      stirs coffee;   ____
      observing whether his hand is above or below the
    line of writing;   ____
      asking with which foot the patient kicks a ball.   ____
53. The patient had a speech disorder.   ____ ____ ____
    If yes, I assessed aphasia by:
      having him write down his chief complaint   ____ ____ ____
      having him repeat sentences   ____ ____ ____
      having him carry out commands   ____ ____ ____
      observing his fluency.   ____ ____ ____

54. The patient had one of the following speech distur-
    bances:
        central aphasia (inability to repeat)   ___ ___ ___
        expressive aphasia (nonfluency)   ___ ___ ___
        neologistic speech   ___ ___ ___
        paraphasic speech   ___ ___ ___
55. I tested the patient for agnosias by:
        writing letters on his hand   ___ ___ ___
        having him identify coins   ___ ___ ___
        having him name his fingers   ___ ___ ___
        having him point to right and left body parts   ___ ___ ___
56. I tested the patient for apraxias by asking him to
    perform imaginary actions such as:
        blow out a match (buccofacial)   ___ ___ ___
        use a hammer (limb)   ___ ___ ___
        swing a baseball bat (body)   ___ ___ ___
        entire act of toothbrushing (ideational)   ___ ___ ___
57. I tested the following frontal lobe reflexes:
        snout   ___ ___ ___
        sucking   ___ ___ ___
        palmomental   ___ ___ ___
        grasp   ___ ___ ___
        glabella   ___ ___ ___
58. I observed the following abnormal movements:
        waxy flexibility   ___ ___ ___
        echopraxia   ___ ___ ___
        perseveration   ___ ___ ___
        forced grasping   ___ ___ ___
        magnet reaction   ___ ___ ___
        mitmachen   ___ ___ ___
        gegenhalten   ___ ___ ___
        negativism   ___ ___ ___
        ambitendency   ___ ___ ___
59. The patient had a disturbance of affect.   ___ ___ ___
    If yes, I tested it by the 10-sentence test.   ___ ___ ___

60. The patient seemed to have pseudo-neurological symp-
    toms.   ___ ___ ___
    I tested his suggestibility by:
       falling backward suggestion   ___ ___ ___
       tired eyelid test   ___ ___ ___
       hand sticking test   ___ ___ ___
       circle test   ___ ___ ___
61. The patient showed intellectual impairment.   ___ ___ ___
    I tested his ability to think by:
       proverbs   ___ ___ ___
       conceptual series   ___ ___ ___
       similarities   ___ ___ ___
       the Kent Intelligence Test   ___ ___ ___
       the multiplication table 2*3, 2*6, 2*12 etc.   ___ ___ ___
       the Mini-Mental State Examination   ___ ___ ___

CHAPTER FIVE

SEVEN STEPS TO MAKE A DIAGNOSIS

6. Diagnoses
Multiple Diagnoses and Diagnostic Hierarchy
Principal Diagnosis
Provisional Diagnosis
Past Psychiatric Diagnoses
Lifetime Diagnosis

7. Prognosis

SUMMARY

Chapter 5 offers seven steps to make a diagnosis: 1. observation for diagnostic clues; 2. screening of the patient's affliction and listing of the differential options; 3. classification into a psychiatric category; 4. assessment of the patient's history and background to confirm the diagnostic impressions; 5. exploration of hidden diagnostic possibilities; 6. formulation of diagnoses; and 7. prognosis.

But where shall the wisdom be found?
And where is the place of understanding?

> The Holy Bible, King James Version,
> Job 28:12

There is no single diagnostic approach that works optimally for all interviewers or all patients. There may not even be one style that is always beneficial or always harmful in every case.

In the following we describe the work of two psychiatric residents whose interviewing styles reflect two extremes on a continuum.

Here is Ken Steiff's highly structured style. After one open-ended question at the beginning of the interview, Dr. Steiff presented the patient with a laundry list of psychiatric symptoms. For this purpose he had prepared about a dozen sheets each with the symptoms of one psychiatric disorder. During the interview he would underline the symptoms that the patient endorsed. If the symptoms fulfilled diagnostic criteria for a disorder, he would mutter to himself: "Wow!" and "That's it! Here we are!"

Then he told his patient: "You see you have somatization disorder; here is the proof. Look at all the symptoms you have."

How did the other residents who trained with Dr. Steiff respond to his interview approach? Even though they agreed with his diagnostic impressions, they felt that such an interviewing style was completely inappropriate. He did not use enough open-ended questions to become gradually more specific. He was not client-centered, i.e., only slowly and cautiously introducing more directive techniques. Instead, he behaved like a computer programmed for symptom checking.

How did the patient respond to Dr. Steiff's approach?

"He really seems to know what he is talking about. I have been with a couple of psychologists before, and all they did was beat around the bush. They did not seem to know what's going on with me at all. That's unlike Dr. Steiff. He really is on top of things."

This was not the only patient who appreciated Ken's style. He developed a following like the other residents. Maybe he had a lower return rate than others, but those who came back seemed to swear by him.

Here is the opposite, an unstructured diagnostic style in an interview which was conducted by Rosa Dahli. Dr. Dahli let her patients talk about what *they* wanted; she tolerated digressions, complaints, praises, gossip, and lengthy chats about God and the world. If a symptom surfaced, she hardly followed up. It took her several visits to come up with a diagnostic impression. Her long-term patients said that she was one of the best psychiatrists they had seen.

If the patient is considered the best judge, we would have to conclude that for any interview style there will be some patients for whom the approach works. Generally, the positive response is based on a good match between the personalities of the patient and the interviewer.

If we use research results, both Ken's and Rosa's styles seem to be justified. Gauron and Dickinson (1966) report:

Two major coordinate axes could be superimposed on the approaches to making a diagnosis. One involved the dimension structured versus unstructured. The other involved the dimension inductive—logical versus intuitive—alogical.

Mendel (1964) divided therapists into hedgehogs and foxes. The hedgehog is a problem solver with a probing, analytic, pragmatic mind depending upon logic (a friend of DSM-III-R we may add), while the fox engages in scattered and diffused thinking, waiting for experiences to take shape in his mind (a critic of DSM-III-R we may suspect). Interestingly, Gauron and Dickinson (1966) found that the same approach was not consistently used in every case by a given interviewer.

These findings remind us of the classic dichotomy between predominantly left-sided versus right-sided brain activity. The ideal approach is clear: use both. Listen to the patient, follow the direction of his thought, see where it carries you (the intuitive method), then analyze your global impression, trace its origins, and test and verify the observations (the left-sided method). Conversely, in some patients start systematically with the chief complaint, include likely and exclude unlikely diagnostic options (left-sided method) and ask yourself what your overall impression of the patient is, how your specific observations fit in. Have you missed the forest because of all the trees (the right-sided approach)?

Like Ken and Rosa, interviewers may be successful despite a one-sided interviewing style if they have a genuine concern for their patient and transmit it well. What Ken's and Rosa's patient responded to was the genuine caring of these interviewers. It seems clear that rapport is more effective than diagnostic style which is why we put rapport first in this book.

How can you determine then which diagnostic approach is right for your patient? The best indication is your results. If he opens up, is interested in the interview, contributes voluntarily, smiles, asks questions, and offers intimate details, you can consider your approach successful, at least in the short run. If the patient complies with your suggestions and treatment, returns for future appointments, and progresses in the solution of his problems, his behavior confirms that things have worked out in the long run.

Set aside personal style for now. There is a surer guarantee you will obtain necessary information from your patient. These are *seven easy, logical steps* or tools which will help you to establish a diagnosis, quickly and reliably.

1. Observation for Diagnostic Clues

As soon as the patient gets in contact with you, no matter what the setting, you have to establish rapport (see chapter 2). This first step allows you to observe the patient for diagnostic clues in his behavior. You also get a feeling for his motivation to see you. All these observations take place before you ever approach his chief complaint.

2. Screening of the Problem

From the beginning of the interview keep a list of all possible diagnoses in your mind. Whenever you make an observation about your patient, or get a report about symptoms or disturbed behavior from him, register these clues and decide at once which major psychiatric, personality, and adjustment disorders are compatible with these clues. Thus you generate a list—we call it list no. 1 of included psychiatric disorders. During the same screening process, you also make observations and obtain clues which exclude other psychiatric disorders. We will call this list no. 2 of excluded disorders.

Besides lists no. 1 and no. 2, you are left with the disorders that you have not covered yet. We will call this list no. 3 of unexplored disorders.

You can conceptualize the diagnostic process as a transformation of a long list no. 3 into a list no. 1, a list no. 2 and a shortened list no. 3.

As you begin, screen the patient's report, chief complaint, and behavioral clues for the main diagnostic areas of psychiatric disorders: psychotic symptoms, mood disturbances, organic factors, irrational anxiety (avoidance behavior or increased arousal), and physical complaints. Add stressors, psychosocial impairments, and lifelong patterns of maladjustment to this catalog. Then organize this information into your diagnostic list no. 1 including a wide variety of major psychiatric, personality, and adjustment disorders or problems of living. Use overinclusive questions for this step, questions that have high sensitivity but comparatively low specificity for psychiatric disorders. List no. 1 has all diagnostic options for the differential diagnosis; it *grows* during the first part of the interview, while list no. 3 of unexplored disorders and problems *shrinks*.

3. Follow-up of Preliminary Impressions

After the patient has revealed his problems, scrutinize list no. 1. Determine the duration of essential psychiatric symptoms or syndromes. Assess their severity in terms of their impact on the patient's life. If you find more than one syndrome, assess their temporal and causal relationship to each other (see below). Check whether the reported symptoms and observed signs satisfy the criteria for one or more disorders—in other words: *Test your diagnostic hypotheses!* Continue to examine one by one all major, personality, adjustment, and atypical disorders, and problems of living in your list, following up and narrowing down. During this third step use questions of high diagnostic specificity geared to identify all essential signs and symptoms of a disorder. The list of excluded disorders (no. 2) *grows* during this process at the expense of list no. 1, because now you exclude by detailed examination the previously included disorders.

4. Getting the Longitudinal View: Confirmatory History

If symptoms, signs, and problems pass the criteria test for a disorder, get more supportive evidence through premorbid history, the course of the disorder, and family history. Exclude medical disorders as the cause of the symptoms. If the problems fail the criteria test for a disorder, eliminate this disorder from list no. 1 and add it to list no. 2, the list of excluded disorders. Thus you *shorten* list no. 1 further in favor of list no. 2. This background information also reveals the impact of the disorder on the patient's life and thus gives a measure of severity.

5. Getting a Rounded Picture: Completion of the Data Base

With step 5, feel compelled to scrutinize list no. 3 again. At this time you go beyond the patient's chief complaint; you don't ask him what *he* wants to tell, but what *you* want to know. Approach the list of unexplored disorders in the light of the new findings.

6. Diagnoses

Organize your diagnostic impressions into a coherent life history. Run your diagnostic impressions through a decision tree to determine present, principal, and past diagnoses.

7. Prognosis

Complete your diagnosis with an explicit prognosis. Factor in the nature of the patient's major and/or personality disorders. Pay attention to how he handles the treatment contract and how he responds to it (see chapter 6). It shows his attitude toward his disorder and gives away his willingness to comply with treatment. For practical purposes, the degree of compliance may outweigh the other factors.

These seven steps are not locksteps—they are not even necessarily consecutive steps with the exception of step 1. These steps are *logical* steps, i.e. at some time during the interview you have to elicit all pathology; at some time you have to determine duration, severity, and relationship of all pathology; at some time you have to get a history; and at some time you have to put it all together into a list of diagnostic impressions. The order in which you do it is often determined by what the patient wants to talk about. As long as his elaborations contribute to any of these diagnostic steps, you may want to follow his leads—a jumpy interview can still produce a complete list of diagnostic impressions.

Besides a stepwise approach, clinicians observe that "sometimes the diagnosis bursts into consciousness before one is aware of the reason why" (Sandifer 1972). However, this intuitive approach—in contrast to systematic interviewing—cannot be taught.

Here is how to apply the seven steps.

1. OBSERVATION FOR DIAGNOSTIC CLUES

Patients need consultation for a number of reasons. Some come to you for administrative reasons perhaps needing a certificate to return to work. Others are ordered by the court. Some need an evaluation requested by a third party, and others come for a second opinion, or advice. In almost all cases patients have some sort of psychological or psychiatric problem. Your initial goal is to help to express that problem.

How do you best proceed? Wasting no time in getting right to the point is risky. The patient may freeze up if you are too direct. It is best to give your patient room and time until you have established rapport, until he trusts you and starts on his own to talk about himself and his problems (see chapter 2).

This first contact where you establish rapport gives you an excellent opportunity to observe your patient's behavior for diagnostic clues that you may want to follow up on. You also may get some feeling for his motivation to consult you at this point in his life.

2. SCREENING OF THE PROBLEM

Even if good rapport is established, some patients will persist with small talk; you may choose to converse until the patient expresses some change or dissatisfaction with his life—then summarize his difficulties for him.

Others may expect that you ask them directly for their chief complaint.

"You should find out what's wrong with me. Isn't that what you are paid for?"

Finally, there is a group of patients who overtly show disturbed behavior during the interview which you may take as an invitation to explore those *signs* closer (see step 1).

Accordingly, you encounter three expressions of a problem:

a. general dissatisfaction
b. circumscribed chief complaint
c. signs

General Dissatisfaction

A patient may appear tense and uncomfortable. He may refuse to talk to you at all, or he may start to talk about other people, about family members with psychiatric problems, or about movies in which a psychiatrist appeared. He may offer his opinions about health care, politics, art, or any topic unrelated to his problem. Or, he may talk about changes in his life, express feelings that "things are not right," but can only poorly describe what is going on. He may only slowly realize that his sleep, appetite, or sex drive have changed, that he avoids people and that his mind is less sharp than a year ago.

You may choose to stay with an indirect conversational approach or probe further by asking him point blank for his chief complaint, to confront him with his behaviors, or to reflect his statements.

As you talk to him, you may first get an idea about his present level of functioning before you find out if he has lifelong or recent problems, and can only poorly describe these changes.

With such a patient, it is your goal to eventually formulate—implicitly or explicitly—the chief complaint for him. If you meet such a patient who is not clear about his complaints, be careful not to scare him away because it may be his first contact with a mental health professional.

Chief Complaint

Most outpatients, especially those who come for treatment in a private practice setting, are cooperative. They expect to be asked why they came to see you, or they may tell you spontaneously. When and if you ask for their chief complaint (see chapter 3), it is helpful to use phrases such as:

"What kind of problems brought you here?"
"How can I help you?"
"Tell me everything that's troubling you."

Give them a chance to express their problems in their own words. Most patients give a chief complaint that involves about one or more of the following four problems:

Symptoms: They are either essential (also known as core), or associated symptoms of major psychiatric disorders.

Patterns of Maladjusted Behavior: The patient describes a lifelong pattern of maladjustment and problems in relating to other people, such as the following case shows. Here is Robert, a 34-year-old, white car mechanic:

"I always mess up just when I seem to establish myself. I'm so impulsive. I get so angry that I destroy what I accomplished. It happened again in the last few weeks."

Stressors: Stressors are generally outside events which have triggered or caused the person's current malaise. As the following example shows, Paul identified a business crisis as the precipitating factor.

"I'm a farmer. Business is bad under Reagan. I'm in debt and I have to work two jobs to get out from under. Now I got that heart attack and I worry. My doctor told me that I can't work the farm any more. I can't sleep because I don't know what to do."

Interpersonal Conflicts: Conflicts with spouse, significant other, family members, boss, or neighbors can be the major factor identified by the patient as the source of his problems.

"Jim, my husband, does not know what intimate is," one patient complained. "He can't give me what I need and I probably can't give him what he needs. We've had no sex for the last three months. If we do it I have to initiate it. But I don't mean that he is not sexual, you know, we are just not intimate with each other. Now, I have met somebody else. I see him every week or every other week but I feel guilty because I'm still attached to Jim and I can't let go."

Signs

A patient may show behavioral disturbances during the first few minutes of the interview which point to a psychiatric problem. Such disturbances may represent signs and clues of a disorder, visible in his mental status.

You may opt to start the diagnostic decision process by confronting the patient with it now, rather than exploring it later:

P: (Talks with a very low voice when he first meets the interviewer in an outpatient clinic.)

I: You talk so softly. Is there a special reason?

P: Yes, I'm afraid somebody from the waiting room is listening outside the door.
   (Register suspiciousness characteristic of paranoid schizophrenia, delusional [paranoid] disorder, paranoid personality but also organic mental disorder, amphetamine psychosis, or psychotic depression.)
or:

P: (Insists on having his wife present at the interview).

I: You wanted your wife to be in here with us. Can you tell me how she can help us with the interview?

P: Yes, she can explain everything better. I have a hard time concentrating. That's why I brought her all the way from X (a town 150 miles away).

(Register dependent behavior as seen in organic mental disorder, depression, avoidant or dependent personality disorder.)

or:

P: (Has rings on *all* her fingers.)

I: You are wearing beautiful rings on each of your fingers.

P: You forgot my thumbs . . . I put them all on when I feel bad but have to go somewhere.

(Register flamboyant behavior as seen in mania or histrionic personality disorder, and also with intoxication.)

These examples are characteristic of a group of psychiatric disorders. Follow up on observed signs if you feel they lead you to the patient's main problems. You have no choice but to confront the patient with his behavior if he refuses to talk to you.

Expanding or Focusing

After you have some idea of the patient's main problem(s), you can pursue one of two different avenues: expand and try to discover more problem areas, or focus on what you have already identified. Further screening of problem areas is useful because it may shed more light on the previous one. Zeroing in on the just explored area on hand may strike the iron while it is hot. Let the patient lead you.

Expanding

If you screen for more problems, use questions such as

"Are there any other problems?"
"Is this your main and only problem?"

The DSM-III-R lists five diagnostic areas that often become the point of origin for a descriptive decision tree:

1. psychotic symptoms
2. mood disturbance
3. organic factors

4. irrational anxiety, avoidance, increased arousal, and
5. physical complaints or anxiety about illness.

In addition, look for

stressors,
lifelong patterns of maladjustment, and
periods of impaired functioning.

Broad, open-ended questions are very useful here. They should have high sensitivity to spot unusual experiences such as ESP (psychosis), or feelings of being on an emotional roller coaster (mood swings), but low specificity for any circumscribed psychiatric condition.

Focusing

If you decide to focus on a problem, encourage the patient with open-ended questions to offer more details. Use techniques such as clarification and continuation to steer him back to his problem when he digresses. Encourage him to elaborate on three areas:

Severity: Do his problems interfere objectively with his life and limit his social effectiveness and/or lead to (subjective) suffering?
Course: How long did he have the problems? Was the onset insidious or sudden, did the disorder become worse or better with time? Was there any particular pattern?
Stressor: Does the patient believe that some outside event brought on his problems?

After you have collected information about these three areas decide whether it points to a major psychiatric disorder, a personality disorder, an adjustment disorder, an atypical disorder, or a problem of living.

Major psychiatric disorders, similar to physical disorders, are characterized by a syndrome of symptoms and signs, or a pattern, or, in some cases, a single symptom such as a chronic delusion, which follows a predictable course, and is often familial.

In contrast, *personality disorders* are chronic, lifelong patterns of maladjusted behavior often without clear onset.

An *adjustment disorder* is an acute, onetime response to a stressor or a set of stressors, and "not merely one instance of a (lifelong) pattern or overreaction to stress" (DSM-III-R).

Atypical disorders (Not Otherwise Specified NOS) are either incomplete major psychiatric disorders, or nonspecific monosymptomatic complaints.

Problems of living may be the result of psychiatric disorders but can also occur in "normal" people embroiled in a complicated marriage, work, legal problems, or other stressful situations.

Differential

What do you do after you have the patient's chief problem? You may find yourself in one of two extreme situations: too little information (situation 1), or (mis)leading information (situation 2). Here are the reports of two candidates who took the National Boards of Psychiatry and Neurology. Their experiences illustrate the two situations:

Situation 1:

After his oral boards in psychiatry and neurology, Dr. Tim R. complained that he must have failed the examination, because his patient did not say much. The patient did not give a chief complaint, answered questions with yes and no only, and used phrases such as:

"They told me to show up here today."
"I guess that's in my record."
"I don't know."
"I forgot."
"Can't remember."

When asked what the patient's differential was, the candidate responded with irritation, "How could I give a differential? I couldn't tell whether this guy was mentally retarded, had an organic brain syndrome, or was severely depressed. I couldn't tell a thing."

"So your patient could have had any of the psychiatric disorders listed in DSM-III-R?" he was asked.

"Sure," the candidate answered, "any or none."

"NONE? You would have had to prove that. But ANY? If you only came up with a list of any disorders—there is your differential! The less you know about the patient, the longer your list of differential diagnoses, the more disorders you may want to discuss with your examiner. Scant knowledge about the patient means that many disorders of adulthood listed on Axis I and II of DSM-III-R can be included in your list."

Situation 2:

Dr. Susan F.: "They gave me this 33-year-old fellow who had a lot of paranoid delusions. I caught that right away. His chief complaint was "My neighbors are out to get me. They bought a TV dish and directed it against my house. That makes me nervous." I thought I lucked out—that's an easy case. What can be easier than a paranoid schizophrenic? So I told them what I thought. The examiners must have read the patient's chart. They asked me again and again what other diagnoses I would consider. I tried my best to convince them that in my book, the fellow has paranoid schizophrenia, but they must have thought that he has something else. I argued for quite a while, but I guess they were in the driver's seat."

"You probably would have passed your examination, if you had followed the *rule of five.*"

"I never heard of such a rule", she said.

"The rule of five means that when you interview a patient, do not decide prematurely on one diagnosis. Challenge yourself, consider at least *five* diagnostic options."

The young lady looked puzzled. "You mean I don't have to figure out what the right diagnosis is?"

"That's right; as long as you include the right diagnosis in your differential. It's better to be overinclusive than overexclusive."

"How could I have found five diagnoses for my paranoid schizophrenic?"

"By looking for them. For instance, what kind of street drugs, if any, did your patient take? Any amphetamines which could produce persecutory delusions?"

"I didn't ask that, because his delusions were so typically schizophrenic that there was not any doubt in my mind."

"Did the fellow have a history of a head injury?"

"He was oriented alright; he could remember four objects after ten minutes and could do similarities fine. So I did not think that he had an organic mental disorder."

"Are patients with an organic delusional syndrome always disoriented or unable to process information?"

"Hmm."

"How was his affect? Was there a history of depression or elated mood?"

"Why should a schizophrenic have elated mood or depressions? And if he does, what's the difference?"

"That he might not be a paranoid schizophrenic after all."

This candidate had tried only to confirm her initial impression, and had collected supportive evidence only for it, while ignoring other options. She was pursuing her goal wearing blinders and elevated a symptom to a psychiatric disorder. Avoid this one-way street trap.

The solution to the diagnostic dilemma of both candidates is the same. Their information should be used to generate a list of all disorders that possibly could explain the patient's complaints and his mental state. On top of that list should be the most severe and devastating disorders, followed by the nonpsychotic, adjustment, and personality disorders, and finally the atypical disorders and problems of living.

Here are three different types of cases you may encounter. If a patient reports depressive symptoms, make a mental list of all disorders that fit this account. Your catalogue could look like this:

Organic affective syndrome
Substance abuse
Alcoholism
Bipolar disorder, depressed type
Major depressive disorder
Schizoaffective disorder
Agoraphobia with secondary depression
Adjustment disorder with depressed mood
Dependent personality disorder
Dysthymic disorder.

If your initial impression suggests a stressor associated with anxious mood, your list should contain:

Organic personality syndrome
Organic anxiety syndrome
Psychoactive substance abuse disorder
Bipolar disorder, depressed type
Major depressive disorder
Delusional (paranoid) disorder
Posttraumatic stress disorder
Social phobia
Panic disorder
Generalized anxiety disorder
Adjustment disorder with anxious mood
Avoidant personality disorder
Dependent personality disorder.

If your initial impression is a lifelong pattern of violent acts, generate a list such as:

Organic personality syndrome, explosive type
Psychoactive substance abuse disorder
Recurrent (hypo)manic episodes
Multiple personality disorder

Intermittent explosive disorder
Antisocial personality disorder
Impulse control disorder

Work with an open mind in assembling these lists. Be over*inclusive* rather than over*exclusive*. Remember that the average patient fulfills criteria for two to three psychiatric disorders during his lifetime (Helzer et al. 1977; Othmer et al. 1981; Powell et al. 1982).

In summary, this step in diagnosis involves two approaches: including and excluding. *Including* supplies evidence to support a diagnosis, *excluding* provides evidence to eliminate a diagnosis. Thus, diagnosing generates three lists: list no. 1 consists of what to include, list no. 2 of what to exclude, and list no. 3 of what is still to be explored.

Both candidates neglected to develop these three lists. Otherwise, the first candidate would have realized that he had a long list of unexplored disorders to be discussed in light of his mental status observations, such as the patient's sex, age, demeanor, comprehension, speech, affect, possibly orientation and short-term memory, and then should have created list no. 1. Our second candidate was not aware that he had a long list no. 1 of disorders which share persecutory ideas.

This section taught you how to screen for psychopathology and problems, and how to make a differential. The next section helps you to verify some and exclude other disorders of your differential.

3. FOLLOW-UP OF PRELIMINARY IMPRESSIONS

At this point you have generated a list of preliminary diagnostic impressions in your mind. Review that list. You may face one of two extreme situations.

First, your list contains mainly disorders that belong to one of the five diagnostic areas described in DSM-III-R, namely psychotic symptoms, mood disturbances, organic factors, irrational anxiety, or physical complaints. For instance, your list contains mainly disorders that have psychotic symptoms in common:

Schizophrenia
Delusional (paranoid) disorder
Organic delusional disorder
Psychosis NOS

Psychotic depression
Paranoid personality disorder
Schizotypal personality disorder.

According to DSM-III-R, you could follow the diagnostic decision tree on p. 378. You would then need to ask questions that allow you to make these decisions in proper order. For example, DSM-III-R recommends excluding or verifying first an organic factor, when you encounter psychotic symptoms. Consequently, you would have to ask for any substance abuse, head injury, and CNS disorder. In addition, you would have to examine the patient for the presence of disturbances usually associated with an organic mental disorder, such as fluctuations in alertness, distractibility, disorientation, amnesia, apraxias, aphasias, or focal neurological signs and others as discussed in chapter 4: Mental Status. If you cannot find an organic factor, next, you would have to ask for the duration of the psychotic symptoms. Did they last longer or shorter than a month? According to the answer, you will branch to the next decision box until you end up at a "leaf," i.e., a "point in the tree with no outgoing branches."

Such a diagnostic interview is, of course, possible but it requires that you as interviewer take over, direct the patient, and structure the diagnostic process: you ask the questions and the patient answers, preferably promptly and to the point.

The pitfalls are obvious. In pursuit of your decision making you will kill spontaneity.

Therefore, postpone the decision making to the end of the interview. Let the patient move in different directions, let him elaborate here and there, and skip while you extract the descriptive features of his pathology.

Second, your list contains a wide variety of major psychiatric, personality, adjustment, atypical, or not otherwise specified disorders (NOS DSM-III-R) and problems of living. A hodgepodge of psychopathology—so to say without any focus on one of the five diagnostic areas. No way can you follow any single one of the five decision trees in DSM-III-R. An interviewer usually does what worked in the first situation (above). He scrutinizes his preliminary diagnostic impressions by determining the following descriptors of the pathological symptom complex:

1. all symptoms that are associated with any given complex;
2. duration of the symptoms;

3. disabling nature of the symptoms;
4. preceeding stressors, if any (posttraumatic stress disorder); and
5. temporal relationship of the symptoms to each other.

For instance, if he finds hallucinations and delusions, he asks:

> "What other symptoms were there together with the hallucinations and delu-
> sions?"
> "How long did they last? Did some last a shorter time than the others?"
> "How much were you affected by these psychotic symptoms? Did you observe
> them with amusement, were they mainly present before sleep, or did they
> occupy all your time and energy?"
> "Was there anything that brought them on abruptly, or did they sneak up on
> you slowly?"
> "How did these hallucinations and delusions relate to the quickly changing
> mood, the sleep and appetite disturbances, the guilt feelings and suicidal
> ruminations? Did they happen in a two-week segment with a six-month
> ordeal of mood disturbances, or did they dominate the picture with depres-
> sion occasionally fading in and out?"

Such an approach usually is understandable for the patient, memorizable
for the interviewer, and provides enough information to allow diagnostic
decision making at a later stage.

In comparison to step 2 which was characterized by questions of high
sensitivity, questions of step 3 usually have high specificity. Apply them
to your preliminary diagnostic impressions formed at the end of step 2.
They confirm or exclude certain diagnostic impressions.

With these descriptive features at hand examine first the major psychiatric disorders of your diagnostic list, then the personality and adjustment disorders. Finally, explore the NOS disorders, and problems of
living.

Major Psychiatric Disorders (Axis I)

How do you interview for major psychiatric disorders?

During my psychiatric residency, one of our teachers impressed us
with his interviewing style. He diagnosed a patient in a few minutes.
"How does he do it?" I wondered. I reconstructed his interviews after
each session . He took advantage of the anatomy of the major psychiatric disorders. First, he asked for the *essential* (core) symptoms and their
severity. Then, he assessed *associated*, i.e., less specific signs and symptoms *only* if the essential ones were present. When the essential symp-

toms were missing he would not waste time completing the catalog of symptoms for each disorder—he avoided redundant exclusions.

Essential Symptoms

Table 5.1 lists essential symptoms for some major psychiatric disorders. An essential symptom is a symptom that is necessary but not sufficient for the diagnosis of a disorder. For instance, you can diagnose alcohol abuse only when the patient drinks, or depression when your patient's mood is low.

Table 5.1 does not contain all DSM-III-R disorders and their subtypes—it is merely a demonstration guide.

The essential symptoms for each disorder refer to the specific psychic functions that are disturbed in the respective disorder: level of consciousness, memory, and intelligence in the organic mental disorders; control over substance intake in alcoholism and drug abuse; perception, logical thinking, and volition in schizophrenia; territorial security in delusional (paranoid) disorder; mood, initiative, energy and risk taking in affective disorders; adaptation to threat in anxiety disorders; control over aggression, sexuality, and hygiene in obsessive compulsive disorder; pain perception and somatic functioning in somatization disorder; awareness about motivation in dissociative disorders; sexual ability, patterns, and objects of erotic arousal in psychosexual disorders; regulation of the sleep-wake cycle in sleep disorders; control of aggression in impulse control disorders; coping with stress in adjustment disorder; information processing in mental retardation; control over food intake in anorexia and bulimia nervosa.

Validated questions to assess the essential symptoms of some of these disorders are listed below (Othmer et al. 1988):

Organic Mental Disorder: 1. What is your full name? I am going to say three words that I'd like you to remember. They are *pencil, car,* and *watch.* Would you say them? Good. I want you to remember the three words. It's very important. I am going to ask you to say them to me in a few minutes. Remember, the words are *pencil, car,* and *watch.*
2. When were you born? What is the date of your birth?
3. What day of the week is today?
4. What month is it now?
5. What is today's date?
6. What year is this?

TABLE 5.1
Essential Symptoms of Major Psychiatric Disorders (Axis I)

Disorder	*Essential Symptoms*
Organic Mental Disorders	Amnesia, disorientation, disordered thinking
Dementia	Amnesia, impaired thinking, spatial constructional difficulties
Intoxication	Maladaptive behavior 2° to drug intake
Withdrawal	Substance specific symptoms
Delirium	Inattention, perseveration, decreased alertness, or hypervigilance, disorientation, amnesia
Amnestic Disorder	Amnesia only (short- and long-term)
Organic Hallucinosis	Hallucinations (often visual) with evidence of an organic factor
Organic Personality Disorder	Personality change 2° to an organic factor
Alcohol Dependence, Abuse	Drinking alcohol
Substance Dependence, Abuse	Substance use for *one month*
Schizophrenia	Hallucinations, delusions, thought disorder for *six months*
Delusional (Paranoid) Disorder*	Delusions without hallucinations
Bipolar Disorder, manic*	Elated or irritable mood for a distinct period
Major Depressive Disorder*	Depressed, agitated mood, loss of interest or pleasure for nearly *two weeks*
Panic Disorder with Agoraphobia	Panic attacks (four attacks in one month, or one attack followed by one month of fear to have another attack) and avoidance
Panic Disorder without Agoraphobia*	Panic attacks (same as above)
Phobia/social or simple	Avoidance
Obsessive Compulsive Disorder	Obsessions or compulsions

Continued on next page

TABLE 5.1—CONTINUED

Disorder	*Essential Symptoms*
Posttraumatic Stress Disorder	Flashbacks of a traumatic event
Generalized Anxiety Disorder	Nervousness, anxiety for *six months*
Conversion Disorder	Physical symptom which is an expression of a psychological conflict
Somatization Disorder	Physically unexplained symptoms such as multiple pain, treatment resistant and medically unexplained dysfunction lasting for several years
Dissociative Disorders	Fugue, multiple personalities, pseudo-neurological symptoms
Psychosexual Disorders	Choice of unusual sex object, disturbed sexual function
Sleep Disorders	Sleep disturbances of more than *one month* duration
Factitious Disorders	Physical or psychological symptoms intentionally produced or feigned
Impulse Control Disorders not elsewhere classified	Uncontrolled impulses harmful to self or others
Adjustment Disorders	Maladaptive reaction to a psychosocial stressor occurring once
Mental Retardation **	Pattern of general intellectual impairment starting before adolescence
Anorexia Nervosa **	Willful starvation, distorted body image, amenorrhea (in females)
Bulimia Nervosa **	Two binge eating episodes per week for at least three months

* If this disorder occurs 2° to an organic factor, the syndrome is called organic mood, organic delusional, or organic anxiety disorder, respectively.

** DSM-III-R lists these disorders as "usually first evident in infancy, childhood, or adolescence." Since all three disorders also affect functioning and adjustment in adult life, they are included in table 5.1.

7. What is the name of this place we are in now?

8. What is the name of the city (or town, district, county) we are in now?

9. Would you tell me the names of two presidents of the United States?

10. Now I am going to say a sentence. When I am through I want you to repeat exactly what I said. Ready, Listen.

   (a) Next week I am going to take a drive in my green car.

   (b) Tomorrow I am going to get some sugar and flour from the store.

11. Would you tell me the three words I asked you to remember? What are the three words?

Alcohol Abuse/Dependence: Has heavy drinking, or drinking, ever caused you problems in your life? (If yes) Has heavy drinking, or drinking, ever been a problem to you over a period of at least a month?

Psychoactive Substance Abuse/Dependence: Have you ever used pot, speed, heroin, or any other drugs to make yourself feel good? (If yes) Have you used any of these drugs more than once over a period of at least a month?

Schizophrenia: 1. Have you ever heard voices or seen things that no one else could hear or see?

2. Have you ever felt your mind or body was being secretly controlled, or controlled somehow against your will?

3. Have you ever felt others wanted to hurt you or really get you for some special reason, maybe because you had secrets or special powers of some sort?

4. Have you ever had any other strange, odd, or very peculiar things happen to you? (If yes) Please tell me what they were.

5. (If yes to any of the above) Did this happen even when you were not drinking or taking drugs?

Mania: 1. Have there ever been times when you felt unusually high, charged up, excited, or restless for several days at a time?

2. Have there ever been times when other people said that you were too high, too charged up, too excited, or too talkative? (If yes) Have you felt this way since you were 15 years old?

3. How long do these mood changes usually last? (If less than 1 week) What is the longest they have ever lasted? (If less then one week) Have these high, excitable moods ever stayed with you most of the time for at least one week?

Major Depression: 1. Have there ever been times when you felt unusually depressed, empty, sad, or hopeless for several days or weeks at at time?

2. Have there ever been times when you felt very irritable or tired most of the time for hardly any reason at all?

3. (If yes on item 1 or 2) How long do these feelings usually last? (If less than two weeks) What is the longest they ever lasted? (If less then two weeks) Have these feelings ever stayed with you most of the time for as long as two weeks?

Panic Disorder: 1. Have you ever had sudden spells or attacks of nervousness, panic, or strong fear that just seem to come over you all of a sudden, out of the blue, for no particular reason?

2. (If yes) Did you have your first nervous attack before you were 40 years old?

3. (If yes on 1) Did you have these attacks even though a doctor said that there was nothing seriously wrong with your heart? (If no) Tell me what the doctor said was wrong with your heart.

Phobic Disorder: 1. Have you ever been much more afraid of things the average person is not afraid of? Like heights, animals, needles, certain small places, thunder, lightning, things like this? (If yes) What were you afraid of?

2. Have you ever been so afraid to leave home by yourself that you wouldn't go out, even though you knew it was really safe?

3. Have you ever been afraid to go into places like supermarkets, airplanes, tunnels, or elevators because you were afraid of not getting out?

4. Have you ever been so afraid of embarrassing yourself in public that you would not do certain things most people do? Like eating in a restaurant, using a public restroom, or speaking out in a room full of people?

5. (If yes to any of the above) When your fears were the strongest, did you try to avoid or stay away from (name feared stimulus) whenever you could?

6. Did this fear (any of these fears) first start before you were 40 years old?

Obsessive Compulsive Disorder: 1. Have you ever been bothered by certain embarrassing, scary, or ridiculous thoughts that came into your mind over and over even though you tried to ignore or stop them? (If yes) Please describe them.

2. Have you ever felt you had to repeat a certain act over and over even though it didn't make much sense? Like checking or counting something over and over or washing your hands over and over again though you knew they were clean?

3. (If yes) Did this problem begin before you were 40 years old?

Posttraumatic Stress Disorder: 1. Have you ever experienced flashbacks, when you found yourself reliving some terrible experience over and over again?

Generalized Anxiety Disorder: 1. Have there ever been days at a time when you felt extremely nervous, anxious, or tense for no special reason? (If yes) Have you sometimes felt this way even when you were at home with nothing special to do?

2. (If yes) Have these nervous or anxious feelings ever bothered you off and on for as long as six months or more at a time?

Somatization Disorder: 1. Have you had a lot of physical problems in your life that forced you to see different doctors? (If yes) Have doctors had trouble finding what caused these physical problems?

2. Did you start having any of these problems before you were 30 years old?

Adjustment Disorder: 1. In the last three months have you been very worried or upset about something that happened to you? Like the death of a loved one, loss of a job, separation, divorce, an accident, serious illness, or that sort of thing?

2. (If yes) Do you feel that you had more trouble handling this situation than most people would have had?

Mental Retardation: 1. While you were in school, did anyone ever say that you were a very slow learner. (If no) Did you ever have to go into a special education class when you were in school?

Anorexia Nervosa: 1. Have you ever deliberately lost so much weight on a diet that people started to seriously worry about your health? (If yes) Were you afraid of getting fat even when other people said you were thin enough?

2. (If yes) Did this first happen before you were 25 years old?

Bulimia Nervosa: 1. Did you ever have a problem with binge eating, when you would eat so much food so fast that it made you feel sick?

2. (If yes) When you were doing this, did you feel your eating binges were not really normal?

3. (If yes) Was the urge to binge sometimes so strong that you could not stop, even though you wanted to?

4. (If yes) After you had binged, did you often feel depressed, ashamed, and disgusted with yourself?"

If you have identified an essential symptom of a psychiatric disorder, establish how long the symptom has been present. For example, has the patient been depressed, tense, and irritable for at least two weeks?

After you have identified essential symptoms and their duration, the next step is to assess severity.

DSM-III-R considers as symptoms complaints that cause distress, or disability, and constitute a behavioral, psychological, or biological dysfunction. A patient who complains occasionally of feeling down but who fully functions at work, in his family, and social life, has a complaint which has not reached the intensity of a symptom. He may be mildly dysphoric but without a psychiatric disorder. Zung (1972) reported on dysphoric mood in the general U.S. population: 48% were dysphoric under age 19, and 44% in the age bracket over 60 had abnormally high Zung Depression Scores. Data from a population of air traffic controllers also showed abnormally high depression scores (Barrett et al. 1978). These groups may not suffer from clinical depression, even though they admit to depressive feelings.

Therefore, if you encounter a symptom, determine whether the symptom interfered with the patient's life; explore, for instance, whether he got into arguments, or spanked his children too much, or was impatient with his customers, has missed work, was criticized by his spouse, lost a friend, needed outpatient treatment, or hospitalization.

Below are eight empirically tested questions to assess dysfunction by social interference. If the patient answers "yes" to one of the questions, in approximately 90 percent of the cases he will also fulfill the associated symptoms of that disorder (Othmer et al. 1981).

1. Has (essential symptom, like drinking, drug use, mood changes etc.) ever interfered with your school, your work, or your job?

2. Has . . . ever caused you any problems with your family, or caused your family to worry about you?
3. Has . . . ever interfered with your social activities or friendships?
4. Have you ever gotten into trouble with the authorities because of your . . . ?
5. Has your health ever suffered from . . . ?
6. Have you ever received medication or treatment for your . . . ?
7. Were you ever hospitalized for . . . ?
8. When you had . . . , were you able to live alone?

Psychosocial impairment is the objective effect, personal distress and suffering are the subjective effects on the patient's life. Personal suffering frequently correlates with objective dysfunction.

Severity of the illness is reflected in a number of areas. The response of the patient's family can be a key indicator. They may criticize, disrespect, and ostracize the patient, or be supportive when the patient's suffering is clearly visible, as in the anxiety disorders.

Severity is also measured by the response of the public. Clearly, when law and order are violated through reckless driving, driving while intoxicated, or disturbance of peace, the patient has a serious problem. Society also looks down upon alcoholism, substance abuse, and may shun persons with other disturbing mental disorders, such as schizophrenia or mania.

Severity can also be determined by the impairment to general health resulting from the disorder as, for instance, in alcoholism, substance abuse, and organic mental disorders.

Severity is determined by the patient's general level of functioning. If you see a patient who has no clear chief complaint and you converse with him instead of exploring his problems, you may get an impression of his level of functioning before you know what factors impair it. DSM-III-R (1987) provides a Global Assessment of Functioning Scale (GAF Scale) which allows you to measure his level of functioning (see below 4. Confirmatory History, Social History).

Associated Symptoms

After determining the essential symptoms assess *associated* symptoms. An associated symptom is one which frequently is present in a disorder but not necessary for its diagnosis. For instance, insomnia is seen in depression, but also in many other disorders such as substance abuse, schizophrenia, bipolar disorder, and anxiety disorders. Associated symptoms are often vegetative, for example, anorexia, hyperphagia, or sexual dysfunction. They may also appear as unexplained pain in the lower back, abdomen, or head; as somatic perceptions such as dizziness, paresthesias, and weakness; or as general psychic symptoms such as lethargy, tension, hopelessness, fear, and discouragement.

The number of associated symptoms for a disorder varies from patient to patient. A minimum number has to be present to fulfill diagnostic criteria for a disorder (see DSM-III-R). Assess them be asking open-ended questions such as:

"What else have you noticed when you get depressed, when you have your highs, your panic spells, and so forth?"

Most patients will list several symptoms. After such a patient-centered question use "disorder-centered" ones to confirm the diagnosis, such as:

"When you get depressed, how is your sleep, . . . your appetite, . . . your sex life, . . . your concentration, . . . your thoughts about the future, . . . and your job performance?"

Make sure all associated symptoms concurred with the essential one at the same *time* period. Find out which symptoms accompanied each other, and which occurred sporadically. The time reference is crucial to verify a past psychiatric disorder. Repeat the essential symptom or chief complaint when you ask for associated symptoms, or ask the patient whether the reported symptoms occurred together (Q. 6):

1. I: What brought you here, Mrs. Holmes?
   P: I'm getting depressed again and cry very easily.

2. I: Can you tell me more about it?
   P: It seems to happen anytime of the day, I get tearful and I start sobbing.

3. I: Have you had any other problems?
   P: Oh yes. I have bursting headaches and my sleep is not good.

4. I: Any problems with eating?
   P: Yes, how do you know? I had a raving appetite and gained close to 60 pounds.

5. I: Any other problems with eating?
   P: Maybe I should tell you about my vomiting. I thought I spit my heart out.

6. I: It is not clear to me whether all the problems happen at the same time.
   P: Oh, is that what you meant? Oh no. I had the problem with vomiting when I was pregnant.

7. I: What about the overeating?
   P: That was three years ago.

8. I: And with your sleep?
   P: That was the worst after I had the baby.

9. I: How is your sleep now?
   P: Oh it's fine. Maybe I sleep too long. I seem to be real exhausted.

10. I: And your appetite?
    P: Right now?

11. I: Yes.
    P: Too good. I even get up at night to get a snack. Can't stay away from that refrigerator.

12. I: Besides your crying spells and sobbing, what else has changed with you?
    P: I worry about my older daughter. She got herself pregnant and my husband is blaming me. I always had problems with my children and my husband.

If the interviewer had not clarified the temporal relationship of the symptoms, he could have mistaken them as associated symptoms of depression. However, the symptoms scattered over time suggested somatization disorder, a diagnosis which he later confirmed.

If your patient reports a sufficient number of associated symptoms to meet criteria for a major psychiatric disorder, you have established the inclusion criteria for that disorder.

Now proceed in the same way for all other major disorders for which essential symptoms are positive.

Exclusion

If you have determined a patient's essential symptoms, their duration and severity, and have a sufficient number of associated symptoms, you can diagnose the disorder but you must keep reservations. You have to await the results of your background exploration (see 4. Confirmatory History below), since medical disorders can mimic psychiatric disorders. The presence of such a medical disorder would exclude the presence of a psychiatric disorder. And, in some cases, the symptoms of psychiatric disorders are also encompassed by some other psychiatric disorders (see 6. Diagnoses below).

Sometimes you encounter essential symptoms of a major psychiatric disorder but they do not interfere with the patient's life. Place the patient under surveillance but defer the diagnosis of a major psychiatric disorder at this point. For instance, a patient may complain about chronic depressed mood, or anxiety, or deep-seated anger but none of these complaints interferes with his work, his family life, or leisure activities. He notices these feelings and has to make an effort to overcome them, or to keep them under control. These feelings have a subjective impact on him but he does not experience any objective impairment.

Essential symptoms can also be too short in duration to meet criteria. If the symptoms are severe, it is best to make the diagnosis anyway, especially when the patient has to be hospitalized. If they are mild, reserve judgment on the diagnosis but follow the patient closely because the symptoms could herald the onset of the disorder.

If essential symptoms are long and severe enough to meet criteria but are not accompanied by a sufficient number of associated symptoms, diagnose an *atypical* (NOS) disorder. One study found such incomplete manifestation of a disorder in 15–20% of patients with positive essential symptoms (Othmer et al. 1981).

Personality Disorders (Axis II)

CAVEAT:

Unlike major psychiatric disorders personality disorders with the exception of antisocial personality are not well established by validation of their diagnostic criteria, follow-up, and family studies. A discussion of these deficits is beyond the frame of this book and can be found elsewhere (Vaillant and Perry 1985). For the purpose of diagnostic interviewing we will treat them as heuristic concepts.

If you try to verify a personality disorder examine whether the patient fulfills the two criteria typical for the anatomy of a personality disorder according to DSM-III-R:

a. trigger-response complex
b. lifelong maladjustment.

For instance, for a patient with dependent personality disorder the loss of a close relationship is a trigger. He perceives the loss as a threat to his lifeline and himself as totally dependant upon this lost nurturing symbiosis. He responds to the loss with a host of depressive symptoms which in contrast to an endogenous depression remit with regaining of support. This trigger-response pattern resurfaces throughout the patient's life. Symptoms of dysphoria and anxiety recur whenever he anticipates a loss. When you observe an anxiety reaction after a loss, you may misdiagnose it as an adjustment reaction, if you don't ask about a lifelong recurrent pattern.

Here is a case example which emerged in a conversation between a resident in psychiatry and his supervisor.

I: Adjustment reactions are rare unless they are superimposed on a major psychiatric disorder or the expression of a personality disorder.

Resident: I can't believe that. My wife cried day and night after we came here from India. She was dysphoric, anxious, homesick, and depressed and did not want to meet new friends. She locked herself in the bathroom. She cried and carried on and often kept the apartment complex awake by hollering and screaming at night.

I: (The interviewer interpreted the departure from India as a threat to the wife's support system. He thought that she showed a maladjusted response to the loss of that support system.)

Your example is indeed very interesting. It does seem to disprove my point. Do you feel comfortable answering a few more questions about your wife?

Resident: Sure, go ahead.

I: Tell me a little bit about your marriage. Was it prearranged by your parents?

Resident: Yes, it was.

I: When you got married, your wife moved into your house?

Resident: Yes, she did. Our wedding lasted three days and then she moved in with me.

I: Can you tell me how she felt when she moved in with you?

Resident: Oh, she cried for the first 2–3 weeks and was depressed.

I: That sounds similar to the reaction she had when she came to the States.

Resident: Hmm . . . I hadn't thought about that. You're right.

I: Do you know any other situations where your wife showed a similar response as when you got married and when you came to the U. S.?

Resident: When we moved away from Delhi, my wife had the same problem. Also her parents told me that she had a hard time adjusting when she went to college.

I: You see? One so-called adjustment problem rarely comes along. Find out what situations or stressors a patient is sensitive to. That will help you to identify the coping deficit and make the diagnosis of a personality disorder. So what do you think is problematic for your wife?

Resident: Well, it seems to be hard for her to get away from her family and friends and adjust to a new environment.

I: Right, that's my feeling too. She seems to be very sensitive to loss of support. You will find time and again that a so-called adjustment problem is just an example in a string of similar problems.

Resident: I understand.

I: Have you noticed that your wife is depressed or discouraged at any other times? Even when there is not a major change?

Resident: Let me see . . . Yes, she had a bad time when her parents could not get a passport in time to come visit. She also cried at her sister's birthday when she could not go back home to be with her. She seems to be easily upset but I never put it together.

The stressor that triggered maladjusted behavior in the resident's wife was the loss of support and familiar environment. The maladjusted response is her inability to overcome or restructure her need for support. This inability will predictably make her seek new dependencies rather than develop autonomy. Her repetitive maladjusted behavior shows a dramatic display of a childlike loss reaction with depressive symptoms which qualifies her for the diagnosis of dependant personality disorder.

Most patients with a so-called "adjustment reaction" to a stressor also show a tendency for repetition, indicating a chronic coping deficit, in other words, a personality disorder. A host of depressive and anxious symptoms accompany such a maladjusted reaction. These symptoms may occur at the mere anticipation of the trigger situation. Therefore whenever your patient reports a maladjustment to a stressor, screen his past for similar reactions and identify the underlying coping deficit. If the patient reports repetitive adjustment reactions, an alarm should go off in your head. Repetitiveness violates the essential criterion of adjustment disorder.

Trigger-Response Complex

First, most patients with a personality disorder show maladjusted responses with persons in three types of relationships: intimate or sexual, or familial; with organized social groups, at church or leisure activities; and with colleagues at work. Therefore, ask the patient to describe his relationship to these groups. Explore whether your patient is callous, suspicious, or exploitative, and whether he fears, or depends on these groups.

Second, a more direct approach is to ask whether there are certain situations that the patient dreads, avoids, or has difficulties handling. He may describe the situations that trigger recurring maladjusted behaviors and reveal a distorted perception of these situations.

"Whenever I meet new people I prefer not to talk to them because I fear they may reject and criticize me."
"People are very critical. They seem to enjoy hurting you. Especially when they find out that you are weak, they take advantage of you. If you stay away from them, they are less likely to bother you." (Avoidant personality.)

The interview itself is often a trigger situation for maladjusted response. Observe if the patient relates to you during the interview in a peculiar way. For instance, he is either blunt in his affect without being depressed or having hallucinations (schizoid personality); or dramatic, self-centered, and flirtatious (histrionic personality); or somewhat anxious, clinging, and asking for reassurance (dependent personality). Address his behavior to detect if the pattern is lifelong.

Lifelong Maladjustment

Some patients do not describe a trigger-response complex but a lifelong pattern of maladjustment, either symptoms or behaviors. Here is an example for lifelong symptoms:

"I'm shy and anxious and easily scared. I would like to be popular but I'm so afraid of being rejected. I'm inhibited and can't speak up for myself." (Avoidant personality.)

When the patient describes lifelong symptoms, link them to a major psychiatric disorder. After remission, major psychiatric disorders can leave some patients with a residual personality disorder (Winokur and

Crowe 1975). Thus, personality disorders can sometimes be viewed as mild forms of the major psychiatric disorders. They can also be precursors of the major psychiatric disorders. The assumed correlation between major psychiatric and personality disorders on the basis of similar clinical features is shown in table 5.2. For a psychodiagnostic interview it is important to investigate such a link.

A growing literature reports the link between the major psychiatric and the personality disorders. It would exceed the frame of this book to review this literature here, but see Koenigsberg et al. (1985).

The patient may report a lifelong pattern of maladjustment and problems in relating to other people.

Sally, a 38-year-old, divorced, childless secretary reported:

"I feel guilty and lonesome when I leave my mother or don't keep her involved. Something bad always seems to happen and I have to come back to her. It makes me feel somewhat depressed that I can't get on my own feet. Whenever I bring home a man that I feel attracted to, my mother doesn't like him. She always seems to favor the older guys who send the flowers, but they bore me to death. I can't seem to get out of this rut."

This example does not describe a symptom, but an entire clinical picture. Get more supportive evidence for lifelong maladjustment by letting the patient describe recurring trigger situations where he was unable to cope effectively. Explore further whether her maladjusted responses are similar in each instance. For example, a person with antisocial personality may be always oppositional, often aggressive, breaking rules, and cunning, but only sometimes dysphoric.

Classification of Personality Disorders

Personality disorders can be classified by one of three characteristics:

1. the situation that triggers maladjusted behavior,
2. perception of the trigger situation and the type of underlying misinterpretation,
3. maladjusted behavioral and emotional response (see table 5.3).

DSM-III-R uses a mixture of these three classifiers, with emphasis on the third. It groups personality disorders into three clusters.

The first cluster, referred to as cluster A, includes Paranoid, Schizoid, and Schizotypal Personality Disorders. People with these disorders often appear odd

TABLE 5.2

Correlation Between Major Psychiatric Disorders and Personality Disorders

Major Psychiatric Disorder	*Personality Disorder*
SUBSTANCE USE	Antisocial Personality or Borderline Personality
	Narcissistic Personality
SCHIZOPHRENIA, PARANOID DELUSIONAL (PARANOID) DISORDER	Paranoid Personality
SCHIZOPHRENIA, UNDIFFERENTIATED (WITH NEGATIVE SYMPTOMS)	Schizoid Personality
SCHIZOPHRENIA, UNDIFFERENTIATED (WITH POSITIVE SYMPTOMS)	Schizotypal Personality
BIPOLAR DISORDER, ATYPICAL (NOS), RAPID CYCLER	Borderline Personality
DEPRESSIVE DISORDER	Dependent Personality
	Passive Aggressive Personality
	Masochistic Personality
AGORAPHOBIA SOCIAL PHOBIA	Avoidant Personality
OBSESSIVE COMPULSIVE DISORDER	Obsessive Compulsive Personality
SOMATIZATION DISORDER	Histrionic Personality

or eccentric. Cluster B includes Antisocial, Borderline, Histrionic, and Narcissistic Personality Disorders. People with these disorders often appear dramatic, emotional, or erratic. Cluster C includes Avoidant, Dependant, Obsessive Compulsive, and Passive Aggressive Personality Disorders. People with these disorders often appear anxious or fearful. Finally, there is a residual category, NOT OTHERWISE SPECIFIED Personality Disorder, that can be used for other specific Personality Disorders or for mixed conditions that do not qualify as any of the specific Personality Disorders described in this manual.

There is great variability in the detail with which various Personality Disorders are described and the specificity of the diagnostic criteria. Disorders studied more extensively and rigorously than others, such as Antisocial Personality, are described in greater detail. (DSM-III-R, p. 337)

When you diagnose a personality disorder, decide which cluster fits best the patient's behavior by using table 5.3:

TABLE 5.3
Personality Disorders as Maladjusted Response to Triggers

Personality Disorder	Trigger	Perception of Trigger	Behavioral Response	Emotional Response
Cluster A				
PARANOID	Close interpersonal relations	"People sneak up on me and harm me."	Guarded distance, secretive, devious, scheming, counterattacking	Suspicious, jealous, angry, hypervigilant
SCHIZOID	Close interpersonal relations	"People are meaningless to me."	Avoids social involvement	Cold, stiff, distant, aloof
SCHIZOTYPAL	Close interpersonal relations	"Others have special magic intentions."	Imagines love or rejection without evidence	Inappropriate excitement, hostile aloofness
Cluster B				
ANTISOCIAL	Social standards and rules	"Rules limit me from fulfilling my needs."	Violation of social rules, standards, and law	Impulsively angry, hostile, cunning
BORDERLINE	Personal goals, close relations	"Goals are good; no, they are not; people are great, no they are not."	Changing goals, ambivalent relations	Labile mood and affect
HISTRIONIC	Heterosexual relations	"I have to show intense emotions to impress."	Flirts, shows exaggerated, nongenuine emotions	Excited by positive, dysphoric by negative response
NARCISSISTIC	Evaluation of self	"I'm the only person that counts."	Self-centeredness, expects recognition without contributions	Labile, grandiose, deflated feelings

Cluster C

AVOIDANT	Close interpersonal relations, public appearance	"People reject and criticize me."	Escapes and avoids social appearances	Anxious, withdrawn
DEPENDENT	Self-reliance, being alone	"I hate to be alone."	Giving up own goals to cling to others (parents)	Anxious, panicky
OBSESSIVE COMPULSIVE	Close relationships, unstructured situations, authority	"My rules must prevail, uncertainty is frightening; feelings interfere with thinking."	Emotional restriction, rigid, angry if his rules are broken; defiance of authority	Anxious, angry, resentful
PASSIVE AGGRESSIVE	Deadlines, demands to perform	"They impose on my freedom, but it is dangerous to resist openly."	Procrastination, broken commitments	Anxious, angry, resentful

Proposed Personality Disorders

SADISTIC	Weak, dependent persons	"I have to show them who is boss; I can make them eat shit."	Cruel, restrictive acts against defenseless people	Pleasure derived from the suffering of others
SELF-DEFEATING	Situations and relationships difficult to master	"I have to endure hardship to prove myself worthwhile."	Enters or creates situations that promise hardship	Indulges in suffering

1. Does the patient tend to be isolated because of socially cold, suspicious, or strange behavior?
2. Does he impose on others; is he dramatic and self-centered?
3. Is he afraid of others, anxious, submissive, or restricted?

CLUSTER A:

During the interview the patient appears suspicious, blunted, odd, or eccentric. He may tell you that others think he is a loner, inaccessible, hard to get to know, and easy to overlook and ignore. He may be described as untrustworthy, strange, and "nutty." He is often suspected of having homosexual tendencies, since he does not assert himself in heterosexual relationships.

During the interview, ask the patient who shows paranoid perceptions whether he has friends he can trust, or whether it is easy for him to open up to others. He may answer that he cannot trust anybody, thus confirming your impression of a paranoid personality.

Ask the patient who appears blunt and disinterested whether he is usually unemotional, or disinterested in other people's feelings. He may answer that he feels as much as the computer he plays games with, thus qualifying for the diagnosis of schizoid personality disorder.

Ask the patient with out-of-body experiences, superstitious beliefs, oddities in dressing, or peculiarities in responding whether he has experienced ESP. His vividly described experiences will help you to establish the diagnosis of a schizotypal personality disorder.

CLUSTER B:

Such a patient appears emotionally labile, or shows excessive emotional responses during the interview. He may report that he is flying off the handle easily, and that others call him unstable and erratic. He may say he cannot establish stable relationships. Check the chronicity of these behaviors. You may ask:

"You seem to be a very emotional person."
"It appears to me that you have stronger feelings than others."
"Do you think that being more emotional has affected your relationship to others?"

Most patients with a cluster B personality disorder admit to this. After you have established hyperemotionality, assess characteristics that differentiate the disorders of this cluster.

Illegal or violent actions that started in the teenage years point to the diagnosis of antisocial personality. This disorder is more common in males.

Rapid mood swings (with or without a history of manic-depressive disorder), self-mutilation, suicide attempts, or even brief psychotic experiences may portray a borderline personality.

Exaggerated, multiple unexplained somatic symptoms are more often reported by females than males. They involve menstruation, sexual activity, and the abdomen. Such complaints may suggest the diagnosis of histrionic personality.

Egocentric and grandiose behavior, with little regard for others, may portend the diagnosis of narcissistic personality.

Similarities in the symptom profiles of these personality disorders with somatization disorder and rapidly cycling manic-depressive disorder are apparent.

CLUSTER C:

A patient in cluster C appears anxious, dysphoric, phobic, or obsessive during the interview. To differentiate the disorders in this cluster, look for the following characteristics:

If he is shy, weighs his words, asks for reassurance, or speaks up reluctantly, consider avoidant personality.

If he is clinging, too dependent, always requiring care, or inviting aggression, consider dependent personality.

If he appears perfectionistic, tries to be precise, is annoyed by unstructured situations, consider obsessive compulsive personality disorder.

If he is unduly demanding, not keeping his promises and not living up to expectations, consider passive aggressive personality.

PROPOSED PERSONALITY DISORDERS:

Some patients appear to be fascinated by physical or mental pain and suffering. They either cause it, or endure it. If you encounter a lifelong pattern of behavior that subjects others to suffering, or on the other hand, seems to seek out very difficult situations almost impossible to handle, predicting failure and pain, consider whether the patient suffers from sadistic or self-defeating personality disorder, respectively.

PERSONALITY DISORDERS NOT OTHERWISE SPECIFIED (NOS):

Sometimes a patient shows a variety of pathological responses, depending on the social situation. He may show dependent behavior toward authority figures, obsessive demanding behavior toward subordinates, and passive aggressive tendencies toward colleagues. This is where diagnosing becomes complex. DSM-III-R allows you to assign more than one personality disorder. This rule transforms the typological into a multidimensional approach.

Table C.1 in appendix C lists DSM-III-R criteria for all personality disorders. It can also be used in identifying features of NOS personality disorders, including those personality disorders that have characteristics of more than one specific personality disorder.

Adjustment Disorders

Establish an adjustment disorder by four criteria:

1. one or more psychosocial stressors;
2. a maladaptive reaction;
3. three months rule;
4. exclusion of major psychiatric and personality disorders.

Stressors (Axis IV)

Acute and severe stressors are usually reported as chief complaints:

"My son committed suicide, and after that happened I cried all the time, neglected my daughter, and became quite irritable with my husband."

Also, patients focus on the stressor, rather than on their reaction to it, when the impact of the stressor is expected to strike in the future:

"My husband told me he wants a divorce."
"My daughter has a boyfriend and I'm afraid they will get married soon. He is a military man, and expects to go to Germany. Since she is my only child and I'm a widow, there will be nothing left for me but my canary."

If a patient talks about a stressor as the cause of his psychiatric problems, investigate such a relationship (Zimmerman et al. 1985).

A stressor (see glossary) may be related to a psychiatric disorder in six different ways:

as 1. time mark
   2. magnifier
   3. consequence
   4. pathological thought content
   5. trigger, or
   6. cause.

If a patient names a stressor, your most conservative assumption is that this stressor is not a true cause but is just a memorable event that coincides somewhat with the onset of a psychiatric disorder; in other words, such a stressor is a time mark. To accept a stressor as more than that, you have to go beyond description—to accept the stressor as cause is an interpretation that cannot be proven with certainty. Here is what you can do: Exclude the possibility that the named stressor is merely a result of the psychiatric disorder rather than its cause as, for instance, a magnifier of the impact, a consequence, or a pathological thought content of the disorder. You also want to exclude a mere trigger function as, for instance, in a personality disorder where similar stressors reveal time and again the same coping deficit.

Maladaptive Reaction

After you have explored the nature of the stressor, evaluate the maladaptive reaction. It may manifest itself in two ways, behaviorally and symptomatically. Behaviorally, the patient may show a decline in occupational functioning, social activities, or in his relationships to others. Symptomatically, the patient may report symptoms and show signs in excess of what you would normally expect as a reaction to stress.

DSM-III-R lists six maladaptive reactions: depressed mood, anxious mood, disturbance of conduct, work or academic inhibition, social withdrawal, and physical complaints. Mixtures among them may also occur.

The reaction should be time limited and not persist beyond six months; otherwise, a diagnosis different from adjustment reaction should be made.

Three Months Rule

DSM-III-R requires that you demonstrate a temporal relationship but not a causality between stressor and response. The maladaptive reaction has to occur within three months of the stressor. This arbitrary rule excludes psychiatric disorders that follow a stressor by a year (anniversary reaction) or more.

Exclusion of Major Psychiatric Disorders

Symptoms of adjustment reactions resemble those of major depression, anxiety disorders, or antisocial personality disorder, respectively. The patient's and family's history and the mental status will distinguish them. Exclude as adjustment reactions psychiatric disorders which fulfill criteria for any other DSM-III-R axis I or axis II disorders. The patient's perception of psychological causality between stressor and response becomes then irrelevant for the diagnosis, but—of course—not for the treatment of the disorder.

Accepting an insufficient number of depressive symptoms as part of an adjustment reaction rather than an atypical depression becomes plausible when the patient has neither a personal nor family history of affective disorder and when the symptom profile is distinct from an affective disorder; for instance, if the patient is distractible, and depressed only when reminded of the stressor, has no vegetative symptoms (such as anorexia or early morning awakening), and is tearful and requests assurance rather than being emotionally withdrawn.

A patient with a personality disorder may develop symptoms under stress. Make sure that the maladaptive response is not just an activation of his preexisting personality disorder. For instance, a patient with antisocial personality disorder may under stress commit unlawful acts, or neglect work and family; a patient with dependent and passive aggressive personality disorder may become dysphoric when deserted, and a patient with avoidant personality disorder may become anxious when asked to appear in public. Such responses are exacerbations of the underlying personality disorder but not indications of an adjustment disorder.

Disorders Not Otherwise Specified (NOS)

When a patient reports a single symptom, try to link it to an essential symptom of a major psychiatric disorder. An effective way is to ask:

"When you have symptom X, what other problems do you notice?"

He may respond with:

> "When I have my low back pain, I wake up too early and feel rotten all day. I just sit around and don't want to do anything, and I hope that nobody will bother me. Wouldn't you feel the same way if you had that kind of pain?"

This answer shows how a patient frequently forms an opinion about his illness, explains a set of symptoms by the presence of others, and reports only the "causative" symptom. The above patient may have an affective disorder in which the back pain becomes the thought content. If you can pair the reported symptom with an essential symptom you have identified it as a possible associated symptom for a major psychiatric disorder.

If you *cannot* elicit any other associated symptoms, investigate the severity of the symptom; does he have to think about it continuously, avoid other people because of it, or is he affected in his marriage? If so, pursue the symptom further.

Isolated signs and symptoms are often physical, such as medically unexplained headache, dizziness, and back pain. There are isolated compulsions such as handwashing, counting, not stepping on cracks; monosymptomatic delusions such as a bad odor (often genital), protruding evil eyes, skin infestation by unidentifiable organisms, or being secretly loved by an important person (erytromania); and isolated mood disturbances such as constant complaining, chronic dysphoria, or silliness.

Here is an example of an isolated delusion. Mrs. Turner is a 49-year-old, white, married woman who accompanies her husband with bipolar disorder to the clinic. She asks to see his physician alone.

I: Mrs. Turner, you wanted to talk to me about your husband's treatment.
P: That's right. I want to impress on you the terrible things that you've done to him.

I: Let me hear about it.

P: Ever since my husband started on lithium, he sweats terribly. The lithium salt must be in his sweat, because it destroys my linen.

I: That's interesting. I've never heard anything like that before. Tell me more about it.

P: I'm also allergic to the lithium. I can't get close to him because of it. We haven't had sex since he started on it.

I: Have you noticed any other changes in you since then?

P: No, not really. Nothing that I can think of . . .

I: Any changes in your sleep, appetite, or general well-being?

P: Oh no. None whatsoever.

I: How are you coming along with your housework?

P: Just fine. I have a job which I enjoy and I get my housework done. My husband tells me what a good housekeeper I am.

I: Can you tell me about your social life?

P: We belong to a church group, we play bridge regularly with friends, I have a girl friend, and my husband has his own friends who come to see us.

I: What have you done about that problem with your husband's medication?

P: I had my own lithium level checked. I have also sent the bedsheets to a lab for analysis, and I've talked to several drug companies that make lithium.

I: Any results?

P: The typical response. Nobody seems to want to make a commitment. My own level was 0.0025.

I: Do you feel people want to mislead you?

P: Oh no, they just don't seem to know. By the way, the real reason I wanted to talk to you is to ask you to stop the lithium. I have heard you are running an experimental program with a new drug. I want you to enroll my husband in this program so that we can have a normal life again.

A diagnostic interview with Mrs. Turner produced no psychopathology other than her monosymptomatic delusion—she had no other delusions or hallucinations, and no history of alcohol, drug abuse, or conversion symptoms. Her affect was appropriate and normal in range. She had normal eye contact, and memory and intellectual functions were intact.

For the diagnosis of an isolated sign or symptom, determine first, whether it is indeed isolated; second, whether it represents a disturbance of thinking, mood, or somatic function; third, which code classifies it the best as an atypical disorder (NOS): psychotic, mood, anxiety, somatoform, or dissociative disorder.

Problems of Living

The chief complaint reflects a problem of living.

Louise is a 48-year-old housewife, mother of three children. She complains about difficulties dealing with her husband. He is too demanding, pushes her too hard, has no understanding for her feelings. Until a few months ago she could keep up with his demands, but lately they became too much to take. She also reports that she does not love her children any more because they are so rebellious.

Such a social conflict may be a problem of living, a major psychiatric disorder, a personality disorder, or an adjustment reaction. Check all four possibilities.

First, examine whether the social conflict is the expression of a major psychiatric disorder. Attempt to translate the conflict into symptoms by temporarily ignoring the content of the complaint and instead focusing on the disturbed psychic functions. Probe for symptoms such as irritability, low energy, decreased sex drive, and social withdrawal. Then search for essential features that are associated with these symptoms. For instance, ask about recent drug or alcohol abuse, or depressed feelings expressed in crying spells, bouts of hopelessness, guilt, and disturbances in appetite and sleep. Find out whether the patient may have obsessive thoughts or compulsions which make her too rigid in dealing with her family, or somatic symptoms which draw her attention to her physical problems and deprive her of the patience necessary to handle her family. If you can translate the patient's social conflict into essential symptoms of a major psychiatric disorder, pursue *that* disorder rather than an adjustment disorder or a problem of living.

Explore whether the problem of living is caused by a personality disorder. If the problem has recurred lifelong, find out whether it arose from a coping deficit in handling certain situations such as living independently, or making and keeping contact with people, or establishing and maintaining stable relationships. A lifelong recurrent coping deficit points to a personality disorder.

Consider an adjustment disorder if you find, however, a onetime stressor followed by some psychiatric symptoms, provided you can first exclude major psychiatric disorders and personality disorders.

If the social conflict cannot be dissected into one of the above, consider a problem of living, a condition that can be treated without being due to a mental disorder. DSM-III-R lists thirteen such conditions:

malingering
borderline intellectual functioning
adult antisocial behavior
childhood or adolescent antisocial behavior
academic problems
occupational problems
uncomplicated bereavement
noncompliance with medical treatment
phase of life problem or other life circumstance problem
marital problem
parent-child problem
other specified family circumstances
other interpersonal problem.

4. CONFIRMATORY HISTORY

The technique to assess the course of a psychiatric disorder, i.e., onset, duration, and severity, differs whether you deal with a major psychiatric or a personality disorder.

Course of Major Psychiatric Disorders

When you probe for the onset of major psychiatric disorders, start with questions such as:

"When did you first experience your present problems?"
"When was the first time in your life that you had problems like this?"
"Do you remember when you experienced this for the first time?"

Check whether the present disorder may have occurred in a different form. The patient who has a current depressive disorder may have started with manic symptoms, the one with schizoaffective disorder may only have had depressed or irritable mood, and the patient with schizophrenia may have shown predominantly catatonic or paranoid symptoms. A patient may not consider these different manifestations as part of his present disorder. If so, educate him about the connection of past and present problems to facilitate communication.

Complement the assessment of onset by questions such as:

"Up to which age were you free of any problems?"

A discrepancy between reported age of onset of a disorder and the age up to which the patient felt healthy may occur in disorders with an insidious onset or a prodromal state.

Steve, a 27-year-old, white, single clerk in a grocery store, demonstrates such a gap between the end of mental well-being and the onset of illness.

I: When did all these problems start?
P: Oh, when I was about 21 years old. I became very depressed, heard voices, and was afraid of women.

I: Hmm.
P: And from then on it seemed to always get worse.

I: Up to what age do you think you were completely well and had none of these problems?
P: Until I was 17.

I: 17?
P: Yes, I remember I enjoyed going out and was even pretty successful with the girls. They seemed to like me then.

I: So what happened between 17 and 21?
P: I don't know . . . something . . . I noticed it first at work.

I: What do you mean?
P: I think people at work didn't really like me.

I: How could you tell?
P: They were talking behind my back. I always had the feeling they were laughing about me.

I: What were they talking about?
P: I don't know, but I thought they were thinking I'm queer or something. I heard them say something about "Another of those homosexuals." I pretended that I did not notice it. But I did not really feel comfortable going out with them. I always had the feeling I had to pretend.

I: Did you hear voices at that time?
P: No, I don't think so. But I sure picked up the remarks these guys made.

This interview exemplifies how the duplicate question of:

"When did your illness start?"
"When was the last time that you were healthy?"

uncovers the period between end of health and onset of illness. This approach will help you decide whether the onset was insidious or acute.

Explore to what extent a major psychiatric disorder interferes with the patient's psychosocial functioning as shown above.

The duration of a major psychiatric disorder may vary from several weeks to a lifetime, and the severity of symptoms (course of illness) may be either chronic stationary, chronic progressive (frequently with exacerbations), episodic, or vascillating. Remissions may be complete or not, leaving the patient with a residual symptomatology or functional deficit. (See figure 5.1).

For instance, in the majority of patients with affective disorder, symptoms cause problems but without long-term deterioration. Symptoms of organic mental disorder, alcohol and drug abuse, agoraphobia and schizophrenia show a characteristic worsening. Symptoms of sociopathy may show gradual improvement over a lifetime due to a "burnout" effect. Symptoms of panic disorder, somatization disorder, and obsessive compulsive disorder show a chronic course with exacerbations.

Help a patient who cannot focus on his condition by a graphic approach. Draw a horizontal time line and tell him:

"If this line represents your life and the beginning represents your birth and the end your present age, where on this line do you think you were first bothered by others and their sneakiness?"

Put each complaint in relationship to the patient's present age and plot them along this time axis.

Course of Personality Disorders

To obtain information about the onset and duration of a personality disorder you need to modify your approach. Personality disorders are lifelong patterns of maladjusted behaviors which are often ego-syntonic. They first become noticeable during the teenage years. You can assess onset and duration by focusing on either recurring interpersonal conflicts or maladaptive personality features.

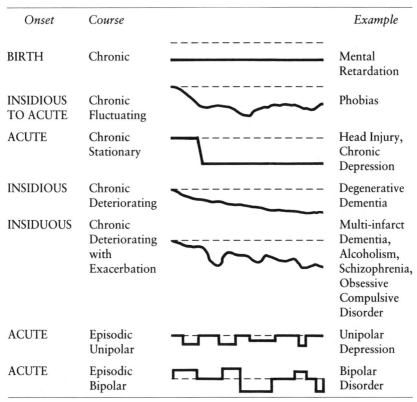

Onset	Course		Example
BIRTH	Chronic		Mental Retardation
INSIDIOUS TO ACUTE	Chronic Fluctuating		Phobias
ACUTE	Chronic Stationary		Head Injury, Chronic Depression
INSIDIOUS	Chronic Deteriorating		Degenerative Dementia
INSIDUOUS	Chronic Deteriorating with Exacerbation		Multi-infarct Dementia, Alcoholism, Schizophrenia, Obsessive Compulsive Disorder
ACUTE	Episodic Unipolar		Unipolar Depression
ACUTE	Episodic Bipolar		Bipolar Disorder

Legend: – – – – – "normal"

FIGURE 5.1
Natural Course of Various Psychiatric Disorders

Track back a *conflict* that the patient has volunteered such as "I have trouble with my husband," and identify the part that the personality disorder plays in that conflict.

A PERSONALITY TRAIT:

Some patients with a personality disorder recognize their maladaptive personality trait such as shyness, perfectionism, or emotionality. Use this awareness to ask for the onset of the personality trait:

"When did you first notice that you were shy, perfectionistic, or overexcitable?"

Expect an answer such as: "As long as I can remember."

Realize that personality features and social conflicts are two sides of one coin: recurring conflicts may express a pathological personality trait and, in turn, pathological personality traits cause recurrent interpersonal conflicts.

Focus on the following key areas to assess *severity:* friends, sexual relationships, family life, work life, bonds in the community, and leisure-time activities. A severe personality disorder affects three areas: work, love, and leisure, while a milder form does not. Another measure of severity is the number of similar conflicts a patient has within a year.

Treatment History

Psychiatric disorders show some evidence of specificity of response to certain drug treatments. Therefore, a detailed history of treatments and treatment responses can serve at least three purposes.

1. It can help to reconstruct what type of diagnoses another psychiatrist may have entertained if records are not available and the patient does not remember his symptoms. For instance, a patient may report that he received 12 ECT's and that he was able to return to work after he was discharged from the hospital. Such a report suggests that the patient's therapist diagnosed an affective disorder.
2. It may help to identify responsiveness to certain treatment modalities. For instance, Keith reports:

    "I took Elavil for three months, and then Norpramine for four months, and I didn't get any better. My psychiatrist drew blood levels and told me that I'm taking enough medicine. But it did not help. My mother went to Dr. J. who switched her from Elavil to Nardil when she didn't respond. Nardil really helped her."

    As interviewer, you know that not only disorders but also response to medication may be partly genetically determined. Entertain a treatment attempt with an monoamine oxydase inhibitor for a patient like Keith.
3. It can help to confirm your own diagnosis. For instance, your patient shows a confusing picture of chronic maladjustment but you are impressed by periods of increased activity and energy followed by social withdrawal and suspiciousness. The patient does not fulfill criteria for bipolar disorder but at best has a combination of a personality disorder and affective disorder, NOS. You decide to treat

this patient with lithium. Two months later, the patient reports that the fights with his wife and children have disappeared, that he got a promotion at work, and that everybody comments on his calmness. He also tells you that the appearance of his desk at work has changed.

"It's not cluttered up any more. All of a sudden I take care of things as they come, I file them, or throw them away. Four years of psychotherapy and many hours reading books of how to manage time have not accomplished what these little lithium capsules do for me. Amazing."

Such a response, even though not treatment specific, may for practical purposes confirm your impression that the patient had an atypical bipolar disorder (bipolar disorder NOS).

For these reasons, a personal and family history of treatment response is important.

Treatments with some specificity for certain disorders are summarized in table 5.4.

TABLE 5.4
Psychotropic Agents and Their Specificity for the Treatment of Major Psychiatric Disorders

Major Psychiatric Disorder	*Psychotropic Agents*
Alcoholism	Disulfiram
Narcotic Addiction	Methadone, naltrexone
Schizophrenia	Neuroleptics
Delusional (Paranoid) Disorder	Neuroleptics
Mania	Lithium, carbamazepine, calcium channel blockers
Depressive Disorder	ECT; antidepressants: tricyclics, mono-, tetra-, and heterocyclics, MAOI's
Panic Disorder with and without Agoraphobia	Propranolol, tricyclics, MAOI's, alprazolam
Obessive Compulsive Disorder	Clomipramine, trazodone
Generalized Anxiety Disorder	Benzodiazepines, buspirone
Somatoform	Tricyclics
Anorexia Nervosa	Neuroleptics, tricyclics

Premorbid Personality

The assessment of the premorbid personality serves three functions in the psychodiagnostic process:

1. It is the baseline for the patient's present functioning. Ask the patient and relatives to what extent the patient deviates from his "normal self."
2. It supports the diagnosis, since some psychiatric disorders are associated with specific premorbid features. For instance, patients with bipolar disorder may show cyclothymic traits, while patients with schizophrenia are often odd and socially isolated prior to the onset of the disorder. If diagnosis and premorbid personality do not match, reconsider your diagnosis.
3. It sets the therapeutic goal beyond which treatment is less likely to produce improvement.

Social History

Divide the social history into its premorbid and morbid part. From the premorbid history assess the developmental milestones and the highest degree of psychosocial functioning. Milestones such as psychomotor and speech development, toilet training, and school performance are especially important when learning disability or mental retardation are complicating factors. Address five areas of school performance:

1. Slow learning, as expressed by repetition of the first grade, and need for special classes or schools, indicates mental retardation or mental dysfunctioning persisting into adulthood. Check for circumscribed deficits such as dyslexia or acalculia.
2. Disciplinary problems, such as lying, stealing, cheating, running away from home, and violent behavior toward superiors, peers, or animals suggest antisocial personality.
3. Hyperactive behavior, which may explain impulsivity and performance failure in adulthood. It may be related to a personality disorder.
4. Phobias (especially school phobia), obsessiveness, or depressive features. They often precede disorders of adulthood such as obsessive compulsive disorder, phobic, or affective disorders.

5. Sporadic school attendance, social withdrawal, isolated antisocial acts, or inappropriate behavior. They may precede adulthood schizophrenia.

Use the patient's work record to gauge whether his past employment corresponds with his intelligence and educational background. Analyze the social interaction with colleagues, superiors, and subordinates. Screen the military record (if applicable) for discipline problems, alcohol and drug abuse, promotion, demotion, and type of discharge.

Compare the patient's highest premorbid functioning in work and family life with his functioning during morbidity. The distance between the two indicates the impact of the disorder on the patient's life, while premorbid functioning sets the treatment goal. Thus, recovery is freedom from symptoms and also return to premorbid functioning. A measure to quantify premorbid, morbid, and present functioning is the Global Assessment of Functioning Scale (GAF Scale, DSM-III-R, p. 12). It allows you to rate global functioning from 1 to 90, 90 being the highest level of functioning. The GAF Scale takes into account the presence of symptoms, their severity, i.e., mild to severe, and their duration, i.e., transient to chronic. It assesses quality of functioning in a wide range of activities, social effectiveness, satisfaction with life, and mastery of problems.

A GAF score assigned to pivotal points of the patient's life illustrates and quantifies the impact of mental disorders on your patient's functioning and allows you to characterize and quantify the natural course of the disorder.

Social history can be used as a detection device for a psychiatric disorder in patients who try to conceal mental problems. For instance, a patient is evaluated for a heart transplant and wishes to get a high priority for the operation. He believes that his past antisocial history, psychoactive substance, and alcohol abuse may deny him a high priority. Therefore, he denies all such symptoms. If you suspect such a simulation, assess a thorough, year-by-year, or even month-by-month social history. Divorces, job losses, arrests, convictions, jail sentences, DWI's, and hospitalizations for injuries in fights are hard to hide. At least, discrepancies and contradictions will emerge which will then lead you to the concealed psychiatric conditions.

Medical History (Axis III)

Physical disorders may complicate or mimic psychiatric disorders. This knowledge can help you avoid a misdiagnosis in two ways.

(a) Medical Disorders as Cause of Psychiatric Symptoms

When you take a medical history, and encounter neurological, endocrinological, metabolic, collagen, cardiovascular, or other medical disorders in addition to psychiatric symptoms, examine whether these disorders or their treatment with pharmacological agents could possibly be responsible for the psychiatric symptoms. For instance, a patient has been diagnosed as having lupus erythematosus. Subsequently, he develops a multitude of anxious and depressive symptoms. His psychiatric personal or family history are negative. Entertain the possibility that these symptoms are due to the lupus and that they may respond to different medication than an affective disorder, for instance to neuroleptics rather than to antidepressants. If you feel that the organic factor is responsible for the psychiatric symptoms you should make the diagnosis of organic anxiety syndrome and organic mood syndrome, respectively, rather than generalized anxiety disorder or major depression.

Table 5.5 shows which physical conditions (left column) are frequently associated with psychiatric symptoms and therefore the cause of an organic delusional syndrome, organic hallucinosis, organic mood syndrome, organic anxiety syndrome, organic personality syndrome, or organic mental syndrome, not otherwise specified (NOS). Consider the relationship especially when you work on consultation service and are called to diagnose and treat psychiatric symptoms in medical patients. Use table 5.5 in the following way:

The patient has one of the medical disorders (rows in table 5.5) known to frequently produce psychiatric symptoms. Then check carefully whether the patient has any of these psychiatric symptoms and consider the diagnosis of an organic mental syndrome.

Neurological disorders may present with psychiatric symptoms. Focal neurological deficits, such as anesthesia and paralysis, or the essential symptoms of an organic mental disorder such as lethargy, confusion, disorientation, delirium, amnesia, or intellectual deterioration give them away. These indicators, however, are missing in the early stages or in mild manifestations of some neurological disorders. A high index of suspicion is then needed to lead you in the right direction.

Endocrine disorders are as often a cause for misdiagnosis as the neurological disorders. Both hypo- or hyperfunction of the thyroid, parathyroid, adrenal cortex, or insulin-producing Langhans cells are responsible for the emergence of psychiatric symptoms.

Electrolyte imbalance, usually a depletion of sodium, potassium, calcium, or magnesium, causes psychiatric symptoms and so can high potassium levels. Serum bicarbonate levels outside of the normal range may also mimic symptoms of depression.

Collagen disease of the vascular system, such as lupus erythematosus, rheumatoid arthritis, periarteritis nodosa and temporal arteritis, can be associated with symptoms of anxiety and depression. Systemic lupus erythematosus can virtually mimic all psychiatric symptoms, including delusions and derealization.

Cardiovascular disorders, especially paroxysmal atrial tachycardia and coronary insufficiencies, can mimic panic disorder, while congestive heart failure and hypertensive encephalopathy may induce delusions.

The remaining physical disorders in table 5.5, such as chronic infections, some carcinomas, some vitamin deficiencies, and some systemic disorders, may occasionally present with symptoms of depression and anxiety but only rarely with delusions.

Usually, a physical disorder is not mistaken for a psychiatric disorder. Occasionally, however, the medical presentation may be preceded by panic, anxiety, or depression. Or, the episodic course of some physical disorders suggests an affective disorder (where an episodic course is typical). Here are nine such disorders:

multiple sclerosis
herpes simplex
encephalitis
pheochromocytoma
systemic lupus erythematosus
acute intermittent porphyria
pancreatitis
systemic mastocytosis
chronic Epstein-Barr viral syndrome.

Often, interviewers associate delusions and derealization so strongly with a psychiatric disorder that they overlook a nonpsychiatric cause.

TABLE 5.5

Psychiatric Symptoms (Columns) Associated with Axis III Physical Disorders (Rows)

	Panic	Anx.	Depr.	Episodic	Del.	Dreal.
Neurological Disorders						
Trans. Cerebr. Ischemia	+					
Cerebral Ischemia		+	+			
Multiple Sclerosis		+	+	+		
Posterolat. Sclerosis		+				
Wilson's Disease		+	+		+	
Huntington's Chorea		+	+			
Polyneuritis		+				
Nieman Pick					+	
Homocystenuria					+	
Brain Tumor			+			
Marchiafava-Bignami					+	
Encephalitis					+	+
Herp. Simpl. Encephalitis				+		
Jacob-Creutzfeldt			+			
Norm. Press. Hydrocephalus					+	
Granulomat. Meningitis					+	
Alzheimer's, Pick's			+		+	
Brain Abscess					+	
Temporal Lobe Epilepsy					+	+
Meniere's Disease	+	+				
Head Injuries		+				
Endocrinopathies						
Thyroid, Parathyroid, Adrenal, Insulin	+	+	+		+	
Pheochromocytoma	+			+		
Electrolyte Imbalance						
Na, K, Ca, Mg, HCO$_3$			+		+	
Collagen Vascular Disorders						
Lupus Erythematosus		+	+	+	+	+
Others		+	+			
Circulatory						
Parox. Atr. Tachycardia	+					
Coron. Insufficiency	+					
Anemia		+				
Congest. Heart Failure					+	
Hypertens. Encephalopathy					+	

Continued on next page

TABLE 5.5—CONTINUED

	Panic	*Anx.*	*Depr.*	*Episodic*	*Del.*	*Dreal.*
Infections						
Tuberculosis, Brucellosis		+	+			
Toxoplasmosis					+	
Malaria (cerebral)		+	+		+	
Viral: Hepatitis, Pneumonia;						
Mononucleosis		+	+			
Subac. bact. endocarditis					+	
Carcinoma						
Oat-cell (Lung)	+	+				
Leukemia			+			
Pancreatic Ca.			+			
Lymphoma			+			
Vitamin Deficiencies						
B_1, B_6, B_{12}, Niacin, Folic						
acid		+	+		+	
Systemic						
Nephritis		+				
Uremia			+			
Early Cirrhosis			+			
Psoriasis			+			
Gout			+			
Amyloidosis			+			
Regional Enteritis			+			
Ulcerative Colitis			+			
Acute Intermitt. Porphyria				+		
Pancreatitis				+		

Legend: Anx.   = anxiety
       Depr.   = depression
       Episodic = episodic psychiatric symptoms
       Del.   = delusions
       Dreal.   = derealization
       +   = present

Note: This table was constructed with the help of information contained in Hall 1980. Dr. R. C. W. Hall gave his permission to quote and abstract from his book.

(b) Psychiatric Symptoms as Indicators of Undetected Medical Disorders

Avoid misdiagnosis when you encounter psychiatric symptoms in older patients with a negative personal and family psychiatric history; when the symptoms occur in an unusual combination; when they show an unexpected course; or when they present at an age for which the onset of the respective psychiatric disorder is rare. For instance, Ronald, a high school teacher in his late fifties, shows symptoms of depression and persecutory delusions for the first time after an episode of indecent exposure at the school's gym. Consider early manifestations of Pick's disease, if you can exclude by laboratory tests or history other medical disorders. Table 5.5 can help you consider and exclude, or verify physical conditions as possible causes of psychiatric symptoms. For instance, the patient has one of the following psychiatric symptoms: panic attacks, generalized anxiety symptoms, depressive symptoms, episodic symptoms, delusions, or derealizations. Find this symptom as one of the headings in table 5.5 (columns). Identify all the medical disorders which can cause this symptom. Then check whether the patient may have one of these disorders. If yes, consider that the patient has an organic mental syndrome.

Your work setting often determines the likelihood of an association between physical conditions and psychiatric symptoms. Consultation psychiatrists, family practitioners, and psychiatrists in rural areas may encounter more frequently physical and pharmacological causes for psychiatric symptoms than those professionals in multidisciplinary settings such as a university outpatient clinic, where mental health professionals often work in a tertiary care function.

The side effects of pharmacological agents (see table 5.6) may be mistaken for symptoms of a psychiatric disorder. Table 5.6 shows most of these agents grouped according to their therapeutic use with a residual category. These agents are not considered psychotropic except for the stimulants, the autonomous nervous system agents, the antihistamines, and some vitamins, especially B_6 which facilitates the metabolism of some monoamine neurotransmitters (Hall 1980).

Psychiatric symptoms due to these agents are not limited to toxic effects or interference with brain metabolism such as delirium, confusion, disorientation, lethargy, tremor, and ataxia. Therefore, you may

TABLE 5.6
Psychiatric Symptoms (Columns) Frequently Associated with Axis III Conditions, i.e. Nonpsychiatric Drugs (Rows)

Drug	D	S	I	R	IN	A	E	H	DL	P	DR	C	DS	L	T	AT
Agents Against Infections																
Sulfonamides	+		+	+						+						
Sulfones			+		+					+						
Anthelmintics			+				(+)			+		+				
Antituberculars	+		+							+		+				
Antimalarials			+							+				+		
Trichomonacides	+		+		+					+		+				+
Antihypertensives																
Rauwolfia Alkaloids	+	+										+			+	
Ganglionic Blockers															+	+
Beta Blockers	+															
Autonomous Nervous System Drugs																
Sympatholytics	+									+					+	
Sympathomimetics				+	+					+					+	
Anticholinergics				+				+		+	+	+	+			
Stimulants																
Amphetamines	+							+	+	+			+			
Phenylphenidate			+		+				+	+						

Continued on next page

TABLE 5.6—CONTINUED

Drug	D	S	I	R	IN	A	E	H	DL	P	DR	C	DS	L	T	AT
Analgesics																
Salicylates		+		+								+				
Acetaminophen, Phenacetin				+					+			+				
Propoxyphen	+						+									
Analgesics, Other	+			+						+		+				
Hormones																
Insulin				+						+		+				+
Oral Antidiabetics				+								+				+
Thyroid Drugs			+		+											
Adrenocorticosteroids	+		+		+		+			+						
Estrogens						+										
Estrog. + Progestins							+									
Diuretics																
Carbonic Anhydrase Inhibitors			+	+									+			
Xanthines			+		+						+					
Diuretics, Other						+						+				
Others																
Antineoplastics	(+)	(+)	(+)	(+)	(+)		(+)			(+)	(+)		(+)			
Cardiac Glycosides	+	+	+	+	+	+		+	+			+	+		+	
Antihistamines				+	+		+	(+)		+	+					
Vitamin B Complex	+	+										+				+

overlook a drug induction unless you ask the patient to bring in all medications he has been taking for the last two months. Ask especially the elderly for whom drugs have a prolonged half-life of excretion. Note that the average geriatric patient takes nine agents daily which may lead to drug interaction and potentiation.

Include in your medical history a list of all hospitalizations and disorders the patient was treated for in his lifetime. Assess the patient's compliance with his past medical treatment and his response to the various agents. Both help to predict compliance and therapeutic response to your present treatment.

Use table 5.6 in two ways:

1. Examine whether a patient who takes any of the medications listed in table 5.6 may have had psychiatric symptoms that coincided with the beginning of that drug treatment.
2. Examine whether psychiatric symptoms that occur in patients without a personal or family psychiatric history, in an atypical form, or at an unusual age are due to medication taken for a physical ailment. With axis III, DSM-III-R offers organic mental disorders associated with physical disorders, or conditions whose etiology is unknown. Tables 5.5 and 5.6 help you with axis III diagnoses.

Family History

Some studies suggest most major psychiatric disorders are familial. Monozygotic twin studies and adoption studies favor the interpretation that the disposition to psychiatric disorders is genetically transmitted, even though the mode of transmission is unknown (Goodwin and Guze 1984; Wender et al. 1986).

Family history can be used to confirm a psychiatric diagnosis and to predict course and treatment response in young patients with their first affliction, especially when making the differential diagnosis of psychotic depression versus schizophrenia, or atypical mania versus schizophrenia. For instance, if your patient has had several depressive episodes but first-degree relatives suffered from manic-depressive disorder, suspect manic-depressive disorder in your patient also. Such knowledge may caution you against the use of antidepressants which could precipitate a manic or hypomanic episode, but suggest a combined use with lithium carbon-

	D	S	I	R	IN	A	E	H	DL	P	DR	C	DS	L	T	AT
Antitussives							+									
Diphenoxylate	+									+						
Diphenidol	+				+		+								+	
L-Dopa	+			+	+		+			+				+	+	+
Vascular Muscle Relaxants	+						+								+	
Antiarrhythmics	+		+	+	+		+	+	+	+				+		
Nicotinic Acid			+	+	(+)											
Hydantoins	+		+				+								+	+
Succinimides					+		+									+
Narcotics	+		+				+							+		
Narcotic Antagonists	+				+		+									

Legend:
D = Depression	E = Euphoria	DS = Disorientation
S = Suicidal	H = Hallucinations	L = Lethargy
I = Irritability	DL = Delusions	T = Tremor
R = Restlessness	P = Psychosis	AT = Ataxia
IN = Insomnia	DR = Delirium	+ = present
A = Anxiety	C = Confusion	(+) = possibly present

Note: This table was abstracted from Hall 1980 by permission of Dr. R. C. W. Hall.

ate. But if first-degree relatives of a patient with major depression have documented chronic schizophrenia, scrutinize your patient's course for evidence of social decline to exclude schizophrenia.

At this point, there are only a few family studies on personality disorders (with the exception of antisocial personality). Since personality disorders appear to be associated with major psychiatric disorders, and since the latter are familial, personality disorders may also be familial. Therefore, ask your patient whether any of his first-degree relatives were in some way either: 1. loners, odd, or eccentric; 2. in social trouble (the black sheep of the family); or 3. somewhat dependent, abused, rigid, or resentful. Such questions may puzzle your patient initially. He may be unresponsive to your questions, only to return later with ample information after he talked to parents and other relatives who had carefully concealed some family secret. Such awareness helps *you* to predict his course and outcome and *him* to understand the nature of his disorder. It reduces his guilt and his unjustified blaming of his parents for their sins committed in his upbringing.

5. CHECKING FOR UNEXPLORED DISORDERS

Suppose that in a town like Vienna the experiment was made of treating a square such as the Hohe Markt, or a church like St. Stephen's, as places where no arrests might be made, and suppose we then wanted to catch a particular criminal. We could be quite sure of finding him in the sanctuary.

Sigmund Freud
Resistance and Repression, Standard Edition, vol. 16:288, 1916–1917

After you have verified some initial diagnostic impressions and excluded others, you are left with a list of psychiatric disorders that are unexplored—list no. 3. Remember, a chief complaint reflects only what the patient chooses to talk about. Therefore, to be comprehensive you have to reach beyond the boundaries of the chief complaint and what the patient volunteers. Use a disorder-oriented approach and explore essential symptoms that the patient does **not** offer. You may be surprised what you find.

> Rachel, a 27-year-old, black, attractive female presented with depressed affect.

P: I'm five months pregnant. While I save for our baby, my husband spends all his money at the races. I just can't take it anymore.

I: You must really feel let down.
P: You better believe it. I cry for hours.

I: How long has that been going on?
P: My husband has always worked long hours, but since I got pregnant with our second child, it's gotten worse. Now he even stays out overnight.

I: You seem to feel stuck.
P: Stuck and desperate. I can't sleep, I lost my appetite, I don't feel like talking to anybody.

The interviewer felt quite empathic and protective of the patient, and in the remainder of the interview stayed within the limits of her spontaneous complaints. His list of diagnostic possibilities included:

> adjustment reaction, depressed type
> depressive disorder
> bipolar disorder, depressed type

Two days after this interview, the patient's aunt called. She complained:

"My niece is still drinking like a hole. She drives her husband out of the house. This poor fellow has tolerated her drinking for the last three years. Isn't there anything you can do about it?"

Rachel had never mentioned her drinking or drug abuse during the interview. When the interviewer confronted Rachel with the aunt's concern, Rachel reluctantly admitted to her drinking but claimed that her husband was exaggerating it. Nevertheless, the interviewer had made the mistake of restricting himself to the patient's initial chief complaint. He never generated a list no. 3, let alone assessed it.

Screen for hidden major psychiatric disorders by asking for their essential symptoms (see table 5.1), especially for memory problems, alcohol and drug use, physical problems, "spells," and avoidance behavior. To screen for personality disorders, ask your patient whether he had a rough life and got into situations that were difficult to handle.

6. DIAGNOSES

Coming up with a diagnosis makes sense out of madness. It labels the disorder, not the patient; it condenses a multitude of data into one term; it serves communication, and allows prediction of treatment response and outcome.

Multiple Diagnoses and Diagnostic Hierarchy

DSM-III-R encourages multiple psychiatric diagnoses on axes I and II. These diagnoses can be specified by terms such as principal diagnosis, provisional diagnosis, or "in remission" (see below). In many diagnostic systems, including DSM-III and DSM-III-R, a hierarchical principle is used to exclude certain psychiatric diagnoses to the benefit of others. Usually, the more pervasive disorder receives priority over the less pervasive disorder.

The hierarchical principle underlying the diagnostic decision process can be traced back to the first attempts by Jaspers (1959) and Foulds (1976). DSM-III-R refers to this hierarchy, but does not use it strictly (DSM-III-R, p. XXIV). The exclusion of one psychiatric disorder by another is limited to two situations:

1. If a psychiatric disorder is felt to be due to an organic factor, then the additional diagnosis of nonorganic psychiatric disorder is not made. For instance, if a patient has major depressive disorder after chronic treatment with reserpine, he will receive the diagnosis of organic affective disorder and not the additional diagnosis of major depressive disorder.
2. The defining symptoms of one disorder are at the same time associated features of another disorder. For instance, a patient has schizophrenia and also reports some depressive symptoms. He will receive only the diagnosis of schizophrenia but not the additional diagnosis of dysthymia since dysthymia is thought to be part of schizophrenia.

In contrast, if a patient has obsessive and compulsive symptoms in addition to schizophrenia, he will receive the diagnosis of obsessive compulsive disorder in addition to schizophrenia, since obsessions and compulsions are not thought to be associated features of schizophrenia (see DSM-III-R, pp. XXIV and 16).

Principal Diagnosis

Assign the *principal diagnosis* to the disorder that clinically most reliably and comprehensively explains symptoms present and which are the focus of attention or treatment (DSM-III-R). For instance, if a patient is presently addicted to alcohol but also reports symptoms suggestive of dysthymia, the diagnosis of alcoholism is undoubtedly reliable and of concern for treatment, while the dysthymic symptoms may be due to patterns of alcohol intoxication and withdrawal and are therefore less reliable. Therefore, the principal diagnosis is alcohol abuse or dependence and *not* dysthymia.

A patient may have more than one principal diagnosis. For instance, he may have experienced obsessions and compulsions for several years which significantly impaired his functioning. For the last four weeks, he became increasingly depressed and for the last two weeks, fulfills all criteria for major depressive disorder. This "new" disorder made him consult a psychiatrist in addition to his psychologist who was treating him with behavior modification for his obsessive thoughts and compulsions. Clearly, both disorders are additive in the impairment of the patient's functioning. They justify two principal diagnoses.

Provisional Diagnosis

It happens that the interviewer can assess some symptoms of a psychiatric disorder but the patient's lack of cooperation does not allow him to investigate the full syndrome. The interviewer has the impression that the patient has all symptoms necessary to make the diagnosis but he lacks documentation. Rather than assigning a not otherwise specified diagnosis (NOS), the interviewer may choose to express the level of uncertainty by using a provisional diagnosis (for further description, see DSM-III-R, p. 17).

Past Psychiatric Diagnoses

DSM-III-R does not use the term past psychiatric disorder. However, it uses the terms

in partial remission
in full remission, and
residual state

to indicate the status of previously experienced psychiatric disorders.

Diagnostic Profile

If a patient has more than one psychiatric disorder, it is helpful to plot onset and end of each disorder on a time line. The zero point signifies the patient's birth, the units of the time line are the years of his life, and the end is his present age. The disorders are indicated with bars above it. On top of the graph are the organic disorders, followed by psychoactive substance use disorders, psychotic disorders, mood, anxiety, somatoform disorders, and so on, as they are listed in DSM-III-R. Such a display of a patient's diagnostic profile allows you to visualize the temporal relationship of all disorders. It presents the most succinct diagnostic summary.

Lifetime Diagnosis

Some authors (Othmer et al. 1981; 1988) use in their diagnostic schemes the concept of a "lifetime" or "final" diagnosis which is thought to explain best all psychopathology ever observed in a patient's life. This approach adheres to the concept of one major psychopathological process, an assumption which becomes increasingly doubtful as empirical studies seem to indicate that multiple psychiatric disorders are common.

The "lifetime" diagnosis still has a heuristic value for administrative purposes, such as charts color-coded according to a lifetime diagnosis in large clinic settings. If you are interested in such a diagnostic system, see the PDI-R manual (Othmer et al. 1988).

During the interview, we recommend that you share your diagnostic considerations and decisions with the patient in the form of a diagnostic feedback. A good way to introduce this topic are statements such as:

"Let me wrap up for you what I found that you have suffered from. And let's see whether you agree with me."

Usually, patients appreciate being included in this process. They are anxious to know what you think about them; they also deserve to be rewarded after they have patiently answered your questions. If you do this patients will often tell you:

"You are the first one who tells me what's wrong with me and why you think so."

7. PROGNOSIS

The feedback of the diagnostic impression to the patient sets the natural stage for the next step—the discussion of the treatment options. More about this in chapter 6.

The patient's response to your treatment suggestions clearly show from a diagnostic point his attitude toward his disorder. It gives you an inkling of his degree of compliance. Together with the nature of his major psychiatric and/or personality disorder, his attitude toward his disorder and the treatment options contribute significantly to his prognosis.

Again, we recommend that you share this outlook with the patient. Tell him whether you think he has an excellent chance for full recovery, or indicate that you are concerned about his low interest in his treatment and that a lack of compliance may lead to a prolonged course and future relapse. These concerns should be expressed as such—and not as threats (see chapter 6). The prognostic feedback rounds off the diagnostic process.

Now you are ready to integrate what was taken apart: *Rapport, techniques, mental status examination, and diagnosing.* You will understand how they interact and develop throughout the seven phases of the interview.

CHECKLIST

Chapter 5: Seven Steps to Make a Diagnosis

Complete this list after an interview.

1. What was the chief complaint?
2. List all psychiatric signs and abnormal behaviors (clues), if any, that you observed during the initial minutes of the interview.
3. List the differential diagnostic options (at least five) that these signs and behaviors suggested to you.
4. Did you address any signs or clues?
5. Give reasons why you treated clues the way you did.
6. Did the observed behavior or the chief complaint suggest a psychiatric symptom, a long-term maladjusted behavior, a stressor, or a social conflict?

7. How did you follow up on the chief pathology?
8. How soon after the start of the interview did you have a list of five diagnostic options?
9. If the patient reported psychiatric symptoms as chief complaint, list all disorders for which these symptoms are
   a. essential,
   b. associated.
10. Did you screen for essential symptoms?
11. Did you screen for a lifelong maladjustment?
12. If the patient reported lifelong maladjustment,
    a. describe the situations he is sensitive to,
    b. list the personality disorders which are associated with your patient's pathology,
    c. list the major psychiatric disorders that could explain his maladjusted behavior.
13. Did you screen for a stressor?
14. If the patient named a stressor, determine how the stressor is related to the disorder: cause, trigger, time marker, magnifier, consequence, or pathological thought content.
15. If the patient described a social conflict discuss whether this conflict was the expression of
    a. a major psychiatric disorder,
    b. a personality disorder,
    c. an adjustment disorder,
    d. a problem of living.
16. List all psychiatric disorders that the chief complaint could
    a. include,
    b. exclude,
    c. be neutral to.
    Separate the disorders into major psychiatric, personality, or adjustment disorders. Make sure you have at least five disorders included.
17. Did you get a description of the premorbid state?
18. List indications for slow learning, learning disability, social isolation, disciplinary problems, phobias, obsessions.
19. In what way did the disorder interfere with the patient's intimate relationships, work, and hobbies?
20. Did you check for unexplored disorders? What type of disorders did you detect? List them!
21. When was the onset of the disorder? Was it sudden or insiduous?

22. Was the course chronic, episodic, chronic progressive? Did it leave a deficit?
23. What is the impact of the disorder on the patient?
24. What was his response to previous treatment(s)?
25. List the medical disorders that could mimic the patient's symptoms.
26. List pharmacological agents the patient is taking which can mimic his psychiatric symptoms.
27. List the psychiatric disorders that occurred in the patient's first-degree relatives.
28. Did any blood relatives commit suicide?
29. Did any of the patient's first-degree relatives have the same psychiatric disorder as the patient?
30. What was the natural history of the patient's disorder in his first-degree relatives?
31. Which psychotropic drug(s) worked and did not work in the first-degree relatives who had a psychiatric disorder similar to your patient's?
32. List all psychiatric disorders for which the patient fulfills DSM-III-R criteria.
33. What is the patient's principal diagnosis?

CHAPTER SIX

SEVEN PHASES AND THE FOUR COMPONENTS: HOW TO PUT IT ALL TOGETHER

1. Warm-up

2. Screening of the Problem

3. Follow-up of Preliminary Impressions

4. Confirmatory History

5. Completion of the Data Base

6. Feedback

7. Treatment Contract

SUMMARY

Chapter 6 shows how to synthesize the four components explored in chapters 2 through 5 in longitudinal progression. It demonstrates how to conduct an interview by simultaneously establishing and maintaining rapport, selecting the most effective interviewing techniques, monitoring the mental status, and progressing in a flexible yet orderly manner in the diagnostic evaluation through the different phases of the interview which are determined by the shifts of the interviewing goals.

A strictly clinical approach will not enable psychiatrists to progress beyond a certain level of accuracy in diagnosis. Until such a time when we are able, in the laboratory, to refine the techniques of psychopharmacological, neurochemical, and electrophysiological investigations of psychiatric disease, dependence upon clinical techniques of diagnosis is necessary.

Eli Robins, 1981

The four tasks of the interviewer—to maintain rapport, to monitor the mental status, to apply the appropriate interviewing techniques, and to propel the diagnostic process—interact with each other throughout the psychodiagnostic interview. Several shifts in goal and topic occur during the course of the interview which subdivide it into seven phases: 1. warm-up, 2. screening of the problem, 3. follow-up of preliminary impressions (hypothesis), 4. history taking, 5. completion of the data base, 6. provision of feedback, and 7. closing of the treatment contract.

The interplay of the four components and the seven phases is summarized in table 6.1. This table does not suggest a straightjacket approach; on the contrary, it should raise your awareness of tasks to be completed in an interview. The order of completion is often determined by the connections the patient makes and not necessarily by the order in table 6.1. For instance, if the patient describes as his chief complaint severe symptoms of depression (phase 2 of the interview) and then makes the connection to his mother's depression and describes her disabilities, you may temporarily shift into assessing his entire family history (phase 4 assessment). This order follows the patient's needs. If this topic is exhausted you may then return to phase 2 and pursue assessment of further symptoms of depression, their severity, course, and the preceding stressors. Thus, you strike a balance between the opportunities that the patient offers and the overall organized interviewing process taught on these pages.

245

TABLE 6. 1
Seven Phases of the Interview and the Four Components

Phase	Rapport	Mental Status	Technique	Diagnosis
1. WARM-UP	Put patient at ease, set limits	Observe appearance, psychomotor function, speech, thinking, affect, orientation, memory	Select productive questions	Note diagnostic clues from patient's behavior
2. SCREENING OF THE PROBLEM	Empathize with suffering, become a compassionate listener	Explore mood, insight, memory, judgment	Open with broad screening questions	Classify the chief complaint; assess symptoms, severity, course, stressors; list differential diagnoses
3. FOLLOW-UP OF PRELIMINARY IMPRESSIONS	Become an ally, make shifts in topics clear	Assess speed of thinking, ability to shift sets	Shift topics, progress from open- to closed-ended questions	Verify or exclude diagnostic impressions
4. CONFIRMATORY HISTORY	Show expertise, interest, thoroughness, and leadership	Evaluate responsibility, judgment, remote memory	Follow-up, shift topics, handle defenses	Assess course, impact on social life; family and medical history
5. COMPLETION OF DATA BASE	Motivate for testing	Test mental status functions	Fill in gaps, follow up clues, reconcile inconsistencies	Exclude unlikely disorders
6. FEEDBACK	Secure acceptance of diagnosis	Discuss mental status findings, explore interest in help	Explain disorders and treatment options	Establish diagnosis and prognosis
7. TREATMENT CONTRACT	Assume the authority role and assure compliance	Make inferences about insight, judgment, and compliance	Discuss treatment contract	Predict treatment effects

PHASE 1: WARM-UP

Goal: Find a relaxed tone and comfort the patient. Take control over aggressive, intrusive, or delirious patients. Establish rapport.

For *rapport,* give the patient time to become familiar with you and the surroundings. Involve him in small talk so he can get used to your voice and the way you talk. Address his apprehension and show concern for his well-being. Put him at ease.

If your patient is aggressive or belligerent, as in the emergency room, set limits. Help him to recognize what you expect from him and what is acceptable to you. Make him aware that cooperation is to his own advantage.

Medicate the very excited or delirious patient. After he is sedated, conduct a modified diagnostic interview (see chapter 8.3: Mania).

Observe *mental status functions* such as appearance, psychomotor activity, speech, and affect during the warm-up. Anxiety (anticipatory and phobic) surfaces frequently here. As time goes on, the anxious patient may gain control over his affect. Therefore, register this initial anxiety for later follow-up. Similarly, look for signs of suspiciousness.

The themes of the small talk in the warm-up phase are not arbitrary. Choose topics that allow you to examine the patient's uncensored mental functioning. Is he oriented? Can he memorize well enough so that history taking will be reliable? Questions such as

"When did you contact this office first?"
"Where did you park your car?"
"How easy was it for you to find the office?"

are nonconspicuous ways to test his recent memory.

Technique: You learn what type of questions are most productive. Do open-ended questions elicit detailed elaborations? Or rambling? Or short answers like

"I don't know."
"You tell me."

What vocabulary does the patient prefer? Visual, abstract, or auditory? Can he comprehend long questions, understand their abstract meaning, and talk about familiar subjects without difficulties?

Diagnosis: Pick up clues of disturbed mental functions. They can be more productive in starting the diagnostic process than asking for the chief complaint. Regardless whether you pursue the clue or not, start forming diagnostic options for your list no. 1 (see chapter 5).

The length of this initial phase depends upon the patient's cooperation. If he is reluctant or hesitant to talk to you, it will take longer to establish rapport than when he volunteers all information. When you both feel comfortable with each other, you are ready for the next phase.

PHASE 2: SCREENING OF THE PROBLEM

Goal: To elicit and collect both essential and associated symptoms and signs of present major psychiatric, personality, and adjustment disorders.

Open this phase in one of two ways. Either follow up on a lead from the previous phase such as disorientation, affect, hallucinations, delusions, or a thought disorder; or ask a variation of the question: "How can I help you? What kind of problems bring you here? Where shall we start?" These questions will assess the chief complaint.

Focusing on the chief complaint opens phase 2 of the interview.

Rapport: In phase 2 you switch from putting the patient at ease to investigating his suffering. Thus, you place your "visitor" in the patient's role. Help him now to express his suffering and respond with empathy. Your compassion as listener deepens rapport. Be tactful and aware that you are dealing with mental pain—not with pieces of a puzzle, or a character in a novel. Interviewing is not just playing detective, or choosing—like a computer—the most efficient algorithms of a decision tree for the patient's problems. At stake in this early phase is the patient's mental anguish and not primarily the interviewer's diagnostic curiosity.

Mental Status: The question for the chief complaint changes the character of the interview from conversation to *exploration*. This switch confronts you with the patient's degree of insight and understanding of his problem. This is very important to establish because insight determines how to approach his psychopathology (see chapter 2). Explore his mental status functions by adopting the patient's view of his problems which will give you better results than remaining an aloof outside observer. For instance, a patient with a drinking problem still drives inebriated in spite of several arrests and two severe accidents, one nearly fatal.

The family judges these acts as irresponsible and almost criminal. However, the patient feels that he cannot overcome his agoraphobic feelings and panic attacks to go to work if he does not have a few drinks. If you adopt the patient's view of his drinking rather than that of his family (or society) you utilize his insight to interview him, which will help your rapport, mental status, and diagnostic assessment.

Technique: The switch to the chief complaint is a shift from small talk to screening for disorders. You initiate it with open-ended, nonstructured questions which become more structured and even closed-ended when you need to pinpoint a symptom. If your patient is reluctant to talk about certain topics, or distorts the facts, recognize his resistance and underlying defense mechanisms and deal with them.

Diagnosis: The assessment of the chief complaint moves the patient's disorder into the center of the interview. The chief complaint confronts you with symptoms, patterns of disturbed behavior, reactions to stressors, and problems of living. Base your initial diagnostic impressions on these reports. Construct and keep track of three lists (chapter 5):

list no. 1 of likely disorders—be overinclusive
list no. 2 of excluded disorders
list no. 3 of disorders not yet checked.

List the disorders according to the hierarchy as outlined in chapter 5, i.e., start with the major psychiatric disorders, followed by personality disorders, adjustment disorders, and problems of living.

The four components of the interview interlock: while you ask for symptoms and problems, you observe at the same time the patient's mental status for emerging signs of disturbed behavior. Their follow-up by confrontation, for instance, fuels the diagnostic process. If these interventions disrupt rapport, identify the mental status functions responsible for the stalling—persecutory ideas or anger, for instance. Then change your technique to revive rapport and the diagnostic process.

Monitor how the patient formulates, how he thinks, and how he processes information. Analyze what type of questions help him to open up and talk about his problems, and which questions distract and confuse him. Adjust your technique accordingly. Redirect when he digresses from discussing his own problems. What can you conclude from these observations for mental status and the differential diagnosis?

PHASE 3: FOLLOW-UP OF PRELIMINARY IMPRESSIONS

Goal: To make diagnostic decisions. Verify the likely and exclude the unlikely diagnoses.

Rapport: Phase 3 is the most taxing for the patient because he has to give you very specific information that allows you to make diagnostic decisions. While the previous phases were patient-centered, allowing the patient to select the topic and describe his pain and suffering, this phase becomes task-centered. The patient has to answer detailed questions which sometimes are difficult and not always purposeful for him. Furthermore, questions may seem to jump eratically from one topic to another. Recognize when the patient becomes puzzled, and explain the rationale for your topic selection and sequencing.

This far into the interview, the patient should be convinced "that you know what you are doing," that you are not only a compassionate listener but also an expert.

Mental Status: During phase 3 you request detailed and precise information from the patient. Thus, you become aware of selected mental status functions, such as thought content, remote memory (symptoms that occurred in the far past), and recent memory, insight, concept of words, goal directedness in thinking, tightness of associations, and speed of thinking. Since you may switch topics quickly, you can also judge the ease with which the patient can shift sets.

Technique: Since during this phase you seek specific information that allows you to make specific diagnostic decisions, you use a variety of steering techniques: curbing when the patient becomes too detailed about a topic, accentuated or abrupt transitions when you need to cover different topics and to check out your diagnostic options. Since you are more active during this phase than in the previous one, you may encounter resistance and defense mechanisms that you have to handle.

Diagnosis: You check out the disorders on list no. 1. Verify or exclude them. Decide whether the patient's's complaints fit best a major psychiatric, or a personality, or an adjustment disorder. Frequently, you find a combination of one or more major psychiatric disorders with a personality disorder. Try to separate them and follow each of them up. This process shortens and solidifies list no. 1, the likely disorders; it lengthens list no. 2, the excluded disorders.

As in phase 2, there is no diagnostic progress without your simultaneous rapport, your continuous monitoring of the patient's mental status, and your fine tuning of assessment techniques. If the interviewer neglects any of these four components, he will miss information to support his diagnoses. Or he may not be able to make one at all. Insensitivity to mental status and rapport may put the whole interview in jeopardy; the result—premature termination.

PHASE 4: CONFIRMATORY HISTORY

Goal: To get the history, the course of the disorder, the premorbid personality, the psychiatric family history, the medical and social history to confirm the diagnosis.

Rapport: While assessing the patient's history your expertise will show. Understanding the patient's problems establishes it. Thoroughness and interest in his problems will intensify rapport.

This phase is easy for the patient, because you cover territory known to him—the patient has given a history to health professionals before. However, there are obstacles to rapport in this phase: embarrassing topics—being fired from a job, imprisonment, drug abuse, venereal disease, unfaithful behavior, and so forth.

Mental Status: Phase 4 gives ample opportunity to test the patient's remote memory. His past actions reveal his social responsibility. Extend the social history by exploring his future plans, which will give you a feeling for his judgment.

Technique: Your goal during this phase is to keep the patient animated to give you a detailed history of his psychiatric disorders. Find new angles to help him view his past. Generate new insights. Sudden transitions in topics revive the interview. Pay attention to his reality distortions and his resistance to give certain information. Identify his defense mechanisms, and handle them cautiously if they obstruct the diagnostic process. If this is your first contact with him, you may bypass them (see chapter 3).

Diagnosis: Determine the duration of the patient's problems and their course. Were they episodic, chronic, or deteriorating? Major psychiatric disorders appear to be associated with specific personality disorders; be aware of this relationship. Schizophrenia, for instance, may be preceded by a schizoid or schizotypal personality disorder.

The patient's social history shows the impact of the illness's effect on the patient's's life.

The medical history may contribute to the psychiatric diagnosis. For instance, multiple unnecessary surgeries point to somatization disorder; endocrinological disturbances have possibly triggered or complicated an affective disorder. Seizures or head injuries may have predisposed the patient to an organic mental disorder.

Finally, screen his first-degree relatives for evidence of psychiatric disorders. Manic-depressive disorder, schizophrenia, or alcoholism in one or both parents may increase your diagnostic certainty and you may get a glimpse of what the future has in store for your patient.

Phase 4 solidifies the diagnostic impressions on list no. 1. When you review premorbid personality and history and find a chronic course where you had expected remissions, you may detect a previously overlooked personality disorder. Add it to list no. 1 and scrutinize it.

Phase 4 is not rigidly separated from the preceding phases. Historical data may emerge earlier, and aid your diagnosis. Favor a natural flow of information over a rigidly systematic approach. As long as the patient gives you pertinent information, let him lead you through his past; give him the chance to explain his history to you like a museum guide.

PHASE 5: COMPLETION OF THE DATA BASE

Goal: To fill in gaps in the mental status assessment and to test some functions. To follow up on clues noticed during the interview, and to clarify inconsistencies in the history.

Rapport: Master two rapport-related tasks during this phase:

1. Motivate the patient to take some tests. Testing taxes rapport because it may activate performance anxiety. It reminds him of a student role. If rapport is fragile, he will refuse testing (like May in chapter 8.). To assure cooperation explain each test carefully. Emphasize that, unlike in school, there is no failing of the test; it serves to help and not to grade or degrade him. Provide him with immediate feedback about the results and how they support the diagnosis.

2. In the case of inconsistencies, confront the patient gently with them. Such a confrontation may arouse anxiety, suspicion, or anger. Therefore manage this phase with tact, emphasizing that *you* did not understand, that *you* are confused, rather than implying that he misinformed you.

Mental Status: You may spot some gaps; you may have a vague notion about the patient's concentration, recent memory, and intelligence from the interview, but you feel you need quantitative data to clearly support your preliminary impression. Now is the time to test, just before the "Feedback" phase, while testing may have interrupted the flow of information earlier.

Technique: This phase may be opened with an accentuated transition. If you found inconsistencies, tell the patient that *you* don't have a clear picture about some events in his past, or that *you* need some help to reconcile A and B. If you have some clues, follow up on them by making the patient aware of your observations. Don't threaten him, but communicate that it is in *his* best interest that you understand the background of these inconsistencies or of that clue.

Diagnosis: Phase 5 completes the collection of evidence for your diagnostic impressions, your list no. 1. This phase also offers the last chance to go beyond the chief pathology and screen for so far unexplored disorders, list no. 3. Screen especially for alcohol and drug abuse which can imitate—during intoxication and withdrawal—a host of psychiatric symptoms. Thus, you reduce list no. 3 in favor of lists no. 1 or no. 2.

Clues not yet explored should be dealt with now. For instance, perhaps the patient looked at his watch repeatedly and polished his glasses eight times during the interview. Or perhaps he used the same phrase over and over such as

"Typical for the government," or
"And then the usual thing happened again."

Now is the time to clarify inconsistencies between the patient's psychiatric history, your diagnostic impression, and previous treatment. For instance, explore whether the depressed or anxious patient who was treated with neuroleptics ever heard voices or had delusions that would justify such treatment. Or explore a mismatch of an event and his age, or of his schooling and his occupation.

Again, during this phase, the four components of the interview are interrelated. Your diagnostic impression will help you to decide which mental status tests to select, which gaps in history to close, which behavioral clues to follow, and which inconsistencies to reconcile. Your rapport and mental status findings will guide you in your technical approach.

PHASE 6: FEEDBACK

Goal: To explain to the patient what is wrong with him and how he can be treated.

Integrate all observations about rapport, mental status, and history. You should have a working diagnosis after 30 to 45 minutes of interviewing. Share some of the results of this integrative process with the patient. Interviewers frequently fall short of this task, either by oversight, or by attempting to maintain professional secrecy. If you want the patient to comply with your treatment, give him feedback.

Technique: Open the feedback phase by telling the patient something like:

"I have asked you a lot of questions and we have discussed many points. Is there anything you would like to ask me?"

After you have answered him, tell him what you have learned about his problems. Tell him *how* and *why* you think he is suffering. Link his suffering, symptoms, and the nature of his illness. Discuss in lay terms your working diagnosis. However, delay the disclosure of your diagnosis if it may affect him negatively. Explain *what* can be done to alleviate his suffering and to control (or cure) his disorder.

Rapport: Your feedback should have two effects:

1. to give the patient confidence in your understanding of his problems, and make him accept you as an expert;
2. to give the patient confidence in your treatment recommendation, and make him accept you as an authority.

Your roles as expert and authority intensify rapport and may bring out his personality traits. The dependent patient may glorify you, while the narcissistic personality may try to dismantle you of your authority. To stay in control, recognize his personality traits. Register changes in attitude. If a negative interplay develops, address, discuss, and interpret it.

Mental Status: The patient's response to your feedback highlights three mental status functions: cooperativeness, insight, and judgment. They reflect how serious he is about seeking help. Disinterest in treatment may be an alarming clue for suicide potential. Listen carefully. Patients who have concealed their suicidal tendencies throughout the interview will admit their hopelessness if you address their disinterest in help at this point. Consider then hospitalization.

Feedback enhances the patient's understanding of his condition. You learn how well he accepts his disorder and the treatment options. His acceptance of them improves his prognosis.

PHASE 7: TREATMENT CONTRACT

Goal: To select a treatment plan and to agree on a treatment contract.

Rapport: Your role as authority peaks during this phase. The more the patient recognizes your competence during the interview, the easier he will accept and follow your treatment recommendations.

Mental Status: The patient's comprehension of your treatment plan and insight into his problems become apparent; but after a comprehensive interview you should encounter no surprises with respect to disturbed functions anymore.

Technique: Discuss in- or outpatient care, the pro's and con's of different modes of therapy available, such as types of psychotherapy, pharmocotherapy, or a combination thereof, or electroconvulsive therapy, cost, time involvement, and outcome measures. Point out that the treatment plan will be tailored to his needs; that every detail will be considered. For outpatient care, indicate how often and how long he has to be seen.

If you recommend pharmacological treatment, discuss type of medication, dose, timing, efficacy, and side effect profile. Be detailed about all possible adverse effects so the patient feels completely informed. Tell him what to do if they surface. Only then discuss the beneficial treatment effects.

Avoid raising false expectations about treatment success. Prepare him for possible changes in the treatment plan. Explain what the prognosis is with and without treatment. If and when he accepts your treatment plan and promises to comply with the details, you know that (for now) he may have accepted your authority.

After the discussion of an individualized treatment plan, the patient may assume that you are the therapist. In spite of this assumption, discuss this point explicitly. If you feel competent and are willing to treat him, tell him so; otherwise recommend a referral. Give him the option, whether he wants *you* to treat him or not. He may feel that a therapist of a different gender may be more acceptable, or a therapist who lives closer to his home. Your charges may be too high; he may want to use a mental health center. Before you initiate treatment, be sure that the patient fully accepts you as his therapist and that he made this choice in the face of alternate options.

After the patient has understood and agreed to the treatment plan and has accepted you as his therapist, close the treatment contract. Take every detail seriously and let him agree to all terms: how often and how long you will see him; how much you will charge for regular and broken but uncancelled appointments; who will cover for you when you are out of town; how he can reach you after hours. Tell him under which circumstances you expect him to call. The more explicitly he agrees to all terms, the more he will feel obliged to keep his part of the contract.

At the very end of the interview you may want to ask the patient how he felt at the beginning of the interview and how he feels now. Indicate to him that you are looking forward to seeing him again. Express a justifiable degree of optimism about the future visits and the anticipated progress.

CHAPTER SEVEN

PHASES AND COMPONENTS APPLIED TO TWO INTERVIEWS

SUMMARY

Chapter 7 analyzes two interviews. The first one is an average interview with a mostly cooperative patient; the second one deals with a resistant patient. Both interviews are analyzed with respect to the four components outlined in chapters 2–5. The first interview is relatively short and complete since it shows the seven phases (see chapter 6). The second interview is somewhat longer, yet incomplete because the interviewer has difficulties in establishing rapport and in motivating the patient to cooperate fully.

Suicide is not an isolated event, but rather the last link in the chain of increasingly mortal symptoms.

Eli Robins, 1981

1. FIRST INTERVIEW

Most psychiatric patients are cooperative. They answer questions to the point and engage in the interview either spontaneously, or at least after a brief warm-up period.

We have reproduced a typical interview with a hospitalized, 29-year-old, white female. We edited it by numbering all questions, modifying others, and adding several questions (Q.) and answers (A.) to illustrate what we discussed in chapters 1–5. We also divided it into seven phases to show how each phase contributes to rapport, mental status, techniques, and diagnosis. Important questions are italicized.

Phase 1: Warm-Up

In an intensive medical care unit, the patient is sitting up in her bed in a hospital gown. Her ashblond hair is unkempt, showing half an inch of new brown growth at the roots. She wears no makeup to camouflage the greyish color of her skin.

She glances at the psychiatrist when he approaches her area which is separated from the neighboring beds by a partly drawn curtain. She licks her dry lips; her lower lip is bruised and swollen, presumably from the intubation two days ago. She looks older than her stated age. She swallows when the interviewer is ready to address her.

1. I: Hello, Mrs. Goodman, my name is Dr. O. Has Dr. M. told you that he wanted me to see you?
   P: Yes, he told me that.

2. I: Do you feel comfortable talking to a psychiatrist?
   P: Well . . . I don't know what good it can do . . . just asking a bunch of stupid questions isn't going to help me a bit. But I guess you do what you want to anyway, no matter what . . . (Patient speaks hesitantly.)

3. I: If you talk to me we may be able to understand what got you here.
   P: I know that anyway. I don't need you for that. (The patient slumps back into her pillow and turns to the side away from her interviewer.)

4. I: Gee, you must really feel pissed that you bite my head off before I have even started to talk to you.
   P: Darn right.

5. I: Being that pissed . . . you sound as if you've gone through hell.
   P: (Slowly she turns around and looks at the psychiatrist.) I'm sorry . . . if I sound rude . . . I just can't help it, I'm so keyed up . . . any little thing makes me fly off.

6. I: Maybe you can get some things off your chest . . . and, of course, if you feel too bad and if you can't take it just say so . . . and we can continue later.
   P: Hmm.

7. I: How have you been treated here?
   P: Oh, I can think of a better place.

8. I: How long have you been in the ICU?
   P: For the last two days. I came here Saturday night.

9. I: Can I do anything for you before we start . . . (waiting) like getting you something to drink?
   P: A glass of ice water would be fine. (The interviewer goes to the nursing station to get it.)

Q. 1–9:

Rapport: The patient rebuffs the interviewer's opening remarks. Right away, he addresses her despondent attitude toward him and shows sensitivity for her discomfort. He penetrates her territorial defense ("the patient turns away") with strong language to match her affect and to get her attention. He activates her guilt feelings when he confronts her with her hostility. When she shows regret, he quickly responds to her verbal signal ("keyed up") with empathy.

She puts him in the role of overwhelming authority (A. 2) which he mollifies by telling her that he can continue the interview later if she so desires (Q. 6). But he takes care not to encourage her so that she can escape the interview, thus maintaining his role as authority.

He shows concern for her well-being and tries to put her at ease by getting her something to drink. From a psychoanalytical point of view, he offers to gratify oral needs believed to be activated during a depressive state.

Mental Status: Observation yields an alert, white, slightly disheveled female who looks older than her stated age. She does not maintain eye contact; she shows some evidence of psychomotor retardation. Her affect appears sad, irritable, despondent, and depressed; she does not smile when the interviewer walks in. She shows reactivity in her affect when he evokes guilt feelings.

Conversation reveals that the patient is alert and comprehends the questions. Her speech is goal-oriented and fluent but slow with increased latency of response. She elaborates on the closed-ended Q. 1 and 2 rather than limiting herself to yes/no answers. She is oriented to place, person, and time; her short-term memory is grossly intact (she remembers correctly the time of admission).

Technique: Initially, the distractible and hostile patient resists talking and is unwilling to cooperate with the interviewer. Her unprovoked hostility permits him to answer in kind by using slang to get her attention. Even though he is aware that this confrontational approach may provoke more hostility, he feels it is important to quickly put her in a responding mode. As soon as he has her attention—because she answers him, and also to the point—he attempts to replace the hostile interchange by an empathic approach. This works because it activates her guilt feelings. A. 9 concludes the warm-up phase; the patient appears to be at ease; she accepts a glass of water from him.

Diagnosis: The mental status findings and the admission to the ICU suggests for list no. 1, the included disorders:

affective disorder, uni- or bipolar
somatization disorder
substance abuse
histrionic personality disorder
borderline personality disorder
adjustment disorder with depressed mood.

The mental status findings exclude (list no. 2) as present diagnosis severe organic mental disorder.

Phase 2: Screening of the Problems

Chief Complaint and Symptoms

10. I: What got you here in the first place?
    P: I had problems with my husband—we were arguing and fighting—and the kids got on my nerves. And so I couldn't sleep. On Saturday, I took some pills.

11. I: Took some pills?
    P: Well, I took all the prescription pills that we had in the house . . .

12. I: Hmm.
    P: Because I was tired . . .

13. I: (Just looking at her.)
    P: I just wanted to lay down and go to sleep . . .

14. I: (Still looking at the patient.)
    P: . . . and . . . and not wake up.

15. I: Hmm . . . You must have really felt awful . . . not wanting to wake up.
    P: Yeah . . . I guess . . . I really had it. I felt all worn out.

16. I: So bad that you were ready to die?
    P: I wasn't thinking about it that way . . . at the time. I was . . . just tired of everything—like I said, I just wanted to lay down and go to sleep and forget everything . . . I didn't think about it as killing myself.

17. I: Just to get rid of all those feelings?
    P: Yeah. That's right. To kill all those feelings.

18. I: Do you still feel that way?
    P: Hmm . . . I don't know . . . I guess . . . at times.

Severity

19. I: What happens to you when you are that down?
    P: I don't want to move. (The patient pulls up her cover, turning away to the side) I don't want to see anybody . . . I want to be left alone . . . just have peace and quiet. (The patient closes her eyes.)

20. I: Hmm . . . (The interviewer puts his hand on the patient's shoulder which is covered by the blanket.)
    P: . . . Not answer anything.

21. I: Ah . . . hmm, do you feel like this right now?
    P: Hmm . . . now . . . ? (The patient turns to the interviewer and opens her eyes.) Earlier I guess. Everybody gets on my nerves . . . I want to be left alone . . . everything is an effort.

22. I: I see . . . It must really bother you to talk to me now.
    P: Yeah . . . hmm . . . eh . . . it's all right, I guess. You seem to understand . . . that makes it easier.

23. I: I see . . . so . . . you still feel down?
    P: Yeah, pretty much.

24. I: I'm so sorry that you have such a rough time. Were you so much down that you felt like out of it?
    P: Yeah, like losing my mind.

25. I: Like losing your mind? Like even hearing things?
    P: Yeah . . . I just would . . . like maybe . . . be in a room by myself . . . and I'd think . . . I heard somebody . . . heard somebody call me . . . call my name or something, but I didn't see anybody talking . . . and there wasn't anybody.

26. I: Yes, that happens to people when they feel really depressed . . . tell me more about it.
    P: Just my name . . . maybe two or three times . . . like I was aware of it . . . maybe not like a voice.

27. I: When you felt like this . . . could you get anything done . . . like your housework?
    P: Oh no, . . . everything was too much . . . I couldn't even go to the grocery store—it made me so nervous.

Course

28. I: When did it all start?
    P: I have had those feelings off and on. But it really got worse over the last six weeks.

29. I: Off and on . . . ?
    P: Yes. They hit me out of the blue.

30. I: And you could not go to the grocery store then either?
    P: Oh no . . . That was just in the last few weeks. Before that I was just crabby and bitchy . . . terrible with my kids and with Al (the patient's husband).

31. I: You could work back then?

    P: Yes, I could but I was draggy . . . just not worth a shit. But I guess I looked all right . . . from the outside. And it didn't really last that long.

32. I: And now?

    P: Now? Now that's different. It really hit me for a loop. I haven't had anything like this before.

Stressor

33. I: So it really hit you this time. Tell me what happened, what brought it on?

    P: Hmm . . . I felt pressured. It just seemed everybody was making demands on me . . . more than I could stand. And I felt . . . like I was trapped.

34. I: Trapped?

    P: Yeah, at work. We had a girl at work . . . she was going into surgery . . . and then we had another one going on vacation, and I was taking over both their jobs and mine . . . and I kept forgetting and misfiling things . . .

35. I: Ah, lets look at your concentration and memory a little later . . . Anyway, you said you felt pressured.

    P: Pressured . . . yeah . . . I felt like closed in and trapped. I had to get things done and I couldn't. The more I tried the worse it got. I got all tangled up. That pulled me down.

36. I: (Interviewer frowns.) You felt overworked?

    P: (Irritated.) Yeah, didn't I just tell you?

37. I: Being overworked pulled you down?

    P: Yeah, at my job and at home . . . must have been . . . there wasn't anything else going on . . .

38. I: (Interviewer raising his eyebrows.) Hmm . . .

    P: Don't you believe me?

39. I: (With emphasis.) Of course, I believe you. It must seem that way to you.

    P: What do you mean?

40. I: I mean you felt more pressure because there was more pressure . . . or maybe because you could take *less* pressure.

    P: (Annoyed.) You're playing with words.

41. I: Maybe I play with how one can look at it.

    P: (Patient shakes her head.) You confuse me.

42. I: I'm sorry . . . but let me ask you, has that happened before that somebody was out?

    P: Oh yeah, it happens every year once or twice.

43. I: And then it gets to you?
    P: Hmm . . . hmm . . . no . . . last year I just went to the supervisor. I just told him we were falling behind and he better send somebody else down . . . but Ron (the supervisor) couldn't do that, really. He had a girl answer some of the mail that I thought was important. The rest, he said, just has to wait.

44. I: Hmm . . . and this time?
    P: This time was different. I didn't feel up to it. I felt I had to handle it . . . by myself. I couldn't face him and tell him that I couldn't pick up Rosie's work. So I just drudged along.

45. I: You could not face him?
    P: Oh, it just didn't feel right. I just thought I'm letting her down if I complain behind her back. I couldn't do that.

46. I: So you felt you couldn't let her down?
    P: Yeah, tattle on her.

47. I: How did you feel otherwise?
    P: Crabby . . . down in the dumps . . . I guess.

48. I: So this time you feel different . . . different to begin with?
    P: You mean because I was down I felt that way?

49. I: Yes, that's right.
    P: But what else should have pulled me down?

50. I: Sometimes people feel down without a reason, we'll talk about that later.
    P: But that's crazy . . .

Q. 10–50:

Rapport: Since the interviewer had some difficulties in establishing rapport initially, he delayed the question for the chief complaint (Q. 10). And since rapport is still not stable, he screens the patient's behavior for signs of resistance such as hostile posture, avoidance of eye contact, evasive or short "yes/no" type answers.

He assumes a role as empathic listener (Q. 15, 22, 24, 26, 33). He exercises patience waiting for her answers without pushing to keep her in a spontaneous talking mode rather than in a reactive answering mode, where answers have to be extracted like teeth. He neutralizes her admission of a possibly embarrassing symptom (a hallucination, A. 25) as an experience typical of depression to put her at ease and to encourage her to elaborate on other psychotic symptoms.

A. 33–36 show that the patient interprets her dysphoric feelings as the result of stress rather than as a spontaneous shift in mood, showing that she has only partial insight. The interviewer attempts to challenge her perspective, but she maintains that her disturbed feelings are due to outside stress (Q. 38–41).

Mental Status: During *exploration* the patient reports psychomotor slowing, suicidal ideation, and a fleeting auditory hallucination. She gives detailed responses indicating her cooperation. Her vocabulary expresses at least average intelligence. She interprets her symptoms as a reaction to outside pressure which she feels she should have met. Her interpretation of her disorder seems to show limited insight which is not easily corrected. Her attitude toward work and colleagues reflects a lack of assertiveness, guilt feelings, and low self-esteem. She tries to overcome her inadequacy by obsessive work habits and increased effort, rather than by asking for assistance. Therefore, her approach shows impaired social judgment.

The interviewer prepares the patient for later *testing* of memory in phase 5 (Q. 124).

Technique: Q. 10 is broad and open-ended to allow the patient to select her topic. This question for the chief complaint (Q. 10) is introduced by an accentuated transition which is viable here since the patient does not seem to be anxious or suspicious. The interviewer follows up on the clue ("I took some pills") by echoing (Q. 11), continuation (Q. 12–14), specifying (Q. 16) and summarizing (Q. 17) techniques. With Q. 18 he shifts to the present to probe for persisting depressive symptoms and suicidal ideation as mental status functions.

The smooth transition (Q. 19) aims at the severity of her depressions. Q. 33 introduces as a new topic the precipitating event using another smooth transition. In a subtle way, this question asks for her interpretation. He echoes her interpretation (Q. 34) but starts to question its accuracy, mainly by frowning (Q. 36) and eyebrow raising (Q. 38). The patient notices his doubts and responds with irritation (A. 36, 38, 40, 41). Starting with Q. 39 he suggests by his questions an alternate interpretation, namely that her problems may be due to a decrease in coping ability rather than to an increase in stress (Q. 39–50).

Diagnosis: The interviewer opens phase 2 with a question for the chief complaint rather than following upon behavioral clues noticed during the warm-up phase 1. The patient lists associated symptoms for depression: suicidal tendencies (A. 10), irritability, and social withdrawal (A. 19, 21). Q. 11–17 clarify the suicidal remarks as an intent to kill her depressed feelings rather than herself. Such suicidal gestures (common are also wrist slashing and skin burning) may express one or more of the following:

1. the wish to communicate severe suffering (cry for help);
2. frustration and anger against oneself;
3. an attempt to induce guilt in others;
4. an attempt to get rid of depressed feelings.

In contrast, hanging, shooting and jumping from high places are serious, mostly successful suicide methods.

Q. 24–26 assess psychotic symptoms, hallucinations, and delusions, i.e., severity of the illness. The patient experienced an auditory hallucination of having her name called. She explained this brief auditory experience as due to her nervous condition rather than as the effect of a magical event. Because of her insight, this hallucination is considered a pseudohallucination.

Q. 28: The switch from cross-sectional to longitudinal symptom assessment examines whether diagnostic criteria for depression are met, i.e., duration of more than two weeks which helps to distinguish depression from adjustment disorder with depressed mood, since depression has diagnostic priority over adjustment disorder (DSM-III-R). The patient fulfills diagnostic criteria for major depression.

Q. 33–50 assess as precipitating event the increased work load which the patient attempted to handle rather than negotiating with her supervisors for a better work distribution. Guilt feelings and obsessive compulsive tendencies may have contributed to such a behavior. It is unclear whether guilt and obsessiveness are personality traits magnified by depression, or symptoms of a depressive episode.

From the patient's response which indicates that she could handle similar situations in the past, we can conclude that the increased work load is not a cause for her depression—it is unlikely that it has triggered the depressive episode. The most plausible interpretation is that the patient was depressed to begin with and that her failure to adjust to the increased work load magnifies her decreased coping ability during her depression.

At the end of phase 2, the screening phase, list no. 1 of possible diagnostic options includes:

alcohol abuse
substance abuse
bipolar disorder
unipolar depression
cyclothymia (preexisting)
dysthymia (preexisting)
histrionic personality disorder
borderline personality disorder
obsessive compulsive personality disorder.

All these disorders should ideally be scrutinized in phase 3. This list is not written in stone. As clues evolve during the interview other disorders may be added (see below, panic and obsessive compulsive disorder). List no. 2 excluded psychiatric disorders like adjustment disorder.

All disorders of DSM-III-R not mentioned in list no. 1 or list no. 2 remain in list no. 3, the unchecked psychiatric disorders. They don't surface because the patient's complaints or behaviors give no indication that they are present.

Phase 3: Follow-up of Preliminary Impressions

51. I: Hmm. Let's talk about it.
    P: You know I wasn't sleeping well. That's probably why. I just felt like I had to get out and away from everybody . . . I started to lose my appetite, and you know . . . just evasive things.

52. I: Evasive things?
    P: I don't want to talk about them . . . not now.

53. I: Evasive things . . . (The interviewer looks at the patient but she does not answer). Sounds like you try to push them out of your mind?
    P: Yeah.

54. I: They must still bother you.
    P: It's so crazy . . . well, let's just forget about it now.

55. I: Must be difficult to talk about it.
    P: Yeah, I don't want to think about it any more. I really felt bad.

56. I: Yeah, you felt so bad that it even affected your sleep.
    P: Yeah, it was lousy.

57. I: What kind of sleeping problems?
    P: Oh, I'd stay up til 11:00 or 12:00 at night, and I'd be up through the night . . . and I'd get up around 5:30 or 6:00 in the morning . . . and just go all day.

58. I: And your appetite?
    P: (Does not answer.)

59. I: Did you lose any weight?
    P: Yes, about 30 pounds . . . my clothes were falling off me. Everything looked too big.

60. I: What's your weight now?
    P: (Laughs). I don't want to answer that. (The patient weighs 176 pounds at the interview.)

61. I: Did you want to lose that much?
    P: Yeah . . . but I also did not have any appetite.

Mania

62. I: You say: You feel crabby and down in the dumps now. Have you ever felt the opposite: *Were you ever really up, so people would say: "My goodness, you are high, are you taking diet pills or something?"*
    P: Yeah, like "What happened? Where did you get all that pep to do things, what's going on?" And the next day I'd be so low, you know.

63. I: How long did your longest high last?
    P: About three weeks.

64. I: For three weeks!
    P: Yeah, at least.

65. I: What kind of things did you do during that time?
    P: What do you mean?

66. I: Did you ever do something . . . that you regret now . . . like spending a lot of money, getting involved with something or someone?
    P: No, no, nothing like that.

67. I: What about your energy then?
    P: Oh, that was fine. I just felt contented—and I was pleased with everything around me.

68. I: How was your sleep during that time?
    P: Well, I stayed up late and got up early, but I slept through the night at least. I needed less sleep.

69. I: How was your speech?
    P: I might have talked faster.

70. I: Faster?
    P: Rattling—yeah. (The patient laughs, embarrassed).

71. I: Did others comment on that?
    P: Well, my husband would tell me to shut up once in a while. (The patient laughs again and blushes).

72. I: Does he usually do that?
    P: No, it's just when I got to rattling.

73. I: How often did you have that rattling period?
    P: I don't know. Not real often to that point, to that degree.

74. I: Did you start a lot of projects then?
    P: Well, I liked to be busy.

75. I: Did you get it all done what you started?
    P: Oh sure, it all fell right into place.

Drug and Alcohol Abuse

76. I: *Did you ever take any street drugs to feel that good?*
    P: (Patient gives an empty stare.) No . . .

77. I: Or for any other reason?
    P: No, never.

78. I: What about drinking?
    P: Liquor . . . ? No, I don't like any of it.

79. I: Do you take any pills . . . pain pills? If we looked in your medicine cabinet at home, what would we find?
    P: Nothing now.
80. I: And before that?
    P: Aspirins.

81. I: Often?
    P: When I got headaches, I would. But mostly my husband would take them.

Obsessive Compulsive Disorder

82. I: *Besides these depressive feelings—you described them really well—did you have any other concerns, anything else unusual?*
    P: Like what?

83. I: *For instance, thinking about the same things over and over again, not being able to push a thought out of your mind?*
    P: Yeah, I've had that. I've been struggling with that over the last few weeks.

84. I: What kind of thoughts were those?
    P: Well, about two months ago for one thing, I kept having dreams that my little girl was dying . . . One Sunday morning in church I looked up in front and I could see her playing in her coffin up there, you know. For several days after that, all I could think about was seeing her laying up there. I got kind of panicky to the point where I hated to let her out of my sight. I was afraid something would happen to her.

85. I: Did you ever have the feeling that you yourself would harm her . . . accidentally . . . or even intentionally?
    P: No, like I said, when I could feel myself getting angry, I would send the kids out, because I knew I could get carried away spanking them. But no, I didn't ever really think I'd ever hurt her.

86. I: Did you have other thoughts that forced themselves into your mind?
    P: Yeah, but I don't want to talk about them.

87. I: You don't want to discuss them now . . . (after a pause). Were these types of thoughts only there when you were depressed or were they present all the time?
    P: They were there quite a lot of the time . . . because that's what used to bring me down, you know. I'd be okay, and then I'd start thinking on things and then I would start feeling myself getting down . . . really getting depressed. And then when I was depressed, it was much worse to where it kept me there.

88. I: When did they first start?
    P: Two or three months ago, I think.

89. I: Were these thoughts like visions that would come up in your mind . . . like with the coffin?
    P: Yeah. Like that . . . like visions . . . but sometimes just thoughts.

90. I: Is there anything that you did about it? Any ritual or any kind of procedure to prevent those things from happening? You said, you did not let your daughter out of sight. Did you do any more than that?
    P: No, there was nothing else to do.

91. I: Did you do things like checking . . .
    P: (Patient looks puzzled and frowns).

92. I: Like checking the locks . . . or the fireplace or the gas?
    P: I didn't check anything.

93. I: Did you feel these visions or thoughts were really silly . . . ?
   P: Hmm . . . One scared me. You know, I always felt like I wasn't going to have her until she was grown, from the time she was born, you know. But some of the other ones have been silly.

94. I: Can you tell me a few silly ones?
   P: No.

95. I: You must feel quite embarrassed about them that you feel so strongly about hiding them—any reason?
   P: Many reasons, but I won't discuss them either—you seem to know a lot about them anyway.

Panic Disorder

 96. I: Okay. *You say some of these thoughts scared you. Have you ever felt so scared that you had a spell of panic?*
   P: Yeah, that morning when I saw her up front (in the coffin), I had to leave. I was shaking and crying (little laugh), you know, kind of on the verge of hysterical, I guess.

 97. I: Did you have to fight for your breath?
   P: No.

 98. I: Just describe what happened to you when you had that spell.
   P: I was scared, uptight, my hands were clammy.

 99. I: Clammy? Also tingling?
   P: No, there was no tingling.

100. I: And your vision?
   P: My vision? There was nothing wrong with it, nothing.

101. I: And your heart?
   P: Nothing wrong with my heart, just the same.

102. I: Any pounding?
   P: No, nothing like that.

103. I: How often did you have these types of spells?
   P: Not more than two or three times. It's just really started coming. This was just a couple of days ago.

Q. 51–103:

Rapport: Mrs. Goodman gives a coherent history and elaborates spontaneously, all signs of good rapport. Therefore, further empathic remarks are not necessary. The interviewer continues to challenge her explanation for her depression. However, when she explains her depression as being due to inadequate sleep, he adopts her perspective; he forms an alliance with her without attempting further to correct her level of insight, thus preserving rapport.

She refuses to discuss obsessive thoughts (A. 51–54, 86, 94–95). This refusal may be due to an anxiety of being overwhelmed when discussing them, or fear to be considered "crazy" or "silly." Since her refusal is limited to symptoms not essential for a working diagnosis and immediate management, the interviewer, after repeated confrontation, expresses empathy with her refusal, and decides to abstain from further pressuring her and to bypass her resistance in order not to endanger rapport. She acknowledges his expertise (A. 95) which seems to justify his approach.

Mental Status: The remark about her colleague whom she could not let down represents nearly unrealistic if not delusional guilt. The patient also shows suppression of her possible obsessive thought content which she seems to experience not as an ego-dystonic but as threatening to her integrity. She experiences her aggressive impulses as difficult to control and sends her children outside. This also reflects a need for social withdrawal which she acted out when the interviewer first met her. Spontaneously, she reports classic vegetative symptoms of depression but not clear-cut hypomania or mania (Q. 62–75). She seems to have experienced severe anxiety in connection with the obsessive thought content. During the interview, overt anxiety is not manifest except in her refusal to talk about her obsessions. The anxiety experienced in the past does not appear to be a clear-cut panic attack.

Technique: Q. 56–61 are specifications of symptoms mentioned in A. 51 using specification (Q. 57) and checking for symptoms techniques (Q. 58–61).

Q. 62–75: The interviewer approaches manic symptoms with a smooth transition. He contrasts her present depressive state with its opposite. After she admits to elation but denies unrestrained buying sprees (A. 66), he checks for other manic symptoms (Q. 67–69, 74, 75) with circumscribed open- and closed-ended questions.

After a smooth transition (Q. 76), he screens for drug and alcohol abuse and excludes it.

Q. 82–95: He checks obsessive compulsive disorder with a standard strategy: with broad questions (Q. 82, 83) he screens for the presence of essential symptoms of the disorder. Since the patient refuses to describe her obsessive thoughts, he confronts her with her resistance in Q. 87 and 95. When the patient refuses to discuss the reason for the resistance, he starts to discuss other pathology.

Q. 96–101: With a smooth transition he links the obsessions to panic disorder by picking up on the patient's clue "scared" (A. 93) and continues with open- and closed-ended, symptom-oriented questions.

Diagnosis: The interviewer checks for further symptoms of depression—social withdrawal (A. 51), initial, intermittent, and terminal insomnia (A. 56, 57), and weight loss without body image distortion (A. 59). Q. 62 asks for elation which she endorses and which lasted for about three weeks (A. 63), without imprudent behavior (Q. 65, 66), but increased energy (Q. 67), reduced desire for sleep (A. 68) and push of speech (A. 69–73). These symptoms suggest some elation but it does not interfere with the patient's life. Only her self-report documents it. No hospitalization or treatment was required. These behavioral changes without symptom value may be within normal limits and experienced as a contrast to her depression. However, they should be remembered because they may predict a different treatment response from clear unipolar depression.

Q. 76–81: According to the diagnostic hierarchy, the interviewer could challenge his diagnosis of major depressive disorder by finding severe drug or alcohol abuse. Cocaine, amphetamine, and alcohol withdrawal can produce depressive feelings. Therefore, he rules out alcohol and drug abuse.

Q. 82–95: The exploration of obsessive symptoms yields thoughts consistent with depression (harm may come to her daughter). The patient reports repetitive dreams, one abnormal perception, a visual hallucination or pseudohallucination, and some recurring fears about it. The interviewer explores thoughts of infanticide not uncommon in a depressed mother.

The patient admits also to silly intrusive thoughts but is unwilling to elaborate on them. Since these thoughts appear to be linked to her depressive episode and started relatively late, a preexisting obsessive compulsive disorder is unlikely. Consistent with this is the finding that she has no compulsions.

Q. 96–103: The patient's symptoms are atypical for panic disorder; she is more concerned about her hallucinations than her anxiety. Vegetative symptoms of a panic attack are missing. Since her fears are associated with a depressive episode, even more typical attacks would not establish the diagnosis of an independently existing panic disorder. Therefore, panic disorder is excluded.

List no. 1 of included disorders is:

1. Major depressive disorder
2. Bipolar disorder NOS (Bipolar II)
3. Dysthymic disorder
4. Cyclothymic disorder
5. Histrionic personality disorder
6. Borderline personality disorder
7. Obsessive compulsive personality disorder.

List no. 2 of excluded disorders is:

1. Bipolar disorder (typical)
2. Alcohol abuse
3. Substance abuse
4. Obsessive compulsive disorder
5. Panic disorder
6. Adjustment disorder with depressed mood.

Phase 4: History

Longitudinal Course

104. I: *Were you ever depressed before?*
    P: Yeah . . . off and on for two or three days.

105. I: But did you have any long periods where you had to go for treatment or even be hospitalized?
    P: No . . . not before this time.

106. I: When were you first depressed in your life?
    P: About ten or eleven years ago.

107. I: *Have you also experienced some highs during that time?*
    P: Yeah, I don't know, probably not as much as I was down. I mean, I was just kind of going along evenly and I was probably down more than I was up . . . or else I was just going even, you know, kind of leveled off.

108. I: Did these bad or good days ever prevent you from doing your work or disturb your family life?
     P: Not really, I may have been more irritable, but that's all.

Premorbid Personality and Social History

109. I: *Were you a moody person . . . as a child or a teenager?*
     P: I was usually pretty up, you know. I was pretty happy. I had problems with my mom, but as long as I could avoid her, I got along with everybody.

Family History

110. I: *Was there anybody else in your family who was depressed?*
     P: Well, I have a sister who was in Topeka State Hospital, but I don't know what her problems were. She never talked about them.

111. I: Is she older than you?
     P: Yeah, she's about 14 years older and she's just had her problems in the past couple of years.

112. I: Is she completely well now?
     P: No, she's still seeing a psychiatrist fairly often.

113. I: Is she taking any medication?
     P: Last time I knew she was.

114. I: Do you know what kind of medication?
     P: No.

115. I: Does she have a family?
     P: Yeah, she's got two kids, one is out of high school and the other is a junior this year.

116. I: How many brothers and sisters do you have?
     P: Three brothers and three sisters.

117. I: How are they . . . does any of them have any problems?
     P: Well, I have another sister (the patient laughs), she said if she ever went to a doctor, they'd probably lock her up. But she won't go. . . . she has her down days.

118. I: So you have three sisters—that means there are four girls in the family and three boys. Three of you girls have some problems, but the fourth one has no mood swings or problems?
     P: I don't know, I'm not around her.

119. I: What about your brothers?
     P: They all seem okay; they usually get along fine.

120. I: What about your children? They are young, aren't they? Anything un-
     usual?
     P: No. My oldest one just had a few problems in school picking up stuff
     like her math, but you know, that's just kids. I don't think there is
     anything to worry about. My other children, too, they are lively, they
     pick up things and I think they are okay.

121. I: How many children are there altogether?
     P: Three.

122. I: What about your parents—were there any kinds of problems, psychiatric
     problems, nerve problems?
     P: No. They were never treated for anything anyway.

123. I: Any drinking problems?
     P: No.

124. I: Your mother had several babies. Did she have problems after the deliv-
     ery? Like did she feel unusually blue or did she have to stay longer in the
     hospital than usual? With any of them?
     P: No. She was in kind of bad health, she had heart problems. With my
     older brother she had a heart attack just after he was born. Outside of
     that there wasn't any problems.

Medical History

125. I: *Did you yourself have any medical problems so far?*
     P: Not up till now.

Q. 104–25:

Rapport: Rapport is good. The patient answers to the point; she
elaborates without prodding and does more so as the interview goes on;
she feels comfortable enough to reveal some intimate and embarrassing
symptoms. Now, she clearly assumes the role of "carrier of an illness"
with some distance from her disorder which makes it easy to interview
her about herself and her family. She does not indulge in suffering, or
strive to be treated as a VIP.

Mental Status: The patient gives a consistent and detailed history
which tells us that her remote memory is intact even though her data are
not yet confirmed by outside sources. She appears to have more insight
into her past mood disturbances as endogenous mood swings. She also
seems to understand the mood disturbances of her family members as
disorders and not as environmentally determined reactions, even though

she interprets her present mood disturbance as a reaction to outside events. She may not be aware of this inconsistency because she experiences her present mood disorder as ego-syntonic. It will be the therapist's task to create more cognitive distance to her present depressed feelings.

Technique: The interviewer uses both smooth (Q. 104, 125) and more accentuated transitions (Q. 109, 110) to introduce new topics. The patient's goal-oriented answers show that she tolerates all transitions well. Q. 104 shifts from a cross-sectional to a longitudinal view with a smooth transition to keep the patient focused on her depressive symptoms. Q. 107: The interviewer chooses another smooth transition to assess the history of depressive and manic symptoms. More abrupt transitions (Q. 109 and 110) introduce the assessment of the premorbid personality and family history. They indicate to the patient that the interviewer is changing the topic.

Diagnosis: The history of the present disorder reveals that it is episodic in nature and that the present episode is the first one severe enough to require treatment (A. 105). The proportion of elated feelings to depressed periods—fewer elated than depressed days—concurs with clinical expectations (A. 107).

Q. 109: The interviewer explores the patient's premorbid personality. She seems to have been outgoing and popular which is consistent with an affective disorder but may exclude obsessive compulsive personality disorder. Q. 110–15: One out of three sisters of eleven first-degree relatives has a psychiatric disorder which was remitting and did not affect the marriage. This history is consistent with pure familial affective disorder.

A. 125 indicates medical good health and *excludes* somatization disorder.

List no. 2 of excluded disorders is:

1. Bipolar disorder (typical)
2. Alcohol abuse
3. Substance abuse
4. Obsessive compulsive disorder
5. Panic disorder
6. Adjustment disorder with depressed mood
7. Obsessive compulsive personality disorder
8. Somatization disorder.

Phase 5: Completion of the Data Base

126. I: You told me a lot about your problems. That helps me to help you. There are a couple of things left that I would like to test. Is that alright with you?

    P: Yeah, that's alright.

127. I: You told me that you started to forget things at work. Therefore, I'd like to test your memory.

    P: Okay.

128. I: I would like you to repeat four words: Grey, watch, daisy, and justice. Can you do that?

    P: Grey, watch, daisy, and justice.

129. I: That's fine. Try to remember these words. I will ask you to recall them a little later.

    P: I'll try.

130. I: While we are at it, let me ask you to do some calculations for me.

    P: (With a smile) I was never too good at math, but I'll try.

131. I: I like you to subtract seven from one hundred, and then keep doing it, always subtracting seven from the remainder. Let's start. What's hundred take away seven?

    P: 93—86—79—72—63—oh no, it's 65—58—51—54 sorry, 44 —37—30—

132. I: That's fine.

    P: No, I don't think so . . . I have trouble remembering the number that I have to subtract from. It confuses me.

133. I: Let's try some other things. How about some multiplication. Like 2 times 48.

    P: Oh no . . . 2 times 48? 86. No, I'm sorry, 96.

134. I: 2 times 96.

    P: That's . . . 180 . . . 192.

135. I: 2 times 192?

    P: That's 400 . . . 300 . . . and 84.

136. I: Very good. Let me go back to a couple of things that you said earlier. You took too many pills . . . Did you ever try to harm yourself before?

    P: No, that was the first time.

137. I: Did you ever think of harming yourself?

    P: (Raises eyebrows.)

138. I: When you were sad . . . or angry at somebody . . . or frustrated with a situation?
     P: No, not really. I could have kicked my husband a couple of times when he got me upset, but I usually just shut up or screamed . . . but then later we'd talk about it.

139. I: So this time was really the first time that you tried to harm yourself.
     P: I really felt bad then and I still do.

140. I: You said you had some down periods before and it started eleven years ago. What's the longest that you felt alright in between.
     P: Maybe two to three years.

141. I: I hope we can stop these moods swings for good. Now let's go back to the four words I asked you to remember. Can you remember them?
     P: Watch, daisy, and justice. Well, there was another one. Let me see, what was it? It was before watch, I think. Hmm . . . Yes, that's it—grey.

142. I: You are really doing fine.
     P: But that's pretty simple stuff.

143. I: Not for everyone. But you did fine. Before we close, are there any questions that you would like to ask me?
     P: No . . . they will probably come later . . . after you have left.

144. I: How did you feel during the interview?
     P: Oh, . . . it was okay. I feel you understand what's going on with me . . .

Q. 126–44:

Rapport: To submit to testing requires that the patient trusts the interviewer. Therefore, he prepares her for it and asks for permission (Q. 126). He also prepares her for memory testing (Q. 127) and gets her permission. She agrees without hesitation to be tested which confirms that the interviewer and the patient have good rapport. A. 144 assures the interviewer that the patient experiences him as an empathic listener and expert.

Mental Status: Even though the patient shows by the way she reports her history that she has adequate concentration, memory, normal sentence structure, and flow of speech, indicating at least average intelligence, the interviewer decides to obtain some quantitative measures of functions to document her baseline performance. The patient can repeat four words immediately and recall them after a few minutes. Her series seven backwards shows some mild difficulties with concentration; she makes two mistakes but immediately corrects them herself. Her IQ according to the RAIT is in the normal range.

Technique: The interviewer introduces phase 5 by summarizing what he has learned and what he is missing, thus preparing her for testing. He justifies testing by referring to her earlier remarks about her forgetfulness (Q. 126–27).

At the end of this section, the interviewer asks the patient about her feelings during the interview. This shift from data collection to rapport serves two purposes: it concludes the interview, and gives the patient a chance to reflect about it (Q. 144).

Diagnosis: At the beginning of phase 3 the interviewer had excluded substance abuse, alcoholism, obsessive compulsive, panic, and somatization disorder. He ponders whether besides borderline, or histrionic personality disorder, cyclothymic disorder may have preceded her more severe depression. The patient's report of at least two-year intervals between mild but noticeable symptoms of depression exclude however cyclothymia. Her stable marriage and absence of repeated suicide attempts exclude both personality disorders.

Phase 6: Feedback

145. I: Let me tell you then what I have learned so far. What you described to me sounds like depressive episodes. They seem to get longer and more severe as time goes on. Does that make sense? Do you have any questions about that?
   P: I understand that. But what brings them on? Why do I have them?

146. I: You think it is your work and what happens at home, or your poor sleep. But what makes you sleep more poorly in the first place?
   P: Hmm . . . , but there isn't anything . . . maybe my thoughts . . .

147. I: Yes, maybe they change also because you get depressed.
   P: But why do I get depressed?

148. I: I really don't know. All we know is that depression runs in families.
   P: The children learn it from their parents?

149. I: Well, we don't think so. Even when parents with this disorder have their children adopted at birth by another family, these adopted children can develop the same disorder as their biological parents.
   P: Hmm, I see.

150. I: Adoptees from healthy parents don't have that risk. Therefore we believe that a disposition for psychiatric disorders is inherited.
     P: So, it's all inherited?

151. I: That's probably not the whole story. The environment, such as the upbringing, may contribute to the outbreak and the severity of the disorder.
     P: So, what can you do for me if I was born with it?

Q. 145–51:

Rapport: Phase 6 reveals that the patient accepts the interviewer's expertise. She shows interest in his explanation of her disorder which may lower the risk for suicide. Toward the end of the interview, the interviewer challenges again the patient's insight into her disorder and attempts to use educational therapy for the understanding of her disorder. This improved insight may assure cooperation with treatment.

Mental Status: Mrs. Goodman's partial insight can be corrected by educational efforts which shows that she is not delusionally fixed.

Technique: The interviewer gives a comprehensive, easy-to-understand explanation of the patient's disorder in the hope that this explanation will aid in her cooperation with treatment. He finishes his explanations with questions that invite her to ask questions of her own so that he can check her understanding of his clarification. This technique works; the patient responds with several questions (A. 145, 147, 148, 150, 151).

Diagnosis: Her interest in her treatment may be considered a good prognostic sign, since major depression shows good response to treatment if the patient is compliant.

Phase 7: Treatment Contract

152. I: There is medication that helps you to overcome your depression faster; you may have heard the name of some of these drugs. They are called antidepressants.
     P: I don't know ... sounds familiar. Does that mean I have a chemical imbalance? That's what one of my friends was told who had depressions.

153. I: Some psychiatrists feel that there is an imbalance, since drugs work on depressive disorder.
     P: What should I do?

154. I: I'm worried about your overdose ... I'm also concerned that you still feel pretty bad. You also appear worried and puzzled, even though your thinking is pretty clear and your speech sounds good to me. Therefore I would really like you to stay in the hospital for a while, relax, and have us take care of you. Since I'm in the hospital all the time, I could also see you in the morning and evening to get a feeling for your daily mood swings.

    P: Do I really need to stay in the hospital?

155. I: Here we can better watch out for you, we also can give you a higher dosage of medication at the beginning. Hopefully, this will make you feel better faster. That's really what I would recommend.

    P: If you think so, I'll do it.

156. I: That's the right first step in my opinion. As we get on with your treatment I will tell you more about your condition, the medication, and its side effects, and we will also talk about some other problems that you may have.

    P: OK. I'll go along with it.

Q. 152–56:

Rapport: The interviewer explains the treatment plan using an educational approach which will help to establish his role as expert. But he also talks about his concerns for her and what steps should be taken. Specifically, he recommends extended hospitalization and justifies it by pointing out the advantages for the patient. Thus, he asks her implicitly to accept his *authority* by following his advice. For a patient with some insight into her condition, a good justification for the treatment plan is to inform her about its advantages. Her response shows that she is willing to accept the plan.

Mental Status: The patient has insight and is interested enough in her health to agree to the treatment plan. Her judgment is functioning so that the prognosis for her cooperation with treatment is good.

Technique: In phase 7 the interviewer explains the treatment plan but makes sure that the patient stays in a questioning mode as an indication of her interest. He expresses personal concern for her well-being (Q. 154), thus motivating her to agree to the treatment plan.

Diagnosis: The patient's collaboration with the treatment plan improves the prognosis for her condition. Her lack of histrionic display during any interview phase excludes histrionic personality disorder which was initially suggested by her overdose. At the end of the interview, list no. 1 of included disorders is:

1. Major depressive disorder
2. Bipolar disorder NOS (bipolar II)

List no. 2 of excluded or unlikely disorders is:

1. Bipolar disorder
2. Substance abuse
3. Obsessive compulsive disorder
4. Somatization disorder
5. Panic disorder
6. Adjustment disorder with depressed mood
7. Dysthymic disorder
8. Cyclothymic disorder
9. Histrionic personality disorder
10. Borderline personality disorder
11. Obsessive compulsive personality disorder.

Case Summary

Identifying Data

This is the first psychiatric admission for Mrs. Goodman, a 29-year-old, white female who was brought to the emergency room by her husband because of an overdose.

Informants: The patient, who is reliable and cooperative.

History of Present Illness: The patient has experienced mood swings of short duration and mild intensity, separated by several years since her late teenage years. Episodes of elated mood, reduced need for sleep, increased energy and talkativeness alternate with short periods of depression, irritability, and social withdrawal. None of these mood swings impaired the patient either in her normal functions or to such an extent that treatment was necessary.

Approximately six weeks ago, the patient was put under increased pressure at work. At this time she experienced family problems, irritability, insomnia with early morning awakenings, anorexia, weight loss of 30 pounds over six weeks, obsessive worries, brief auditory hallucinations of somebody calling her name, and social withdrawal. Her feelings of depression became so intense that she overdosed on aspirin in order to get relief from these depressive feelings. The overdose led to the present hospitalization. The affective disorder was not complicated by alcohol or drug abuse.

Medical History: Negative, except for occasional headaches.

Social History and Premorbid Personality: The patient was an outgoing and popular student with average scholastic accomplishments and without disciplinary problems. She completed high school successfully. She is currently married but experiences discontent in this marriage.

Family History: The patient has eleven first-degree relatives. Only one of three sisters had a psychiatric hospitalization which was followed by apparent recovery.

Mental Status: At the time of the interview the patient is a slightly disheveled, 29-year-old, white, alert female who is initially hostile but cooperates later and is concentrated throughout the interview, showing good comprehension. She is fully oriented, with recent and remote memory intact. Her speech is goal-oriented. Her affect and mood are depressed, appropriate, and stable, with restricted range of affective expression.

Past auditory and visual hallucinatory experiences were of brief duration with some insight into their morbid nature. Some obsessive worries and fears may still be present, but the patient refuses to elaborate on them.

The patient is not homocidal or suicidal at the present time.

She has partial insight; it is somewhat impaired concerning the impact of her job on her depression. Her judgment seems to be adequate at the present time.

Impression: Major depression.

Differential Diagnosis: Rule out bipolar disorder NOS.

Treatment Plan: Because of good premorbid personality, remission of symptoms is expected as a result of treatment with antidepressants. Marriage counseling is advisable to determine to what extent the affective disorder contributes to marriage difficulties.

Prognosis: Excellent for symptom remission.

DSM-III-R Coding: Major depressive disorder single episode, moderate 296.22. Depressed mood is present for at least six weeks; also loss of appetite, insomnia, agitation, diminished ability to concentrate, indecisiveness at work, and a suicidal gesture (criterion A). There is no evidence for any organic factors or uncomplicated bereavement (criterion B), no evidence for mood-incongruent delusions or hallucinations (criterion C), schizophrenia, schizophreniform, delusional disorder, or psychotic disorder NOS. Therefore, criteria A–D of DSM-III-R for major depressive episode are satisfied.

The longitudinal course of the illness appears to be episodic which is consistent with an affective disorder. Furthermore, there is no evidence of any other disorder which could challenge the diagnosis, such as organic mental disorder, drug or alcohol abuse. The obsessive features mentioned by the patient are not sufficient to make the diagnosis of obsessive compulsive disorder but could be followed up further. The anxiety feelings represent, at best, an isolated panic attack NOS during a depression, rather than an independent disorder.

2. SECOND INTERVIEW

This interview is with Miss Kelly Jasmin, a 19-year-old, white, slender female. She was referred for a diagnostic evaluation by another psychiatrist in whose office the interview takes place. This office is adjacent to a psychiatric hospital. It is 8 o'clock on a Monday morning in St. Louis, Missouri; the interviewer is aware that he is tired, which affects his interview.

The patient sits slumped over her crossed legs in the waiting area and does not look up when the interviewer enters. She wears a long-sleeved blouse over skintight pants tucked into boots—all black. Necklaces with big pendants and oversized rings decorate her. Her black hair is spiked, colored red at the tips, and shaved around the ears—completing the punk look.

She looks up only after the interviewer addresses her. Her face is white with makeup; her eyebrows are plucked to a thin line.

Phase 1: Warm-up

1. I: Hi, Miss Jasmin. My name is Dr. O. I'm glad you came over this morning.
   P: Hi.

2. I: (While walking with the patient to the interviewing room.) You are still over in the inpatient unit, Miss Jasmin?
   P: No.

3. I: Oh?
   P: (Gives a hostile look.)

4. I: I thought you were still on the inpatient unit and came over here on a pass.
   P: No.

5. I: So Dr. A. must have discharged you after I talked to him last.
   P: He discharged me last Saturday.

6. I: (Entering the interviewing room.) Please come in and have a seat.
   P: (Patient sits down without a word.)

7. I: Can I get you anything, a coffee maybe?
   P: No. (At this point the interviewer notices that the patient has placed an open coke can on his desk which she must have held in her left hand when he approached her from the right in the waiting room.) May I smoke?

8. I: Sure, go right ahead. Here is an ashtray.
   P: Thanks.

9. I: Before we start, what would you like me to call you?
   P: Kelly is fine.

Q. 1–9:

Rapport: The interviewer notices the patient's inattention and indifference when he enters the waiting room. He decides not to confront her with this displayed lack of interest, nor to address it indirectly by asking her, for instance:

"How did you feel about Dr. A. asking you to come over here this morning?"

but to wait until he can decide whether the patient's indifference results from being initially uncomfortable with him, from having a negative transference to him, or from a major psychiatric or personality disorder. Instead of a confrontation, he attempts to warm up the patient by reviewing the circumstances of the referral. Unfortunately, he is not up-to-date, prompting the patient to correct him with a minimum of words.

Rapport is not improved when the interviewer offers her a beverage because he had overlooked the patient's coke can on his desk. Thus, his offer appears to be routine rather than genuine concern for her comfort.

Not being up-to-date on the patient's status and the oversight of the coke would not matter if the patient is eager to talk about her problems. However, this is not the case. It remains the interviewer's task to establish rapport by tapping her suffering.

Mental Status: Observation of the patient's attire suggests that she attempts to set herself apart from mainstream teenage fashion, possibly protesting against social norms and/or searching for her identity. This may indicate that her social judgment is impaired, or that she belongs to a subculture where a punk look is the accepted uniform.

Her psychomotor movements appear normal except for the lack of a reactive movement—such as looking up—when the interviewer enters the small waiting area.

During the brief conversation it becomes apparent that she understands all questions, and answers them appropriately, indicating adequate information processing, and without any indication for a thought disorder.

Her affect appears to be restricted because she is indifferent to the interviewer and the topic of the interview, merely going through the process without being emotionally engaged.

She comes for the appointment unescorted and she recalls her discharge day which is incompatible with severe anxiety, gross uncontrolled psychotic excitement, and disorientation to time and place (list no. 3).

Technique: The interviewer goes through the formalities of introduction. He reviews the circumstances of the referral and asks the patient how she wants to be addressed.

Diagnosis: The patient's attire together with her lack of a reactive movement when the interviewer enters the waiting room and her emotionally restricted response during the warm-up period suggest, besides situationally determined poor rapport, several psychiatric disorders for list no. 1:

Major psychiatric disorders:

Drug intoxication or withdrawal
Schizophrenia
Bipolar disorder, depressed
Major depressive disorder

Personality disorders:

Paranoid
Schizoid
Schizotypal
Antisocial
Avoidant.

It excludes (list no. 2) possibly:

Bipolar disorder, manic
Dependent personality disorder.

Phase 2: Screening of the Problem

10. I: Has Dr. A. told you what this visit with me is all about?
    P: Yeah. (Looking at the interviewer with a blank facial expression.)

11. I: What did he tell you?
    P: Just what you think about me (blank look).

12. I: Think about . . . (waiting)? Think about what?
    P: (The patient answers quickly without a change in tone) About me cutting myself.

13. I: Yes, he told me he was puzzled.
    P: (The patient shrugs her shoulders and looks down at her knees.)

14. I: What do *you* think about it?
    P: (With a blank facial expression.) Nothing.

15. I: Would you like to talk about it?
    P: (Shrugs her shoulders.) It's OK, I guess.

16. I: When was the last time that you did it?
    P: (Patient looks up at the interviewer.) Wednesday, the day before I came to the hospital.

17. I: Why don't you tell me all that happened during the day when you cut yourself?
    P: I got mad at myself. (No change in facial expression, posture, gestures or intonation.) I was angry.

18. I: Angry. . . ?
    P: Yeah.

19. I: Angry about what?
    P: About not getting anywhere.

20. I: Hmm . . . Sounds like (pause) . . . you felt stuck?
    P: Yeah. (The patient looks bored.)

Q. 10–20:

Rapport: To establish rapport, the interviewer probes whether the patient has been adequately informed about the reasons for the referral (Q. 10–12). This topic does not establish rapport. At this point the interviewer could have continued to ask the patient whether she thought Dr. A.'s idea to seek a second opinion was a good one. This might have caused her to ventilate her feelings about the present interview and to possibly open up. Instead, the interviewer assumes that the patient's cutting is her chief complaint and the center of her suffering. Therefore, he focuses on the emotions that may underlie her self-mutilation. He echoes her emotion (Q. 19) and gives a summarizing interpretation (Q. 20). However, the patient's affect remains restricted and her verbal elaborations scarce.

Mental Status: The patient is cooperative enough to talk about herself, which allows a progression from conversation to exploration of her current and past problems. Her verbal production shows poverty of response without prolonged latency. Her affect as expressed in face, gestures, and intonation remains restricted.

Technique: The interviewer uses four open-ended questions (Q. 11, 12, 14, 17) which are all answered with a short sentence or a single word. When the patient expresses a feeling (A. 17), he echoes this feeling in a client-centered manner (A. 18, 19) and attempts an interpretation. These techniques do not initiate a spontaneous free flow of information.

Diagnosis: The interviewer decides not to address any of the three diagnostic clues (attire, lack of reactive movement, restricted emotional response) observed during the warm-up period. Instead, he attempts to tackle the patient's chief complaint which appears to be wrist cutting. As we shall see later, wrist cutting is more of concern to the referring psychiatrist than to the patient. However, at this point, the interviewer does not pick up on this, mainly because wrist cutting impresses him, too, as significant psychopathology. The fact of wrist cutting supports two diagnostic options considered above (list no. 1):

bipolar disorder, depressed
major depression with suicidal ideation

It adds two other diagnostic options:

adjustment disorder
borderline personality disorder,

and excludes none of the disorders considered above.

21. I: Can you tell me more about it?
    P: I don't know. Just with my grades in college.

22. I: Your grades in college . . . which college do you attend?
    P: The XXX community college.

23. I: Hmm . . . What's your major?
    P: I haven't declared one.

24. I: What do you take?
    P: Sculpture (pause). . . , painting (pause). . . , writing . . .

25. I: And what kind of grades do you get?
    P: A's and B's.

26. I: Sounds pretty good to me.
    P: I got a C in weaving. (The patient draws down the corners of her mouth.)

27. I: How did you feel about that?
    P: Fine, I guess. (The patient shrugs her shoulders.)

28. I: (Displaying surprise in his voice and facial expression.) What did you expect to get?
    P: At the beginning, a C is fine. There's a lot of technique involved (in weaving).

29. I: So you are really doing all right?
    P: (Silence.)

30. I: Then . . . what made you cut yourself?
    P: Just . . . in general.

31. I: I don't understand. Can you explain?
    P: (No change in voice or facial expression.) I was just mad.

Q. 21–31:

Rapport: The interviewer tries to bring to light frustrating situations that may result in the patient cutting herself, thus getting to the core of her despair. But he draws a blank. No emotional outpouring occurs. Instead, she gives some longer but mainly factual answers. He attempts a positive feedback by telling her that he thinks her grades are good (Q. 26). But the praise yields merely the report of a C in weaving. Overall, her answers express reluctance, without overt resistance or refusal to speak.

Mental Status: The patient shows ambivalence; she expresses concern about her college grades, but then contradicts herself and reports good grades and satisfaction with a C. This ambivalence reveals an illogical aspect of her judgment. Eugen Bleuler (Bleuler 1972) considered ambivalence as a symptom of schizophrenia which is, however, not empirically established.

Technique: Open-ended Q. 21 produces only a vague answer. Follow-up results in a nonconvincing series of answers which does not explain satisfactorily her wrist cutting. Thus, the fact-oriented questions produce diagnostically useless results, yet the interviewer pursues them in the expectation of hitting on a topic that might help to initiate a more spontaneous and productive flow of information. Positive feedback (Q. 26) and two open-ended questions (Q. 27, 28) directed at assessing her feelings about a mediocre grade in school, followed by summarizing of her feelings, leave the interview on the one-sentence answer level. Probing for the motifs of her cutting (Q. 30, 31) produce only superficial answers not revealing a plausible motif. In full circle, the interviewer returns to the topic of cutting without having learned anything significant about the underlying psychopathology.

Diagnosis: The patient's answers do not point to any stressor necessary for the diagnosis of adjustment disorder. Her reluctance to volunteer information may suggest the presence of passive aggressive personality disorder. Her ambivalance about her grades underscores as diagnostic options schizophrenia, and/or any of the personality disorders of cluster A in DSM-III-R.

Phase 3: Verification of Diagnostic Impressions

32. I: Any other feelings?
    P: No.

33. I: Did you feel, in any way, down?
    P: No.

34. I: Any other problems?
    P: I don't know.

35. I: How was your sleep during that time?
    P: Okay.

36. I: And your appetite?
    P: Fine.

37. I: Any problems with eating at all?
    P: Sometimes

38. I: What kind of problems?
    P: Sometimes I eat too much.

39. I: Do you do anything about it?
    P: Like what?

40. I: Did you ever try to starve yourself?
    P: Maybe for a day or so.

41. I: Did you ever do anything else—like trying to vomit?
    P: Yeah, a couple of times but it didn't work.

42. I: What types of things do you eat when you eat too much?
    P: Pretty good food. Lots of fruits and vegetables.

43. I: So you ate all right and slept fine when you cut yourself.
    P: I guess.

44. I: Was anything else going on?
    P: (Just looks at the interviewer, then takes out a cigarette and lights it.)

45. I: Anything with your friends? Or your boyfriend?
    P: No, we were fine.

46. I: What were you then thinking when you were cutting yourself?
    P: I was just mad. (No change in tone of voice or facial expression.)

47. I: Mad? Mad enough to die?
    P: No. Just to cut myself.

48. I: Do you have any idea why you did it?
    P: I was angry.

49. I: About. . . ?
    P: Myself.

50. I: So you cut yourself when you are angry about yourself?
    P: Yeah, and about others too.

Q. 32–50:

Rapport: The interviewer resigns himself to assessing symptoms of major psychiatric disorders that could explain the cutting in the hope that he would hit on symptoms which would mobilize the patient's emotions and help to improve rapport. Neither the topics of depressive symptoms and eating disorder nor open-ended questions enhance rapport and induce more spontaneity.

Mental Status: The patient reports her arm cutting in a matter-of-fact way. Her affect appears blunted; she displays an inappropriate distance to her maladjusted behavior. She indicates overeating and an attempt to induce vomiting. However, unlike a patient with bulimia, she is not eating junk food but "lots of fruits and vegetables." Overeating on those appears to be bizarre and points toward an ambivalence about her eating habits.

Technique: The interviewer checks out whether depressive symptoms were associated with the wrist cutting. If he keeps the symptom-oriented questions open, the patient makes him specify (Q. and A. 39), or answers them with yes or no as if they were closed-ended (A. 32, 35, 36, 45). The two summary statements (Q. 43 and 50) are met with vague consent which leaves it doubtful whether these summaries establish any facts.

Diagnosis: The interviewer is aware that the patient is only reluctantly cooperative with him and shows no spontaneity. He decides to verify or exclude some diagnostic options which may be associated with the self-mutilation. First, he focuses on depression; however, most depressive symptoms are denied for the time of the last arm cutting, excluding depressive disorder as an explanation. The interviewer branches into the assessment of bulimia nervosa. A. 36–43 exclude that disorder.

During this section, the interviewer notices that the patient's affect appears most consistent with schizophrenia, and/or any of the personality disorders of cluster A in DSM-III-R.

51. I: Tell me what you do when you are angry.
    P: I take a razor blade and keep cutting myself.

52. I: And then?
    P: (In a matter-of-fact way.) Then I clean the wounds.

53. I: Yes. . .?
    P: With alcohol.

54. I: Yes . . . ?
    P: I sometimes put some Band-Aids on.

55. I: Hmm . . .
    P: Or I just roll down my sleeves.

56. I: How do you feel then?
    P: I don't know.

57. I: Do you feel any different afterwards?
    P: (Without displaying any emotion.) A little better, maybe.

58. I: Is this like punishing yourself?
    P: Getting rid of the tension.

59. I: And does it work?
    P: A little.

60. I: Can I see your arms?
    P: (Patient rolls up her left sleeve exposing the forearm. One red scar down along the forearm is visible besides seven or eight pale old scars. The patient points at the red scar.) That's where I cut myself last.

61. I: Hmm . . . I see some other scars too.
     P: I have some on the other arm too. (She rolls up her right sleeve and exposes a forearm covered with scars running 2 to 3 inches in length.)

62. I: You must really go through a lot, that you feel you have to cut yourself so often.
     P: (No answer and no change in posture, gestures, or facial expression.)

63. I: How do you feel about that?
     P: (Patient shrugs her shoulders.)

64. I: How often does it happen?
     P: About every two months. (Her face remains motionless; the inflection of her voice does not change.)

65. I: Since when have you been doing it?
     P: For the last two years, since I was 17. (Throughout, the patient's face remains expressionless and she reports her self-mutilation in a matter-of-fact way.)

Q. 51–65:

Rapport: The interviewer switches from assessing the motivation for the cutting to the process of the cutting per se. But the patient's report does not revive anger, pain, hurt, guilt or satisfaction. Her report remains factual and emotionless.

Mental Status: The patient's affect is blunted which, in isolation, could be interpreted as *la belle indifférence*. However, a dramatic presentation of life events, ill fate, or other symptoms which usually are associated with *la belle indifférence* is missing. The patient shows no psychomotor retardation; she talks and moves at normal rate.

Technique: The interviewer stays with the topic of arm cutting. By continuation technique he assesses the temporal course of an isolated cutting, the pattern of cuttings over a longer time period, and the associated feelings. He expresses empathy at the end of this assessment (Q. 62); but both techniques fail to induce spontaneous elaborations.

Diagnosis: The interviewer remains impressed by the patient's blunted affect. He considers whether this nonchalant attitude is an expression of true blunting, or a displayed, so-called *la belle indifférence* which is sometimes described as characteristic of hysteria (somatization disorder in DSM-III-R), or histrionic personality disorder. The pattern of frequent arm cutting, whenever the patient feels frustrated and angry, supports the previously considered presence of a borderline personality disorder.

66. I: You must really go through a lot of tension.
    P: Just normal.

67. I: Have you ever cut yourself when you have problems with your boy-friend?
    P: Yes. With my last one.

68. I: When was that?
    P: About nine months ago.

69. I: What happened then?
    P: We broke up.

70. I: How did that make you feel?
    P: Bad.

71. I: Who broke up?
    P: He did.

72. I: And why?
    P: He said, he has to get clear with himself and he doesn't want to have the responsibility of a girlfriend.

73. I: How did you feel then when he said that?
    P: (Emotionless.) Devastated.

74. I: Were there any other changes?
    P: I slept more.

Q. 66–74:

Rapport: The interviewer attempts to improve rapport by expressing empathy for the patient's assumed suffering (Q. 66). Obviously, he does not tap it; the expression of empathy does not improve rapport—interviewer and patient stay aloof. Up to this point, none of the interviewer's techniques has established emotional rapport: open-ended questions, reflection on, echoing of the patient's feelings (Q. 18–20), positive feedback (Q. 26), or expression of empathy (Q. 62 and 66).

Mental Status: Neither the expression of empathy nor the review of a stressful life event expand the patient's restricted affect. No increase in latency of response occurs which could indicate psychomotor retardation and depressed mood rather than blunted affect.

Technique: The interviewer makes a smooth transition; he focuses on the patient's relationship with her boyfriend to evaluate its intensity. She appears to have intense feelings for at least one of her boyfriends; however, the assessment of this emotionally laden topic does not result in a spontaneous verbal eruption.

Diagnosis: Following up on the impression that the patient may have a borderline personality disorder, the interviewer focuses on her intense and unstable relationship with her last boyfriend. However, an emotional ambivalence in the present relationship (which is thought to be a characteristic of borderline personality disorder) is not apparent.

The previously discarded option of an adjustment disorder resurfaces for the time period of the breakup with her last boyfriend (A. 73 and 74). However, it cannot explain the repeated self-mutilation which is more consistent with a major psychiatric disorder or a personality disorder.

75. I: Were you down so much that you started to hear things that were not really there?
    P: (Patient hesitates.)

76. I: Like voices?
    P: A couple of times, maybe.

77. I: Can you describe them?
    P: Somebody called my name a few times.

78. I: Any other voices?
    P: Maybe.

79. I: Hmm . . .
    P: Just my thoughts.

80. I: Do you hear them now?
    P: They are just inside my head.

81. I: Do they sound like a voice?
    P: Just like my own.

Q. 75–81:

Rapport: The patient neither hesitates nor appears embarrassed when she talks about her voices. This suggests that she is as open as her emotional disturbance permits her to be, and that it is this disturbance which prevents her from being emotionally more engaged, or more detailed about her problems.

Mental Status: The patient admits to having phonemes which are voices inside her head. They seem to occur only occasionally without being intrusive.

Technique: The interviewer checks for psychotic symptoms associated with the breakup of her relationship.

Diagnosis: The interviewer probes whether a major depression was associated with the breakup. The breakup could either have been caused by a depressive episode, or could have been a precipitating event for a depression. The interviewer focuses on hallucinatory experiences because, if present, they would clearly exclude an adjustment disorder. Indeed, he gets a report of some hallucinatory experiences. It is, however, not clear whether these experiences were associated with the breakup and therefore indicate a brief psychotic episode, or whether they were related to a major depression, or are even present on a more permanent basis as in schizophrenia or borderline personality.

82. I: When this happened, did you take any street drugs?
    P: Not lately.

83. I: And before that? What did you take?
    P: Everything.

84. I: Like what?
    P: Oh, speed, pot, downers, hashish, crystals, bennies, heroin, cocaine, mushrooms.

85. I: Yeah . . .
    P: Lots of alcohol too.

86. I: For how long?
    P: For a few months or so.

87. I: When was the last time that you took it?
    P: Not since I broke up with my boyfriend. He was very much into that.

88. I: Did you like any of these drugs more than others?
    P: I liked them all.

89. I: Do you do any with your present boyfriend?
    P: No.

Q. 82–89:

Rapport: In this section the interviewer does not make any effort to improve rapport. He stays with a symptom-collecting approach which enables him to include and exclude disorders without the benefit of the patient's spontaneity and a genuine affective expression of her suffering. He enjoys a rapport comparable to that of a computer program which checks off symptoms and diagnostic criteria.

Mental Status: The fact that the patient took different types of street drugs indiscriminantly in the past but not at present—because her former boyfriend was a drug abuser—underscores her field dependence and her vulnerability to being influenced by others.

Technique: The admission of psychotic symptoms leads the interviewer to assess possible causes for the hallucinations. Therefore, he assesses essential symptoms of drug and alcohol abuse.

Diagnosis: The patient admits to a period of indiscriminate polydrug abuse. Her former boyfriend seems to have exposed her to street drugs which the patient did not continue to abuse after she broke off with him. Her drug abuse is therefore a *folie à deux* and reveals more her dependency on and suggestability by others than an autochthonic abuse disorder. Her wrist cutting is not limited to the periods of substance abuse; therefore, the abuse is not responsible for the cutting.

90. I: How are you getting along with him?
    P: Fine.

91. I: Can you describe this relationship?
    P: We are getting too close.

92. I: Do you love him?
    P: Yeah.

93. I: Do you have any other feelings for him besides love?
    P: (Takes a puff from her cigarette and then swallows.)

94. I: Do you fight?
    P: We argue a lot.

95. I: Have you ever hurt each other?
    P: Not physically.

96. I: Are you jealous of him?
    P: Only if he is jealous of me.

97. I: You said you were too close?
    P: Yeah, we were together all the time. We did not see anybody else.

98. I: And?
    P: We are going to change this now. We are going to meet other people.

99. I: Do you usually have more than one boyfriend?
    P: Yes, I do. Three or four.

100. I: Do you sleep with them too?
     P: No. Just with my main boyfriend. I don't believe in sleeping with anybody else.

101. I: Has your boyfriend also girlfriends other than you?
     P: Usually not.

102. I: And if he does?
   P: It hurts a little . . . but not any more.

103. I: Not any more?
   P: No, I do the same thing.

104. I: Is there a reason why you like more than one boyfriend?
   P: I'm getting too close if I have only one. I can't handle it.

105. I: Have you ever cut yourself because of your boyfriend?
   P: Yes, two months ago.

106. I: Would you like to talk about it?
   P: No, not really.

Q. 90–106:

Rapport: The interviewer talks about her relationship with her boyfriend. This potentially personal and intimate topic does not engage her emotionally. Notice that the patient does not treat the interviewer as an empathic listener in whom she confides, nor does she treat him as an expert who can help her fix what's wrong. She relates to him as if he is a hostile, interrogating authority with whom she has to comply.

Mental Status: It appears that the patient can become very dependent on a boyfriend, and is also capable of developing an intense relationship. She seems to be unable to handle the intensity of these feelings and escapes into alternate relationships without becoming promiscuous.

Technique: The interviewer makes a smooth transition from past to current drug abuse which she denies. He invites her to describe her relationship with her current boyfriend but ends up with a one-sentence answer. Frustrated, he continues to get a feeling for this relationship by using closed-ended questions. Interviewing a patient about a close relationship often results in emotionally laden verbal outpour, but not so here.

Diagnosis: Up to this point the patient shows an acceptable college record. Her drug abuse is limited to the duration of the relationship with the last boyfriend only, and she denies promiscuity. All three facts seem to exclude antisocial personality. The interviewer explores whether the patient is predominantly involved in intense but ambivalent heterosexual relationships which would point to borderline personality. The patient admits indeed that she gets very close to her partners and may get so angry that she cuts herself. This report is however obtained in a piecemeal fashion; it lacks spontaneity to be taken as a testimony for an intense ambivalent relationship. Therefore, it remains questionable whether the patient's behavior indeed fulfills criteria for borderline personality disorder.

107. I: I notice that most of the time you just answer my questions, but you don't want to talk about it on your own.
      P: That's right.

108. I: How does it make you feel talking to me?
      P: Just nervous and tense.

109. I: Yes, I noticed that. Is there any reason why you feel so tense when you talk about these things.
      P: I don't know, I just don't like it, I guess.

110. I: Anything that concerns you?
      P: Yes.

111. I: What is it?
      P: I'm not getting anywhere. I wiggle all the time. I cut myself. And I get those downs.

112. I: So that is what you are concerned about?
      P: My mother is.

113. I: How are you getting along with her?
      P: Fine.

Q. 107–13:

Rapport: The interviewer confronts the patient directly with her unwillingness to talk about her problems and tries to assess the reason of her resistance, but the patient does not come up with an explanation. From an analytical point of view, her admission of nervousness and tension would suggest that defense mechanisms are at work. From a descriptive point of view, it may indicate that a major psychiatric or personality disorder interferes with rapport (see below).

From a role point of view, the interviewer attempts to shed the role of an interrogating authority by confronting the patient with her resistance, hoping she may accept him more as an empathic listener, but he fails to bring about this transition.

Mental Status: The patient describes that she is nervous and tense which may contribute to her guardedness. She first reports that she is concerned about wiggling, cutting, and having downs, but quickly assigns these concerns to her mother which shows that she is ambivalent about her problems and has only partial insight.

Technique: The interviewer confronts the patient with her resistance to elaborate freely (see *Rapport*).

Diagnosis: The patient's downs introduce a new diagnostic element. Depressive disorder was already excluded previously as a sufficient reason for the cutting. But the patient's report of downs raises the possibility of depressions occurring independent from the cutting. This possibility warrants further follow-up.

114. I: Do you also think there is anything wrong with you?
     P: Maybe the lows. I don't like the lows.

115. I: Has anything helped you with the lows?
     P: Maybe the Tofranil a little.

116. I: When you are low, in what way are you changed?
     P: I sleep more. Don't want to do anything.

117. I: Anything else?
     P: That's it.

118. I: Do you still care what you look like when you are down?
     P: Usually not.

119. I: Anything different with your friends when you are low?
     P: I don't think so.

120. I: Do you stay away from them?
     P: No, not really.

121. I: Do you still enjoy sex?
     P: Yes.

122. I: Even when you are down?
     P: (Emphatically.) I enjoy it a lot.

123. I: Do you care for other people when you are depressed?
     P: Yes, I do.

124. I: Who are you close to?
     P: My mother, my sister, my stepfather, and my real father.

125. I: Anybody else?
     P: (Shrugs her shoulders.)

126. I: You did not mention your boyfriend.
     P: (Patient swallows.)

127. I: I notice you swallowed.
     P: (Blushes.) I just didn't get around to him.

128. I: Hmm. How do you feel about him now?
   P: I'm a little mad. But it's really okay.

129. I: How are you getting along with your stepfather?
   P: I stay away from him.

130. I: Hmm.
   P: I stay away from him. He is an alcoholic and he shouts a lot.

131. I: Has he ever abused you?
   P: No, just screamed a lot.

132. I: How about your real father?
   P: He's in Austin.

133. I: When did he last live with you?
   P: When I was real little.

134. I: You say you have some lows. Does anybody else in your family have lows?
   P: My mother does.

135. I: Anybody else?
   P: (Patient shrugs her shoulders.)

Q. 114–35:

Rapport: The interviewer attempts to get the patient's view of her disorder (Q. 114). This question produces a two-sentence answer, an admission that she suffers from lows. However, the follow-up does not induce the patient to elaborate spontaneously, nor to become emotionally involved. Instead, she returns to short, one-sentence answers.

Up to this point, the patient's lack of emotional involvement suggests three interpretations:

1. The interviewer has not tapped the patient's suffering—probably because he mistook her initial report of the cuttings as her true chief complaint, and therefore, he has no access to material that is of emotional importance to her.
2. It is possible that the subject of cutting is emotionally highly charged and anxiety-provoking for the patient. Therefore, she uses the defense mechanisms of denial or isolation to defend herself against feelings that would otherwise overwhelm her.
3. The patient has a disorder characterized by a blunted affect (see below *Diagnosis*).

Mental Status: The patient shows an emotional response when she emphasizes that she enjoys sex even when depressed. She also shows an affective change when the interviewer confronts her with not mentioning her boyfriend as a person she cares about. This reveals that she has some emotional engagement in her main heterosexual relationship.

Technique: The interviewer, frustrated with the patient's short answers attempts again (Q. 116) an open-ended question followed up with "anything else?" (Q. 117). But the patient replies "That's it." To get more data the interviewer resorts to symptom-oriented, circumscribed even though open-ended questions. They produce short, appropriate answers limited to a minimum of information, making the interview boring and dry; every detail is pried out of the patient.

Diagnosis: The patient admits to low mood, low energy, hypersomnia, some neglect in dressing and hygiene, but no decrease of sex drive or social withdrawal. The interviewer does not assess enough symptoms to establish the diagnosis of major depression, over dysthymia. He obtains some evidence for a positive family history of a mood disorder in the patient's mother.

136. I: I asked you a lot of questions. Is there any question that I can answer for you?
     P: (Patient leans forward, emphatically.) Yes. Can Dr. A. or you ever diagnose me? (With emphasis and determination in her voice) I want to know what my diagnosis is. Do you know?

137. I: Very good . . . So you would really like to know what we think about you.
     P: (The patient's facial expression appears animated, and with her left hand she taps on the desk.) Oh yes, very much. Can you tell me what you think about me?

138. I: Well, I don't know enough about you yet, but if you help me . . . You said already that you have some lows and that you don't like to have them. I have no idea how long they last.
     P: (Quickly.) Oh, up to several months. Are those real depressions?

139. I: I don't have any idea how bad they really get.
     P: Pretty bad. I feel silly, I can't do anything. I can't put my mind to anything . . . I tried to kill myself twice and I ended up in the ICU twice—I took an overdose.

140. I: We would call that a depresssion. You seem to suffer from real depressions. But I don't know whether you have real highs also.
     P: Yes, I do. They last a short time and they are not real highs. I'm full of energy, my thoughts are real fast, I can't keep up with them and I talk too fast. I don't sleep a bunch but I don't feel real good. Are these real highs?

141. I: Real negative highs! That's what a patient of mine calls them—negative highs. You seem to have them . . .
    P: That's exactly it—that's a good word.

142. I: So—experts call your condition a bipolar condition where you have both, highs and lows, but I don't really know when you have those highs.
    P: Both before and after my lows.

143. I: Besides your bipolar or manic-depressive problem, there may be something else going on. . . . But I don't know enough about it. You did not tell me enough about it . . . (Pause.) Your cutting and your getting so angry and your relationship to your boyfriends, they seem to be intense. But it doesn't seem that it is all love. Do you have some other feelings?
    P: Yes, my boyfriend—I hate it. I hate it that I get so close to him.

144. I: Hmm.
    P: I have no control over my feelings. They just come and make me do things. They make me do things that I don't want to do.

145. I: I don't know how long that has been going on.
    P: All my life.

146. I: For your diagnosis, we would probably say that you also have a personality problem, especially with your cutting.
    P: (Patient shakes her head.) But I'm not worried about my cutting. That's not my worry. I just have to stop it.

147. I: Can you?
    P: I just have to. Dr. A. told me he will put me into a State Hospital if I don't stop.

Q. 136–47:

Rapport: The interviewer asks whether the patient has any questions for him. And she does. Her first question verbalizes her worry whether the interviewer can diagnose her. This question shows that she struggles with a valid evaluation of her behavior. She experiences herself as "normal" except for the depressive episodes—but her mother criticizes her and points to her pathological features. This discrepancy between her experience of herself and her mother's criticism is the true point of suffering. As soon as the interviewer identifies this point, rapport changes dramatically; the patient spontaneously elaborates on her answers, and begins to ask questions—rapport is finally established.

What has happened? Here is an observation that Jamie Smith, ski teacher and member of the Jane Gang at Winterpark, Colorado, reported on working with children and teenagers. While riding up the Challenger skilift at 5 degrees Fahrenheit we compared notes on the teaching of nonlinear processes.

"I can't teach children and teenagers skiing until they are ready," he said. "I just ski with them, get them through the bumps, and hope that they will imitate me. Finally, they start to ask questions—How do you go so fast?—How can you turn so easy?—How do you do it? Then I know they are ready, I have their attention, they are open to listen, and I can teach them."

Jamie Smith refers to the same strategy that is so important for interviewing patients: you have to find their point of suffering. With the statement: "Do you have any questions for me?" the interviewer had tapped the patient's true point of suffering:

"What is wrong with me? Am I normal, or not?"

Retrospectively, it becomes clear that the interviewer had taken the self-mutilation as the chief complaint when it first emerged but he failed to confirm this with the patient. He mistook pathology impressive to him but not to her for her chief complaint and ended up in laborious data collection not fueled by the patient's emotional engagement.

To keep the patient aware that a diagnostic evaluation is only possible if she engages herself in the process, the interviewer introduces several of his questions with the phrase "I don't know enough about you" (Q. 139, 140, 141, 143, 144, 146). This humble reminder of his need for her cooperation stabilizes his rapport with her.

From a role point of view a transition has occurred. The interviewer is no longer treated as the interrogating authority to whom the patient was referred by her psychiatrist who in turn was backed by her mother, but as an expert who can give her some understanding about herself. Through his role as expert, he can also gain footage as empathic listener.

Mental Status: This segment shows that the patient is capable of detailed and goal-directed verbal elaboration without thought blocking, circumstantiality, or flight of ideas.

Suddenly, she shows appropriate changes in posture, gestures, facial expression, and intonation. One single question has brought about that change which shows how much she is field-dependent.

This section shows that the patient has difficulties with insight. She recognizes her mood swings but she considers only her lows as a disorder.

Technique: Often, interviewers use the technique of having the patient ask questions at the end of an interview. Here, it is used in the middle to mobilize the patient's interest in the interviewing process and to break the monotonous "short question–short answer" format. And the technique works—the patient herself starts to ask questions (A. 136–38, 140). The interviewer keeps her in this questioning mode by making statements about her which he introduces with the phrase "I don't know" which appears to animate her. It works because the interviewer has hit upon the patient's interest in the interview, her point of suffering. She is now interviewed from *her* point of view.

Diagnosis: Her true chief complaint emerges—not the cutting but her question about her normality:

"Am I crazy or not?"

She describes spontaneously (A. 139) a host of depressive symptoms of sufficient duration (A. 138) to support the diagnosis of major depression. Furthermore, she gives enough evidence (A. 140 and 142) for mania, which may precede or follow a depressive episode.

A. 143–46 suggest the possibility of borderline personality disorder supported by the ambivalent relationship to her boyfriend and by her cutting.

An alternate explanation for the cutting is that this act represents an impulse control disorder NOS. This diagnosis is suggested by the patient's statement that she feels many uncontrollable impulses; the cutting seems to be the dominating one. The interviewer has learned so far that the patient usually is angry prior to the cutting, that she feels some relief afterward and that the impulse is ego-syntonic. However, he fails to assess whether this impulse is irresistible. Also, he has not ellucidated other impulses that the patient has difficulty controlling.

148. I: So cutting does not worry you. What worries you then?
     P: That I have delusions and hallucinations.

149. I: What kind of hallucinations do you worry about?
     P: My voices.

150. I: I don't know enough about your voices to give you your diagnosis. You said before it was just your thoughts—so I don't know.
     P: No, it is like a voice that comes from the back of my head and it tells me what to do and what not to do. Is that crazy?

151. I: Hmm . . . Does it also tell you to cut yourself?
     P: It does. But that's the least that worries me. That's just one of many things. It tells me all the other things to do or not to do.

152. I: Can you turn it off?
     P: No. It's there all the time. All I can do is try to ignore it but I cannot turn it off.

153. I: Usually people can turn off a thought. So your voice is more than a thought? Is it your own voice?
     P: It is, because it comes from the inside of my head. But it does not sound like my voice.

154. I: What does it sound like?
     P: It sounds like a neutral voice. Not male, not female. It has no sex and it has no age. So it isn't really my own voice, is it?

155. I: Hmm . . . Is it there at any time of the day?
     P: Yes, mostly.

156. I: Is there more than one voice?
     P: At times there are. Then it is as if you argue back and forth with yourself. But there are many parts and they all talk back and forth. Isn't that crazy?

157. I: I don't know whether you can control them.
     P: No, they just happen to me. Should I be able to control them?

158. I: Well, are there any times when these voices occur more frequently?
     P: Yes, they are all there when I have my highs.

159. I: And when you are in a low?
     P: Then I hear my name called once or twice. That's all.

160. I: I don't know whether you have any other hallucinations besides the voices? Do you also see things?
     P: Yes.

161. I: Like what?
     P: (Puffs on her cigarette.) Funny faces.

162. I: How does my face look to you?
     P: It moves. It makes grimaces. Things pop out. Your mouth pops out. Sometimes I think I can see the atoms of everything and how they move. Everything is changing. I see movements. I can feel my thoughts. They are like electric shocks flashing through my head. Is this normal?

163. I: I don't know how bad it gets. For instance, have you ever seen blood coming out of people's faces?
     P: (After a long pause.) No, I don't think so, just parts of the face popping out.

164. I: So you have visual distortions. What happened to these distortions when
     you took street drugs?
     P: With most drugs they became more intense. Especially with acid. With
     acid things become real bright and real loud—real brilliant colors.

165. I: You also said you had delusions? What do you mean by delusions?
     P: All the time I think I will be famous one time in my life. Very famous.
     I thought this as long as I can think back. I was always convinced that
     at one time I will be famous—that I'm special. I'm convinced that I'm
     a genius. Do you believe that I'm a genius? Or is this a delusion?

166. I: Why do you think this is a delusion?
     P: My mother says so and Dr. A. thinks so. Do you think so too, or do
     you think I'm a genius?

167. I: I don't know enough about you. What do you think?
     P: I just don't know. I had these voices all my life; I had these visions all
     my life. I don't know any different.

Q. 148–67:

Rapport: This remains excellent during this section; the patient continues to elaborate freely. Spontaneously, she reveals her hallucinatory
experiences and talks about her grandiose delusions, while the interviewer displays expertise in asking the right questions which may or may
not be noticed by the patient. She appears to become more trusting in
the interviewer's expertise, as evidenced by the many questions that she
starts to ask. Her formulations and lack of guardedness suggest that now
she experiences him also as an empathic listener.

Mental Status: At present, the patient has auditory hallucinations and
visual illusions if not hallucinations. The hallucinations are congruent
neither with a depressive nor a manic mood, even though they increase
during a high. However, during a high period the patient seems to have
more hallucinatory experiences than during relative normality, or during
a depression. She has permanent grandiose delusions mood congruent
with mania. Presently, the patient is not manic. Therefore, it appears
that her hallucinations and delusions are somewhat permanent and not
limited to periods of affective disturbances. Furthermore, this section
shows her partial insight into her hallucinations and delusions which she
has difficulty in accepting as part of an illness. Her grandiose delusions
affect her judgment and impair her social adjustment and future planning.

Technique: Since the patient's interest has been tapped, as noticeable by her frequent questions (A. 150, 154, 156, 157, 162, 165, 166), open-ended questions that did not work before now produce spontaneous elaborations. Since the patient is now spontaneous, the interviewer can stay with the problems that she introduces. First, he follows up on her auditory (Q. 149–59) and then on her visual hallucinations (Q. 160–64). Thereafter, he returns to her delusions (Q. 165–67).

Diagnosis: Manic and depressive mood disturbances together with mood incongruent hallucinations fit best the diagnostic criteria of schizoaffective disorder, bipolar type. However, there exists a controversy whether this diagnosis predicts a more chronic schizophrenic-like disorder, or a more episodic, affective-like disorder. Since the bizarre thoughts and hallucinatory experiences reach back to her childhood, a personality disorder may have preceded and may underlie the schizoaffective disorder. So far, the interview reveals some evidence for a borderline and/or schizotypal personality disorder. Her intense and intimate relationships exclude schizoid personality disorder. The patient also reports neither severe jealousy nor suspiciousness which excludes paranoid personality disorder.

The patient's initial reluctance to communicate freely with the interviewer had also suggested avoidant personality disorder. But since she opened up after the interviewer tapped her source of suffering, and since he found no evidence that she is afraid of being criticized, the diagnosis of avoidant personality disorder is unlikely.

The only other coexisting disorder may be impulse control disorder NOS which would account for her arm cutting.

168. I: Artists sometimes seem to have different experiences. Vincent van Gogh, for instance, painted things as if he could see them grow. Maybe he really saw them growing. He seemed to be fascinated by light and bright colors.
    P: I see things move, move all the time. Am I a genius?

169. I: I guess when you can express how you see things so that others can see it too and can feel how you feel, you may have some part of a genius.
    P: I can express it sometimes. I have to learn more about it. I take creative writing next term. I am all excited about it.

170. I: Van Gogh hurt himself too, he cut off his ear. But I think there is one thing that bothers you about your experiences. You cannot control them.

They make you do things that you don't want to do. So, therefore, we would call some of your experiences hallucinations. Has the medicine helped with them?

P: A little.

171. I: Which one? The Tofranil or the Stelazine?

P: I don't know.

172. I: You can express your visions and your feelings sometimes?

P: Yes, sometimes.

173. I: How?

P: With my sculptures, with my poems, and maybe with paintings.

174. I: When you feel your tension coming on, when you want to cut yourself, can you put this tension on a canvas rather than on your forearms?

P: I can try.

175. I: I'm interested in how well you can express yourself. Can you bring me your poems and your pictures and whatever you think is the best you have done, where you think you have expressed yourself?

P: I will bring them.

176. I: There have been artists like van Gogh who had depressions and had to go to an asylum, and there were also psychiatric patients who often lived in mental institutions who could express their visions. Have you ever seen those paintings?

P: No.

177. I: I will bring some along and show them to you, if you like.

P: I would love that very much. (Patient smiles.)

178. I: I would like to know more about you to answer your question about diagnosis. Would you like to meet again?

P: Yes. I would like that. I would like to talk about my experiences and get your opinion about it.

179. I: That's great, Kelly. I would like to meet with you again.

Q. 168–79:

Rapport: This remains good, since the patient is interested in the artwork that the interviewer introduces toward the end of the interview. He brings up the topic of art in an attempt to show expertise in her problems by linking her experiences to her need for artistic expression. Since she feels her hallucinations and delusions are part of her existence of an artist, this topic is concordant with her level of insight. The interviewer is capable of understanding the patient's view of herself. He can adopt a vantage point that allows him to interview her from *her* viewpoint, rather than from that of an outsider who makes it apparent that whatever she reports is abnormal from his point of view. Since the patient has some interest in expressing herself artistically, the interviewer attempts to channel her impulse to cut herself into a more sublimated "acting out" in her artwork.

At the end of the interview the patient indicates that she would like to meet again. The interviewer has turned a reluctant patient—who had only followed the pressure of her referring psychiatrist to see him—into an engaged, cooperative patient.

From a role point of view, the interviewer attempts to establish himself as an authority knowledgeable in art and in the artistic expression of unusual experiences which the patient seems to accept. At the end of the session, rapport in its different aspects is established, even though the diagnostic interview is not completed with all its phases.

In an interview, you can postpone the completion of the phases and the diagnostic process at any time, but you cannot postpone the establishment of rapport, simply because the patient may not return. Therefore, if you meet a resistant patient, attempt to establish rapport within the first session even if you have to compromise the completeness of your diagnostic assessment.

Mental Status: This section highlights further the patient's impaired reality testing, her inability to judge what is a disorder and what is not, and to evaluate her creative potential.

Her punk look appears to be an attempt to establish her identity as an artist. Her ambivalence about her school record expressed at the beginning reflects her doubts about that identity. She probably compensates for her lack of success in her artistic work with an "artistic life-style."

Technique: The interviewer establishes a link between the patient's hallucinatory experiences, her need to express herself artistically, and the painter Vincent van Gogh who presumably also had a mood disorder with psychosis. This link fits well into the patient's present level of insight, where she cannot acknowledge her voices as being the expression of an illness, and where she has no distance to her grandiose ideas (see *Rapport* above).

Diagnosis: The patient seems to be cooperative and motivated to learn more about her condition. These factors affect her prognosis positively.

No new diagnostic information emerges in this last section; therefore, the diagnostic considerations given previously may suffice.

Epilogue

Since the interviewer could only obtain the patient's emotional engagement in the last third of the session, this interview is incomplete as far as the phases are concerned. The diagnostic impressions are not substantiated by sufficient examples and details; therefore, phase 3 is incomplete. Phase 4, the longitudinal view with social, medical and family history, is nearly missing in its entirety. Phase 5, the completion of the data base, is missing; tests of handedness, attention, and concentration are desirable. Phase 6, the feedback phase, has been touched upon and is merged with the latter part of phase 3. This merger was induced by Q. 136. Phase 7, usually dedicated to a treatment contract, is reduced to an agreement on a return appointment.

The interview with Kelly Jasmin shows the main point of this book: interviewing is a nonlinear process—many events occur simultaneously. The phases are of heuristic value; they indicate what type of topics have to be covered in a complete interview. When you master these topics, feel free to jump back and forth from screening to family history to feedback and to verification of impressions as the patient's responses urge you to do.

CHAPTER EIGHT

DISORDER-SPECIFIC INTERVIEWING: MAJOR PSYCHIATRIC DISORDERS

SUMMARY

Chapter 8 shows how to modify interviewing strategies for symptoms, signs, and behaviors that interfere with rapport and the information-gathering process for some major psychiatric disorders. These modifications may help you to overcome some typical problems emerging with these diagnoses.

The first step towards a knowledge of the symptoms (of mental disease) is their locality—to which organ do the indications of disease belong? What organ must necessarily and invariably be diseased where there is madness?

Physiological and pathological facts show us that this organ can only be the brain.

Wilhelm Griesinger, 1845

The "standard" interview is appropriate for patients who have enough insight into their symptoms to decribe them (see chapter 7). Their symptoms are "ego-alien" and usually do not interfere with the interview process. This type of interview is therefore feasible with patients who suffer from milder forms of mood disorder, anxiety disorders, obsessive compulsive disorder, panic disorder, somatization disorder, substance abuse disorder, or sexual dysfunctions.

You must modify your interview for major psychiatric disorders if the patient's pathology interferes with either rapport or the diagnostic assessment process. For example, when you encounter the following:

1. perplexity and memory problems, as seen in organic mental disorder,
2. deception as seen in alcoholism,
3. hyperactivity as seen in mania,
4. suspiciousness as seen in delusional (paranoid) disorder,
5. avoidance as seen in phobia,
6. disbelief and embarrassment as seen in panic disorder,
7. persecutory ideas as sometimes seen in mental retardation.

These seven pathological features are not disorder-specific; for instance, hyperactivity, besides occurring in mania, can occur in organic states and intoxication. However, they are core pathology typical of major psychiatric disorders. Similar characteristic features exist for personality disorders. We will describe how to interview for both sets of features in the next two chapters.

We will point out for the disorders discussed what to look for and what special tactics to choose to establish rapport, assess mental status, keep the interview going, and with it the diagnostic process.

The format we use to highlight our method is a running commentary which we insert at key points to emphasize the four components of the interview.

1. PERPLEXITY AND SUSPICIOUSNESS IN ORGANIC MENTAL DISORDER

To diagnose advanced dementia is easy, even for the novice. The patient is disoriented; he is unable to memorize three words, to count, spell, or name all months of the year backward (see chapter 4: Mental Status).

In contrast, beginning dementia (due to mild diffuse cortical lesions—especially of the nondominant hemisphere) is considerably more difficult to spot. A key sign for these lesions is perplexity. The patient is bewildered by everyday situations because he cannot understand them. For him, everyday events roll by like isolated still frames of a movie. He perceives the pictures but cannot connect them, and therefore cannot comprehend the intent of the actions. He recalls elements of situations without integrating them logically. For instance, he may not understand what happened when he and his family left the house in the morning. He did not grasp where and why things were placed in a certain way. He is perplexed by the unfamiliar look of the house when he returns in the evening. He often explains the "newness" in a persecutory manner:

"Things are strange. I can't figure out what's going on. I have to be on the watch out to protect myself."

Therefore, if you detect signs of perplexity or suspiciousness in an older patient, either in his history or during the interview, add organic mental disorder to your differential diagnoses.

In interviewing such a patient, the tactic is to recognize his perplexity and accept his misinterpretations without challenge. Do not scare him or arouse his suspiciousness. Let him describe in detail his observations and show your interest in them. Carefully explore how he interprets events. Express empathy for his struggles. If you can win his trust, he may become less guarded toward you. Don't examine him as if you doubt his reports and explanations. Avoid distancing yourself from his account. For instance, a question such as

"What did this mean to you?"

implies that it means something else to you than to him.

"How did that make you feel?"

implies that you might feel differently. Alienation may result and the patient may stop cooperating. Ask instead:

"What were they up to?"
"What did you do?"

Also, use short sentences, because the patient may not remember long ones. Use simple, concrete words. Use *his* vocabulary, and connect questions by smooth transitions, so that he can follow your train of thought without becoming irritable or frustrated. If he shows signs of becoming tired, stop the interview and continue later.

Mrs. M., a 60-year-old, black, widowed female, is presented by a female social worker who is concerned that the patient might be exploited by her relatives. According to the patient, her relatives go through her belongings in her absence. They leave the house in disarray, and sometimes take her checks and money. The daughter reports that her mother was harder to deal with during the last two years and that she accused family members of robbing her.

When the patient enters the room, she grabs the arm of the social worker who accompanies her.

1. I: Hi, Mrs. M., your social worker, Dr. B., has told me about your problems. (The patient looks at the social worker and smiles.) I would like to learn more about them. How long have you been coming here?
   P: Oh, I started about nine months ago. (Information is correct.) I could not get along with my daughter any more.

2. I: How often have you been coming?
   P: About every other week. (Information is correct.)

3. I: Did you miss appointments sometimes?
   P: No, I don't think so. I keep good track.

4. I: So, you have a good memory. You always know what date it is?
   P: Sure.

5. I: Let me see, what date is it today?
   P: (She gives the correct date.)

6. I: Who brings you here to the clinic?
   P: Sometimes I come alone. But mostly my daughter or my son-in-law brings me.

7. I: They bring you?
   P: Yes.

8. I: Who tells them about your appointment?
   P: I do. I call them up and tell them.

9. I: Do they have the time to do it?
   P: No, not really. My daughter takes off from work.

Rapport: The presence of the social worker relaxes the patient because she considers her an ally.

Mental Status: The interviewer starts small talk which *seems* to explore only the peripheral circumstances of the clinic visits and the patient answers openly without suspiciousness. What the interviewer actually does is use *conversation* as a tool for the examination of the patient's recent memory and orientation (the clinic visits can be verified from the record). Both appear to be intact. The interviewer does not pick up on the clue in A. 1 (difficulties with her daughter) because he expects this topic to resurface later.

Diagnosis: The patient's grossly intact memory excludes the diagnosis of advanced dementia (list no. 2).

10. I: So your daughter brings you here. She seems to be concerned about you.
    P: I'm not sure. She seems to keep track of me.

11. I: How's that?
    P: She wants to know where I'm going.

12. I: Has she always done that?
    P: I don't know. It just dawned on me. I just found out about it.

13. I: Can you tell me what happened?
    P: One time when I went out, things did not look the same when I came back to the house. One of the tiles in the ceiling seemed to be removed. Somebody had tampered with my closet. They didn't even close it. And I could not find my money. They must have taken it.

14. I: What did you do about it?
    P: I tried to hide it, so they cannot find it. But then it is gone anyway.

15. I: Why does your daughter do it?
    P: I don't know.

16. I: Do you have any other examples?
    P: Yes. Things never look the same when I come back home. I can tell—somebody is tampering with my things.

17. I: Do you know who?
    P: Only my daughter has a key.

18. I: What did you do about it?
    P: I asked her to give it back. I asked her not to tamper with my things. She looked at me kind of strange. And she lied to me. She lies and says she is not doing it.

Rapport: The patient is neither guarded, nor delivers angry and revengeful tirades; instead, she levels with the interviewer and shares her concerns, which is contrary to a patient with paranoid disorder.

Technique: With a smooth transition, the interviewer reintroduces the subject of the patient's daughter but challenges the patient by stating that her daughter seems to be concerned about her, in opposition to what the patient had said in A. 1. He uses this technique to stir up an emotionally charged response necessary to explore her feelings about her daughter (Q. 11, 13, 16) with factual What? How? Why is it done? questions (Q. 13–15).

Mental Status: Mrs. M. is perplexed; she misperceives and suspiciously misinterprets events.

Diagnosis: The persecutory feelings are of recent onset. They do not show a depressive or manic flavor or an organized paranoid system, such as the belief that she is singled out and discriminated against. Instead, the persecutory ideas reveal bewilderment and mild derealization (A. 13, 16, 18), suggesting impaired information processing.

List No. 1: Included Disorders:

1. Onset of primary degenerative dementia of the Alzheimer type with delusions
2. multi-infarct dementia
3. psychoactive substance-induced organic mental disorder, unspecified
4. organic delusional disorder.

List No. 2: Excluded Disorders:

1. mood disorder with pseudo-dementia
2. schizophrenia, paranoid type
3. delusional (paranoid) disorder.

19. I: Are there any other things going on?
    P: Strange things.

20. I: Can you tell me about that?
    P: Yes.

21. I: Okay?
    P: It is with my grandchild. He likes to come to my house. After his visit I took him to the door and a yellow car was stopping. It stopped right at the corner.

22. I: What did this have to do with your grandson?
    P: Well, he went over there and they talked to him.

23. I: What else happened?
    P: They talked to him and he got in their car.

24. I: Did you know the people?
    P: No, I haven't seen them before in my life.

25. I: What happened then?
    P: I was scared. I thought they had kidnapped him.

26. I: Did you do anything about it?
    P: I called my daughter. I told her about it and she just laughed. I felt like they are tricking me.

27. I: Hmm.
    P: Later I called again and they denied it. They said he was already home. They said a friend's daddy had brought him home.

28. I: Was he home?
    P: They somehow got him. They must have.

Rapport: The patient supplies the interviewer with desired details without censoring.

Technique: The interviewer explores perception and ability to interpret everyday events. The patient tells her story in short segments. She has to be prodded to elaborate. Three types of questions help: time-related questions, e.g., "What happened then?" (Q. 23, 25, 27); questions that tie elements of the story together, e.g., "How is A related to B?" (Q. 22, 28 and 32); and questions that ask for more details, e.g., "How did it look?" "What do you know about it?" (Q. 24). These questions reveal whether she can interpret an event accurately as a chain of cause and effect.

The most powerful of these questions address the patient's interpretation:

"Why did that happen?"
"What does this mean?"
"What did you do about that?" (Q. 26).

Mental Status: The patient could not grasp her grandson's new social relationship. This reveals a deficit of her recent memory not apparent from the initial assessment of her orientation and memory. The patient can reproduce the sequence of events, but misunderstands their social significance.

Diagnosis: The patient's impaired learning points toward an organic process. A depressive disorder in an elderly patient could explain such a deficit, if attention and concentration were disturbed and if psychomotor retardation and social withdrawal were present. In their absence, an organic process is the more likely culprit.

29. I: Why?
    P: They let me talk to him. But his voice sounded strange.

30. I: Sounded strange?
    P: Yes.

31. I: Did those things happen again?
    P: Another time the same car came by and stopped. They picked him up again.

32. I: Was the car waiting?
    P: No, it was just driving by.

33. I: How did they know when your grandson leaves your house?
    P: Oh, they must have known. He must have called them. I heard them whispering on the telephone.

34. I: Did you ask him?
    P: No, I did not want to. I just wanted to see what happened. And there the car came again and picked him up.

35. I: What do you know about the people in the car?
    P: Nothing. But they already had another kid in the car and they let my grandson in too.

36. I: Could he be a friend of your grandson?
    P: No, I don't know him. My daughter says he is, but I don't know. I think something is going on.

37. I: Do you have any idea what that could be?
    P: No, not really. It's just strange.

38. I: Do you feel they are after you?
    P: I don't know. I think they might be. But I'll be on the watchout. And I have my windows nailed down and bolts installed on the doors.

39. I: Would there be any reason why they would be after you?
    P: No, I have not done anything.

40. I: What are they after?
    P: Maybe my money.

41. I: Who would they be?
    P: Oh, I think maybe my daughter and maybe the people in the car.

Rapport: The patient trusts the interviewer. She reveals her fears, concerns, and feelings of insecurity.

Technique: The interviewer focuses on the patient's interpretations of events (except Q. 31, 35), which reveal the patient's intelligence, but also her delusional thinking.

Mental Status: The patient continues to interpret events in a persecutory manner, delusional not organized. For instance, she cannot explain why the parents cooperate in the kidnapping of her grandchild. The patient also perseverates on the theme that these people and her family are after her money.

Diagnosis: Adequate verbal production, together with a deficit in recent memory and understanding of social situations, and the presence of nonorganized persecutory delusions support the diagnosis of an organic delusional syndrome.

In the remainder of the interview the interviewer excluded the presence of depressive symptoms, alcohol abuse, and use of any medication known to interfere with mental functions such as anticholinergics. Further mental status examination revealed also that the patient had difficulties interpreting proverbs, counting backward by two, and copying a cube (see figure 8.1).

These results plus further workup—including an EEG, brain scan, Wechsler Intelligence Test, Shipley-Hartford Test and Hallstead-Reitan Neuropsychological Test Battery which together confirmed an organic impairment—supported the initial impression of an organic delusional syndrome DSM-III-R 293.81.

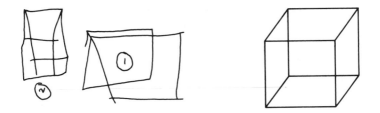

FIGURE 8. 1
Organicity: Draw a cube

2. DECEPTION AND DENIAL IN ALCOHOLISM

There are a number of presentations of alcoholism which seem to appear over and over again:

1. The skid row alcoholic who openly admits his drinking. Often he checks into a hospital for detoxification in exchange for food and housing but refuses to give up his drinking. He often brings contraband to the ward and drinks secretly.

2. The younger sociopathic alcoholic who reports truancy, bad school and work habits, violent behavior, lying, stealing, multiple traffic tickets or a police record. The sociopathic symptoms may overshadow the drinking.

3. The middle-class female alcoholic with a history of affective disorder who reveals her depressive symptoms, but downplays her drinking.

4. The middle-aged professional or executive alcoholic who continues to fulfill his social functions, lives with and is morally supported by spouse and children, emphasizes stress but denies excessive drinking.

While the first two types are easy to interview because they admit their drinking, the latter two have an active interest in concealing their alcoholic dependency.

To overcome these obstacles, you first have to detect the patient's drinking in spite of his denial. You should therefore look for:

1. a past history or family history of drinking, alcohol abuse, or alcohol addiction;
2. a history of frequent short-term illnesses and absenteeism; and
3. signs of intoxication or withdrawal during the interview.

If you suspect alcoholism, but your patient denies it, pursue it. Insist on this topic tactfully, but frequently. Bring it up again and again to make him admit little by little the full story.

Be careful not to make the patient lose face by being caught lying or by accusing him of misleading you. Understand his motivation for lying: an alcoholic usually has the perception that he is not truly an alcoholic; that he could indeed stop drinking if he seriously wanted to; that his spouse, employer, and physician unfairly exaggerate and overemphasize his drinking habit in a dogmatic, nonunderstanding way. He may claim that he drinks for relaxation which he is entitled to in order to compensate for the pressures of his family and job.

Second, when you have established a drinking pattern, discuss the advantage and disadvantage of drinking. Induce him to admit to its good and ill effects so that you can fully explore the impact of the alcoholism on his life. Work toward this goal by asking him whether any family member, colleague, or friend considers him an alcoholic. He may grudgingly admit to such criticism. Then ask him whether he can see the critic's point of view. He may get angry, defend himself, and quote examples of skid row alcoholics whom he considers true alcoholics who should be criticized. It may take more than one interview to get to this stage.

Even when a patient admits that he is an alcoholic and assures you that he is serious about getting on the wagon, expect secret denial. Translate his "cooperation" into its real meaning:

"You expect me to admit that I have a drinking problem. I am willing to admit it, not because I think you are right, but because you don't know any better. When I tell you that I want to stop drinking, I mean: Get off my back. I say I will stop drinking to pacify you but I will hide my drinking better so that people don't get the wrong impression."

If you have collected enough evidence for the patient's alcoholism, there is no use in pressing him to give lip service to the well-known dual therapeutic premise to *admit his alcoholism* and *promise abstinence*. He has to be convinced first that drinking is indeed wrecking his life.

The alcoholic patient is most sensitive to the loss of his support person. If such a loss is imminent, use it to make the patient see the damage drinking inflicts on him. Approximately 25% of suicides are alcoholic; they often follow the loss of a support person (Goodwin and

Guze 1984). If suicide is a gauge for the importance of support, use the support person as leverage in your interview.

Here is an interview with Harold, a 58-year-old professor of economics. Harold had a history of severe alcohol abuse, his wife had threatened divorce, and the dean had reminded him that he might lose his tenured position if he did not curb his drinking. After such warnings—according to the wife—the patient had indeed stopped drinking during the last year. After the wife had returned from a two-week vacation that she had taken without her husband, she found him in an "awful" state when she returned home. He was referred for electro-shock treatment because of severe symptoms of depression.

The patient was sitting barefoot on his bed. He was unkempt, unshaven, and the rancid smell of body odor hung in the room.

1. I: Hi. Dr. A. has asked me to talk to you. (Dr. A. is in charge of the patient's treatment.)
   P: Hi. (Patient avoids eye contact and looks down at his hands. He is sweating. His face is somewhat puffy and blotchy with mild peripheral edema. His hands are tremulous.)

2. I: Did Dr. A. tell you that I was going to see you?
   P: I guess . . . he may have.

3. I: Do you remember what he told you?
   P: Told me what?

4. I: About why I should see you?
   P: I don't know. Maybe something for treatment of depression. (There is no prolonged latency of response.)

5. I: When did he talk to you about it?
   P: Didn't he tell you? You should know. Aren't you the doctor? Why ask me all these stupid questions?

6. I: Well, it is important for me to find out how well you can remember things.
   P: There is nothing wrong with my memory. I'm just sick. Can't you see that? Do I have to tell you what's wrong with me? You should know. (Patient starts trembling.)

7. I: You must feel awful. The way you look tells me that you feel bad; but it's also the way you talk.
   P: What do you mean?

8. I: It seems to bother you to talk with me.
   P: No, that's okay.

9. I: You seem to be irritable.
   P: That's not because of you. Everything just bugs me. Sitting here. Nobody does anything. Nobody cares in this whole damn hospital.

10. I: You must really feel bad.
    P: That's no joke. I don't need any wisecracks. (Patient blushes.)

11. I: Let me get you something that will calm your nerves.
    P: What do you want to give me?

12. I: Just some Librium and a shot of vitamins. (Physican calls the nurse and gives the order for Librium 25 mg and thiamine 100 mg. He takes the patient's pulse. It is 108.) When you have the medication, it will be easier for you to talk to me. You want me to come back in a little while?
    P: No, it's okay. It doesn't make any difference. Let's get it over with.

Rapport: The apparently peripheral questions (if and when the treating physician has discussed the consultation visit Q. 1–4) irritate the patient (A. 5–6). So, the interviewer switches to statements that express empathy for his suffering (Q. 7–12) to find cooperation. The patient becomes less irritable and more agreeable.

Technique: The opening questions assess recent memory. The patient is evasive and resists this line of questioning which prompts the interviewer to assure rapport (see above).

Mental Status: The patient's appearance and poor hygiene suggest either severe retarded or psychotic depression, or—with the background of the history—a withdrawal state. Sweating, puffiness, and fluency of speech support alcohol withdrawal. The patient's irritated refusal to answer questions that assess his recent memory strengthen this impression—so does the elevated pulse rate. Therefore, the interviewer orders Librium to abate withdrawal, and thiamine (vitamin B_1) to prevent Wernicke's syndrome, a vitamin B_1 deficiency.

Diagnosis: The mental status in combination with the history suggests strongly alcohol withdrawal. During this state an underlying depression is difficult to assess.

13. I: When did you come in?
    P: Must have been the day before yesterday.

14. I: Do you know what time?
    P: Must have been in the evening. (Records show that he came in one day ago in the morning.)

15. I: Why did you come in?
    P: My wife and her sister brought me. They must have thought I was sick. I felt sick to my stomach. I was just sitting around. I had not gone to work for a while. They came back from a trip. So they brought me here.

16. I: How well did you sleep last night?
    P: I was exhausted, but I could not sleep. I tossed and turned. I had to get up several times during the night to drink. I drank a lot of water.

17. I: Just last night?
    P: Maybe the nights before too.

18. I: When did you get up in the morning?
    P: Oh, these nurses made me get out of bed and have breakfast. But I was not hungry. I just drank coffee.

19. I: How much coffee did you have?
    P: You mean today?

20. I: Yes.
    P: Eight or ten cups. I don't know. (The nurse brings the Librium 25 mg, water, and the syringe. The patient takes the Librium without any comment and washes it down with a glass of water. He then starts to pull his pants down for the shot.)

21. I: What are you doing?
    P: Didn't you want to give me a shot?

22. I: Yes. You look shaky to me. But don't you want to know why I'm giving it to you?
    P: You do what you want to do in this hospital. What's the sense in asking?

23. I: Well, let me tell you then. I read in your chart that you had a drinking problem. I think you are drinking again and that it's rough for you to get off that stuff. That's why I'm giving you Librium.
    P: What makes you think that? I'm not drinking anymore. I quit.

Rapport and Technique: The interviewer uses the improved rapport to assess some symptoms of alcohol withdrawal in a straightforward checklist manner to prepare the patient for more direct questions about his drinking which he starts in Q. 23.

Mental Status: The patient has some mild disturbances of recent memory and restlessness with insomnia. He is also disinterested in his present treatment but he denies drinking.

24. I: You mean, you have not had a drink recently?
    P: I quit last May, the 18th of May, precisely.

25. I: You mean, you had your *very* last drink then?
    P: Yes, that's when I went to the hospital.

26. I: What happened when you came out?
    P: I was fine all summer. But I did not feel so hot when the semester started.

27. I: What happened?
    P: Well, I just slowly went downhill. My wife thinks I'm depressed again.

28. I: Well, what do you think?
    P: She may be right, I guess.

29. I: So, when you felt depressed, did you take up drinking again?
    P: I could not sleep.

30. I: Does alcohol help you sleep?
    P: Yes, it did in the past. At least in the beginning.

31. I: Did it help this time?
    P: I try not to drink anymore.

32. I: You mean you slowed down?
    P: My wife told me she would leave me if I started up again.

33. I: So you are scared that she will leave you?
    P: I may also lose my job. They may fire me.

34. I: Well, what do you do when you need a drink during the day or when you can't sleep?
    P: I try not to do anything.

35. I: Okay, and if that does not work?
    P: I sometimes go to my study and sleep there.

36. I: In your study?
    P: Yes.

37. I: So you sneak out to your study? Is that where you have your stuff?
    P: What do you mean?

38. I: Well, you told me that you will lose your job, if you are found drinking again and that your wife will leave you. So you have no choice. You have to hide it.
    P: Well, I sleep in the study, so that my wife does not smell it. I have switched to vodka. They say it smells less. But I take it only when I can't sleep, when I need it for my nerves.

Rapport: The interviewer expresses interest in Harold's mental state during the last year and shows empathy in his concern that the patient may lose his wife and job if he is found out drinking again. This concern helps to maintain rapport.

Technique: The interviewer vacillates between collecting the recent history of increased alcohol consumption and expression of interest in the patient's worries (see *Rapport*). This approach keeps the patient talking and slowly admitting his return to the bottle.

Mental Status: The patient's denial melts away.

Diagnosis: The interviewer fills in details of the recent history of alcohol abuse.

39. I: Hmm.
   P: You really don't believe me, do you?

40. I: Well, I am trying to understand you. I know once you start drinking, you need more and more to make it work. And you told me that you started again when the semester began in August. Now it's January. You are right back into it and now it got too much.
   P: You are worse than my wife. You can ask her. She has not said anything about drinking anymore. She has not even talked to the dean. Nobody has said anything about me drinking.

41. I: So what is your main problem?
   P: My main problem is depression. I feel awful.

42. I: I know you do. But I'm afraid we'll do you a disservice by not caring about your drinking problem.
   P: I really don't have that problem anymore.

43. I: Well, you told me you are hiding your drinks now. What do you do when you are at work and your nerves bother you and you feel shaky and can't concentrate?
   P: I told you I have slowed down.

44. I: I know, but when you had a drink in the evening and you feel rotten in the morning, what do you do?
   P: I just have coffee.

45. I: Okay, but if that does not work? Do you have anything in your office for an emergency?
   P: I'm not crazy. I don't want to lose my job. What do you think would happen if they found it?

46. I: So what do you do?
   P: (Silent.)

47. I: I can help you better if you level with me. In the meantime, let me give you the shot. (He gives the vitamin shot.) If you don't want to level with me, why don't you talk with Dr. A. about it.
   P: I don't need anything about my drinking in my chart.

48. I: I won't write anything in your chart. I will just talk to Dr. A. and recommend that we detoxify you. In a few days I would like to look at you again and see how much is left of your depression.

    P: You really don't believe me.

49. I: I know that you are under a lot of pressure, that you are scared you will lose your wife and your job and I don't want you to lose anything. I want to help you as much as I can.

    P: You all say that. But nobody really understands how I feel. Nobody understands the pressure I am under.

50. I: I know you are under a lot of pressure . . .

    P: If my wife sees me having a drink, she exaggerates and thinks I am an alcoholic. And that's the only reason why I hide it. She has not said anything anymore.

51. I: I know. I read the admission note and talked to Dr. A. Your wife did not mention your drinking when you came into the hospital this time.

    P: So don't you believe her?

52. I: I have not talked to her directly.

    P: Why don't you give her a call? She will tell you that I have not touched the stuff.

53. I: Oh, I believe that.

    P: Why is that?

54. I: I think there are some good reasons for her to tell me that.

    P: Why should she? Do you think I hide it that well?

55. I: Maybe. But maybe that's not all.

    P: What do you mean?

56. I: I don't think she wants you to lose your job either.
    What is she going to do when you are out of work?

    P: Why would she bring me here?

57. I: Well, I think she notices your condition. She wants some help for you without naming the problem "drinking." If you don't trust me there is no reason for me to talk to you . . . Although there is . . .

    P: What should that be?

58. I: That I take better care of your interests than you do. You don't gain anything by hiding your problem from your doctor, if you *really* want help.

    P: So what else do you want to know?

Rapport: The interviewer is nonjudgmental and expresses repeatedly that he wants to help.

Technique: The interviewer neither confronts nor interprets Harold's attempts to use his wife as an alibi for his near abstinence to assure his slowing down in drinking. He also bypasses his attempts to downplay his drinking and pursues in detail the patient's recent drinking history, thus wearing down his denial.

59. I: I want to know what you do at work when you need something for your nerves.
    P: You are back on that again.

60. I: If you tell me that, we can drop it for good.
    P: I told you I have slowed down.

61. I: Yes, you slowed down, you try to control it better, and you try to hide it better. So where do you hide your stuff during the daytime?
    P: Oh, just a few days before I came in here. I had one bottle left. After I bought it, I did not want to bring it into the house. So I left it sitting in the car.

62. I: You mean, it just sits in the car so that anybody can see it?
    P: Of course not. I put it where the spare tire is and I wrapped a rag around it.

63. I: So you hide your stuff in your study and in your car.
    P: Not really. My wife often goes into the study. There is not that much room to hide anything.

64. I: Where did you hide it in the past, when you were drinking more?
    P: Then? I had a whole collection in the basement.

65. I: You mean it is all gone now?
    P: Oh no, it is still there. But I have not touched it.

66. I: I understand how you feel and the pressure you are under. I will talk to Dr. A. I think we will give you a few days' rest and good food. Then we will see how your depression is doing. I will give Dr. A. my recommendation.

Rapport: The tactic of extracting the alcohol history little by little prevents the breakdown of rapport. Even though the interviewer is not accepted as an ally during this first interview, he has laid the groundwork for future therapeutic alliance. The task is to achieve the patient's full insight into his drinking problem. With many alcohol and drug addicts this is a long-term rather than a short-term goal which requires prolonged therapy often punctuated by relapses.

The interviewer's active pursuit of the alcohol history places him in an authoritative role which he will give up when the patient has full insight and accepts the goal of abstinence.

Technique: The interviewer's task is to deal with the defense mechanism of denial. In this interview the denial of any drinking was replaced by the admission of drinking a little bit, occasionally, when under duress. Obviously, the patient's withdrawal state contradicts this assertion. However, it is a long process to break down this defense.

Mental Status and Diagnosis: Concerning the present admission, the differential diagnosis includes alcohol abuse and depression. In spite of this patient's denial of drinking, the interviewer assumes that the patient drank heavily ("I had not gone to work for a while") during the wife's absence, but had stopped drinking upon her return to avoid marital conflict. This led to his "desolate state." The essential features of beginning alcohol withdrawal are visible: nausea ("I felt sick to my stomach"), trembling, autonomic hyperactivity (sweating, tachycardia), malaise, depressed mood, irritability, anxiety, and fitful and disturbed sleep. He showed dehydration and a dry mouth (I drank a lot of water). He admits to hiding alcohol at home and in his car to use at work.

The intoxicated alcoholic has often an acute amnestic syndrome which may have been responsible for Harold's inability to recall the time of his admission.

The DSM-III-R diagnosis is 291.80 uncomplicated alcohol withdrawal.

This interview intended only to show one way to deal with the denial by an alcoholic. It did not assess other alcohol- or nonalcohol-related disorders. Such a differential usually poses no difficulty and the format of the standard interview can be applied.

3. IRRITABLE HYPERACTIVITY IN MANIA

Lack of insight, control, and goal orientation, together with elevated drive, all result in irritable hyperactivity and interfere with the interview of the manic patient.

The manic patient's lack of insight prevents you from using rational arguments and confrontation with his altered mood in order to influence him. Handle him like an unpredictable explosive ready to go off at any time.

The lack of insight makes him distractible. A random noise in the corridor may attract his attention. He may be stimulated to excessive monologues by the doctor's tie, or beard, just to comment in the next moment on the nurse's appearance or shape of her legs. From compliments he may switch to profanities. No topic stays in focus. His thinking is unpredictable and erratic.

The elevated drive and disinhibited control make the manic patient talk, shout, persuade, swear, holler, or sing. Blinded by energy, he feels angry, happy, or excited, but above all justified in insisting on whatever he pursues at the moment. Whoever opposes him is his foe. He has some vague feeling that things don't go his way. This ticks him off. The manic cannot realize that his enormous drive is bewildering, frightening, or amusing to the bystander. He has no insight into how he affects others.

How do you interview such a patient?

The best approach is to make his elevated drive work for you. Discern his point of view, identify with his goals, and appear to adopt them. If you help him in the pursuit of his goals, his mood will remain elated. If you oppose him, you arouse his anger and hostility and prevent compliance. If he wants to leave the hospital, you can tell him you want him out even faster but permanently. If he wants to talk to you at this moment, you really wanted to talk to him an hour ago. In short, you agree with him and support him rather than become the obstacle of his goals, forcing you to contradict him, pull rank on him and cross him.

How do you collect the facts to make a diagnosis?

The manic has little insight into his feelings but is aware of his actions. He knows that he is sleeping less, can get into fights and arguments, and realizes that others have brought him to a psychiatrist. Even after remission the manic patient typically talks about his past manic attacks in terms of behavioral (and not mood) changes. He rarely realizes or remembers that he feels or felt abnormally high or elated:

"I wrote more letters, I spent more money than I had; I wrote bad checks; I enrolled in three health clubs at the same time; I bought $6,000 of pottery for my house; I walked out on my girlfriend; I picked up a nurse, a secretary, and a go-go dancer; other people told me to shut up—so I must have talked more; I really don't know how I felt, reasoned, or thought. I didn't feel sick or out of control."

Let the manic patient describe his behaviors but don't expect him to admit that there is anything wrong with him. He feels better than ever. Use his distractibility to redirect him when you reach an impasse. Don't argue and don't try to persuade him, but distract him.

In the following example, the manic patient insists on being discharged (heightened drive). The interviewer agrees with him but lets the patient repeatedly know that he can only be discharged if certain conditions are met. He may tell him that he wants to do more for him than just discharge him: he does not want him to be returned to the hospital. He reminds the patient that he had been readmitted before when released prematurely. If the patient recalls an angry outburst against the police, or the friends who he thought betrayed him, or the doctor who played a dirty game, the interviewer will agree with him and insist that this should never happen again. He tells him:

"I want to help you to cope better with others and not be their punching bag. You see, you shouted and screamed and pushed them, and even struck out at one of them. That's how you ended up in the hospital. I want to help you so that you don't have to scream, shout, and push! Then those people won't bother you anymore."

A description such as "You screamed, kicked, and shouted" is—as mentioned above—superior to an introspection such as "You feel restless, angry, and excited, we have to calm you down," because the patient may not experience himself as restless, angry, and excited. But he remembers that he shouted and kicked.

Clayton, a 38-year-old, white, married patient was transferred to the psychiatric ward from another hospital where he had punched a doctor. His hands and feet were handcuffed to a stretcher. In the accompanying report he was diagnosed as a schizophrenic. "Bizarre actions" and "paranoid delusions" were mentioned, but precise descriptions of the patient's behavior were missing.

a. Establish Rapport

1. I: What happened to you?
   P: (Silent, angry looks, breathing hard.)

2. I: What happened? Why are you tied down?
   P: Screw it. Let me out of here. I'm not talking to you. Just let me out. God will not tolerate it. I want to help mankind, set them all free—we are free creatures—we are equal to God. God will free creatures—we are equal to God. God will see to it. Seeing is believing. I see! I see! Let me out. Now, now, now. Now is now, and now is ever. Now is not never. (Straining on his cuffs.)

3. I: I don't want to keep you here. I want you out, too, after you stop shouting, screaming, and kicking.
   P: Get me out! Get these cuffs off, get them off, off, off! (Shouting.)

4. I: I want them off, too. But I don't want to put them back on again. So when you stop shouting, we can take them off.
   P: Then take them off! Take them off now!

5. I: I will take them off if I don't have to put them back on again.
   P: I want out!

6. I: I want you out too. Understand? You can come out when you talk calmly. I want to know what brought those cuffs on.
   P: I don't want to talk to you. I want out.

7. I: Okay, I'll get you out. But tell me, why are you in them in the first place?
   P: I hit him. I hit that doctor, because he told me I could not get out. He can't do it, he can't do it, he can't do it.

8. I: You will get out. But you are too loud. You shout, you don't talk.
   P: I can talk. Take the cuffs off. (Wriggling on the restraints.)

9. I: I want to take them off, but I don't want to put them back on. I want to make sure that you don't strike out.
   P: Then do it.

10. I: Okay, but I first have to help you talk calmer.
    P: Calm me down? I'm tied down. That makes me shout.

11. I: I will give you a shot so that we can take off the cuffs, so that you don't shout and scream, so that you can talk to me.
    P: I don't need no shot, nobody needs a shot. I'm nailed to the cross. God's son was nailed to the cross, Jesus was nailed to the cross.

12. I: I want you off the cross. Let me help you. Here is the shot so you can get off the cross.
    P: Okay, hurry up. I want out.
    (Interviewer gives the patient a shot of 50 mg chlorpromazine IM without the patient objecting.)

Rapport: The interviewer establishes rapport with Clayton by agreeing with him to have the restraints removed. Since the patient has no insight into his excitability as a symptom of a disorder, the interviewer does not express any empathy with the patient's excited state. In this respect the approach taken with the irritable patient deviates from the second step described in chapter 2: Rapport. Statements like

"It must be awful to be strapped down."

would sound sarcastic to the patient and ignite his hostility rather than kindle rapport.

Technique: The interviewer agrees with the patient's goal but attaches the condition that he has to stop shouting first. He does not present this condition as a restraint but as an assurance that the patient does not have to be put back in handcuffs. He avoids talking about the patient's mental state in which the patient has no insight but addresses only his behavior which the patient can recognize even though he perceives it—unlike the interviewer—as justified.

Mental Status: The patient is alert and shows hostile excitement with thematic perseveration on the goal to be uncuffed. Flight of ideas can also be observed in A. 11.

Diagnosis: All disorders have to be considered that are associated with an excited state such as

organic mental disorder
intoxication with PCP, cocaine, amphetamines
delirious state due to alcohol or sedative withdrawal
mania
paranoid schizophrenia.

b. Rule Out Organic Mental Disorder

13. I: When did you come in?
    P: Too long ago. Two sunrises ago.

14. I: On Sunday?
    P: (Laughs.) It was a Tuesday, not the sunny Sunday. Two days ago was a Tuesday, because today is Thursday.

15. I: Of what month?
    P: Of what month, of what month? I'm not dumb. Leave me alone.

16. I: I will go, but give me the month first. You gave me the day.
    P: I give you nothing. I give you everything. Give, give, give.

17. I: The month?
    P: The month, month, month!
    What is the month?
    Not July, not September.
    But the month in between,
    is what I remember. (Accurate.)

18. I: When did you start to get so restless?
    P: I could not sleep. God wanted me to preach. I want to preach. (Patient stares at the physician.) You are tied down too.

19. I: When did you start to preach?
    P: One and a half weeks ago. I was helping everybody. I was helping mankind, but they caught me. The soldiers of Pontius Pilate caught me.

20. I: Have you preached before?
    P: Two years ago. I was in a hospital. They said they kept me because I was a schizophrenic or something like that. I spent all my money on an invention. I made mock collars and cuffs. Get these cuffs off. (Interviewer orders to remove the cuffs.)

Rapport: The interviewer seems to engage in small talk and gets good cooperation.

Technique: The interviewer explores and tests recent memory, a technique decribed as part of the mental status examination.

Mental Status: Clayton is oriented with intact recent memory. He shows a tendency to rhyme, to pun, and to perseverate on words like "month." His thought content shows religious preoccupation, and the investment in an invention where he lost all his money shows bad judgment.

Diagnosis: Clayton's answers exclude the presence of an organic mental disorder and suggest a recurrent psychiatric disorder, most likely mania, less likely periodic drug intoxication.

c. Rule Out Drug and Alcohol Abuse

21. I: Let's walk around. Let me show you the place.
    P: Doc, you are a nice guy. Let's go all the way.

22. I: Yes. We'll go all around. I want to know more about you. Tell me, when you preach, do you take any drugs?
    P: I never take drugs. I didn't even take what the doctors gave me. I want to be clean. I don't want to be doped. Dopidopidoo. (Starts dancing and singing.) Dopidopidoo.

23. I: Do you drink?
    P: I don't need drinks. I can feel good without them. I feel so good, so good, so good. (Giggles and laughs.)

24. I: What did you do before you came in?
    P: Worked as a tailor. Made good money. But I can do better.

25. I: What do you want to do when you get out of here?
    P: I want to help mankind with my inventions. Nobody has to buy a shirt anymore. They just wear a collar and cuffs.

Rapport: The interviewer offers to walk around with the patient to give him a chance to relieve his restlessness which the patient appreciates.

Technique: The interviewer checks symptoms in a straightforward manner. A more open-ended approach would be less productive because Clayton is distractible and shows flight of ideas.

Mental Status: The patient continues to show flight of ideas with word games. After the removal of the handcuffs the irritable mood is replaced by elation, demonstrating situation-dependent lability of mood. The thought content shows grandiose ideas. Future plans reveal poor judgment.

Diagnosis: All of the above exclude the diagnosis of drug intoxication and support mania.

d. Confirm Bipolar Illness

26. I: You have such big plans now. Have you ever felt discouraged, have you ever felt down?
    P: Have I felt down, down, down? Down in the dumps? Oh yeah. I first worked on my invention and then I go so down, stayed in bed all the time, did not want to move, I felt so bad. (Starts crying.)
27. I: It's all right. You are not feeling bad now.

Diagnosis: A. 26 confirms bipolar disorder. At this point more history can be obtained following the format of the standard interview.

DSM-III-R diagnosis: bipolar disorder, manic, severe without psychotic features 296.43.

4. SUSPICIOUSNESS IN DELUSIONAL (PARANOID) DISORDER

The patient with persecutory delusions experiences life events and everyday happenings as directed against him. He suspects he is persecuted because of his "special knowledge," "insights," or "gifts."

There are two difficulties in interviewing the patient with persecutory delusions:

1. He may become suspicious of you because any of your remarks, gestures, or facial expressions can trigger his feelings of being persecuted

by you. The patient may be convinced that you communicate and collaborate with his ennemies, that you are a member of a secret brotherhood which is out to hurt him. If he decides that you are part of *"them,"* he will become scared or hostile, and stop cooperating. The paranoid patient may not complain openly about your plotting against him; he may hide his suspicions in order not to tip you off that he has found out about you.

2. He fears that you will think him crazy. He may therefore be guarded and withhold information. The giveaway is his interaction with you. He will track you closely with his eyes, give short, vague, and evasive answers with underlying hostility, or reply with counterquestions.

How do you interview such a patient?

The basic strategy in interviewing this patient is to handle his persecutory ideas not as something strange, but share the suffering that these ideas cause him and sympathize with his mental anguish. Treat his delusional interpretations as if they were true. Approach them not from the outsider's but from the patient's point of view.

The novice finds that a difficult task. He is more comfortable with an "outsider" approach which works best with patients who had delusions in the past but are not acutely ill now. Questions like:

> I: "Do you have a tendency to be suspicious?"
> "Do you feel easily harassed?"
> "Are you pretty paranoid?"

will leave you empty-handed with a patient who is presently delusional. Also, neutralizing statements such as:

> I: "Since when have your neighbors, in your opinion, harassed you?"
> "Where else do you believe injustice has been done to you?"

may arouse his anger and lead to objections:

> P: "What do you mean with 'in my opinion.' Don't you think it's true? I don't just believe it; it really has happened!"

Such a response is understandable, since the patient is used to skepticism, ridicule, and rejection by family and friends when he ponders his suspicions.

However, if you convince the patient that you are on his side, he may trust you. When he experiences your empathy, he will become more cooperative and show a need to share his problems with you. Questions that take his suspicious feelings seriously may assure cooperation:

>   I: "How have you been treated by others?"
>   "Have you ever been harassed, unjustly treated, or discriminated against?"
>   "Is it your experience that people don't seem to like you?"
>   "Have you ever been subjected to humiliation?"
>   "Who else did injustice to you?"

This strategy fails if the patient feels "tricked" or "buttered up" and if it makes him feel that you are taking his side in a phony way just to pump him for information and fool him.

Some interviewers resist taking the patient's side. They feel that they reinforce the patient's delusions by pretending to share his poor reality testing and that they violate their professional integrity. If you have such scruples, remember that delusions are fixed, false beliefs that cannot be corrected by logical arguments but only evoke the patient's antagonism and destroy rapport.

Persecutory delusions, like other delusions, mellow with neuroleptic treatment or with time. Their intensity can be measured by the five stages of insight (see 4.3: Exploration—Perception). Adjust your interview style to the patient's stage of insight. At stage V the patient acts on his delusion. Handle the delusion as if it is true. Tell the patient that treatment (medication) is given in order to blunt the effect of those "harassments."

When he does not act on his delusion but merely talks about it (stage IV) or refuses to talk about it any more (stage III) or claims it was only true in the past, but has stopped now (stage II) shows the same distance to the delusion.

Finally, when the patient dismisses his past delusion as factual and recognizes it as part of an illness (level I), express the same view and discuss its morbid nature with him.

Examples: A patient may ask you:

"Do you really believe that my neighbors are after me or do you think it is all in my mind?"

You have several options to respond. If you believe that the patient basically has no doubts in his delusion and is simply testing you, respond like:

"The main thing is that you are convinced that the neighbors are after you. And this conviction of yours is very real for me. I take it seriously. I will help you to deal with it and get you some relief."

If you feel that the patient is starting to question his own delusion and is on the verge of shaking it off, you may proceed by:

"What makes you ask me that question? Are there any doubts in your mind? I'd like you to tell me more about your doubts. Do you feel differently about your past experience now?"

Then help the patient to accept reality and to recognize his past delusion as pathological. However, keep track of the vanishing delusion, because it often returns during a longer follow-up period. Tell him:

"It is not always easy to tell whether one has really been wronged or if one tends to exaggerate because one feels hurt so badly. Therefore, I'd like you to discuss these thoughts right away with me when they appear, so that we both can sort out what to think about them."

The following interview was conducted with Francis S., a 52-year-old, white, female outpatient. She was presented by the social worker who wanted to rule out any psychiatric disorder. According to the social worker the patient had become increasingly discouraged because of difficulties finding a job as executive secretary. Similar to the social worker the resident was not certain whether a psychiatric disorder was present or not. The patient's complaints had been vague. She had said that "the deck of cards was stacked against her," and had refused to elaborate.

1. I: Mrs. S., I have heard from Dr. A. (social worker) and Dr. B. (resident) that you had some problems finding a job. I understand that you are very discouraged about that.
   P: Yes, it does not seem to work out anymore.

2. I: How do you support yourself?
   P: I have some savings. They may last for another two or three months and then I'm finished.

3. I: What will you do then?
   P: I'll just be finished. I can't do anything.

4. I: That sounds real bad.
   P: Well, it is.

5. I: When you say you are finished, what does that mean?
   P: I don't know. It's just over with.

6. I: Do you plan to do anything about that?
   P: I have thought about it.

7. I: Like what?
   P: Like jumping. Just smash myself.

8. I: Are you at this point now?
   P: Not now. But in two months I will be if things don't change.

9. I: That sounds very depressing to me.
   P: Well, it is. I keep on fighting. But I have a feeling that it is coming to an end.

10. I: That must be on your mind day and night.
    P: Well, it is.

Rapport: The interviewer takes three opportunities (A. 1, 4, 10) to express empathy and win the patient's trust.

Technique: Francis' chief complaint (she cannot find a job) suggests a problem of living which can be approached by exploring why the problem developed and what the expected outcome might be. The interviewer chooses to explore the patient's expectations and future plans to get a feeling for her judgment.

Mental Status: The patient's expectation about the future is negativistic and her judgment appears impaired, since suicide does not appear to be a rational solution.

Diagnosis: Disorders with suicidal ruminations or behaviors have to be considered (list no. 1, see chapter 5), such as:

major depressive episode
bipolar disorder, depressed
alcohol abuse
other psychoactive substance use disorders
somatization disorder
dependent personality disorder
passive aggressive personality disorder
borderline personality disorder.

11. I: Does it affect your sleep?
    P: My sleep is alright. I forget it all when I'm asleep.

12. I: And your appetite?
    P: I'm cutting back because I don't have the money. But I like to eat.

13. I: Well, I'm sure Dr. A. can help you to get some money from our social
       worker, from Social Security, or the Welfare Office.
    P: Really?

14. I: What you really need is a job.
    P: That's right.

Diagnosis: Affective disorder is one of the most common psychiatric
disorders in middle-aged females. Therefore, the interviewer explores
vegetative symptoms of depression but comes out empty-handed.

15. I: Tell me what happened at your last job interview.
    P: I came in for the appointment and the secretary was real nice. But I had
       the feeling it won't work out.

16. I: This must be terrible to know already that it won't work out and you
       still go through the motions.
    P: Yes, it is.

17. I: How do they ruin it for you?
    P: They don't give me the job.

18. I: Do you have any idea why they did not give it to you?
    P: No. Not really. I don't know.

19. I: Well, what's your feeling? Is there anything going on?
    P: I don't know. It happens too often.

20. I: You mean it happens over and over again?
    P: Yes.

21. I: I admire you that you still keep trying.
    P: Well, yes. I hope some employer may not know and will hire me.

22. I: You say may not know?
    P: Hmm.

23. I: Can you tell me about that?
    P: Well, I don't know. But I think it has to do with the computers.

24. I: What do you know about these computers?
    P: Well, they are everywhere. If you go on a bus trip, they put your name
       on a computer. When you book an airline ticket, they put your name on
       a computer. They store all the information about you on a computer.

25. I: Hmm.
    P: They have (with emphasis) everything on a computer.

26. I: And why don't they hire you?
    P: Because I know about their computers . . . that's their way to get back at me.

27. I: That puts you in an awful bind. You know about it, but you still need a job from them.
    P: Yes.

Rapport: Again, the interviewer expresses empathy with the patient's situation in order to maintain rapport (Q. 16, 21, 27). When he hits on some persecutory thoughts, he puts himself in the patient's shoes and explores details from her vantage point (Q. 17, 19, 24, 27).

Technique and Mental Status: The interviewer probes for details of the patient's job interview and invites her to speculate about the reasons of her rejection (see chapter 3.1: Complaints). Presumably, since he expressed compassion for her situation, the patient reveals her persecutory delusional explanation for her rejection. Otherwise, she may have been more guarded, since patients with persecutory delusions are exposed to disbelief and ridicule and learn to hide their delusional beliefs.

Diagnosis: The persecutory delusions add to the list of included disorders (list no. 1, see chapter 5):

organic delusional syndrome
schizophrenia, paranoid type
delusional (paranoid) disorder.

The interviewer has excluded another option, namely the presence of a depression with persecutory delusions, by showing the absence of vegetative symptoms of depression (see Q. 11, 12).

28. I: You always have to fill out an application and they put that on the computer. They know everthing about you. Tell me, when did you notice it first?
    P: Oh, that was still when I was in Junction City. I made an appointment with an employer and I went in to see them, but I did not get the job. They already knew about me.

29. I: Was that the very first time?
    P: Yes.

30. I: So everything was fine before you came to Junction City. Where did you live before that time?
    P: We were in Arizona and lived in Phoenix. I was still married then.

31. I: Did anything happen in Phoenix?
    P: No, everything was fine.

32. I: And you had a good job in Phoenix?
    P: No, I really didn't.

33. I: But did you find one eventually?
    P: No, not really. Maybe it was in Phoenix when all this began. This was 18 years ago.

34. I: Tell me about it.
    P: When I came to Phoenix I made an appointment for an interview and when I got there the boss was not even there.

35. I: So he was out of the office?
    P: Yes, and all of a sudden I knew there was something fishy going on and it never stopped thereafter.

36. I: You lived with your husband before it started?
    P: Yes.

37. I: How was your marriage?
    P: Not very good. He was under the influence of his mother.

38. I: Did she live in Phoenix?
    P: No, that was in Illinois. Before we went to Phoenix we lived with his folks in Illinois.

39. I: What happened?
    P: His mother was always against me. She did not say anything, but I felt it. And I told her that I knew. So it did not work out and my husband and I went to Phoenix.

40. I: And that's where it started with the job problems?
    P: Yes. Whenever I applied for a job, they ran my name through a computer and they knew who I was and that I know everything about their computers. So, they got back at me by not hiring me.

Rapport: Since the interviewer continues to interview Francis from her point of view without expecting her to have any insight into the falsehood of her beliefs, he maintains good rapport.

Technique: The interviewer uses continuation and smooth transition techniques to explore the beginning of her delusional thinking and he is able to trace back her delusions until at least eighteen or more years ago.

Mental Status: The persecutory delusion appears to be well organized and long-standing. During the course of the conversation she shows no evidence of formal thought disorder. Everything she says is logical if her delusion were true.

Diagnosis: This segment reveals suspiciousness about the mother-in-law. The long-standing nature of the delusion further supports the notion that an affective disorder is probably not responsible for its occurrence. The persisting delusion also excludes any of the above-mentioned personality disorders as reason for the patient's problems since personality disorders by themselves do not produce delusions or hallucinations.

41. I: You have gone through a terrible ordeal. It must be awful to know that they won't give you a chance. Does your mood ever get affected by this?
    P: I get angry, but I try to show them that they can't wear me down.

42. I: Do you ever hear them talking about you?
    P: No, but I know they are there.

43. I: Have there been times when they haven't bothered you?
    P: No, it's there all the time. I try to ignore it, but I don't seem to get the job that I should.

44. I: You did not tell all this to Dr. B.?
    P: Well, I thought she would think I'm paranoid.

45. I: Is that what people think?
    P: Yes, they think I'm crazy.

46. I: What do you think?
    P: I don't think—I know it's true and they are wrong. They just cannot understand it. You are the first one who seems to believe me. You don't talk to me as if I'm crazy.

Rapport and Technique: The interviewer uses a smooth transition from Q. 40 to Q. 41. Again, he expresses empathy for the patient's ordeal (Q. 41) to maintain rapport and to prevent his becoming part of her delusional system.

Mental Status: The interviewer excludes auditory hallucinations (Q. 42) and documents further a lack of insight on the patient's part.

Diagnosis: The absence of hallucinations and a formal thought disorder allow the interviewer to exclude paranoid schizophrenia.

47. I: Thank you. I'm glad that you feel I understand what you went through!
    P: You can say that!

48. I: When you were under so much stress did you find that any kind of medication or even a glass of alcohol would help you or relax you?
    P: Why do you ask this? Do you think I am a drunk?

49. I: No, I don't think you are a drunk. But when people feel under stress like you do, they sometimes try to do something about it—they may drink a glass of wine and feel relaxed.
    P: I don't like alcohol.

50. I: Have you ever taken any other kinds of drugs?
    P: Like what?

51. I: I'm interested in any kind of drugs and the problems you may have taken them for.
    P: Maybe an aspirin for headaches or so.

52. I: Were there ever times when you had to take something to stay awake?
    P: No, I may drink a cup of tea, I don't even like coffee.

53. I: Have you ever had a problem with your weight and taken something for it?
    P: You mean amphetamines or so?

54. I: Hmm.
    P: I don't like drugs, okay? And I don't like your questions either. I don't like to be accused!

55. I: You are right, you went through enough without me making it worse for you. But I don't mean to accuse you. If it sounded like that I have to apologize.
    P: I don't understand why you think I abuse liquor or take uppers. I don't know what you are driving at.

56. I: Maybe you can tell me why these questions bother you.
    P: You think I'm paranoid from drinking or taking uppers.

57. I: You are right, when you take uppers regularly they can make you sensitive to rejection and can make you suspicious.
    P: Do you think I'm suspicious and paranoid?

58. I: You said employers are against you even before they really know you—just through the computers. Sometimes uppers can make you feel that way.
    P: I'm not taking any uppers. What I feel is real.

59. I: I believe you, I believe it feels very real what you went through. I believe you that you do not take any drugs. I believe also that you went through a lot, and I want to help you!
    P: Then stop accusing me!

Rapport: Rapport deteriorates when the interviewer explores alcohol and drug use. Smooth transitions do not prevent the patient suspecting that the interviewer interprets her problems as a result of drug or alcohol abuse. It makes her aware that he does not believe in her delusional explanations. This stirs her anger and distrust. The interviewer's confidence in his rapport with her is shown to be wrong. When you neglect the patient's stage of insight and express indirectly or directly any doubt in her perception, the suspiciousness of the patient with paranoid disorder can emerge at any time. If you fail like the interviewer did, save the situation, assure the patient, as shown above, that you believe her, that you are on her side, and that you want to help her.

Let's rescue the interviewer—from 20/20 hindsight. A more intuitive interviewer may have used the patient's delusional system to explore alcohol and drug abuse. Let's replay Q. 48ff.:

48. I: All these employers seem to check with the computer. Is there anything put into that computer record to harm you?
    P: Must be. Otherwise—why wouldn't they give me a job?

49. I: Do you have any idea what that could be?
    P: No. But maybe something about me knowing about computers . . . that I can't be fooled . . . that I may be dangerous to them.

50. I: Could there be anything else? Something to badmouth you? Something like dealing with drugs or cocaine, or taking it, or maybe secretly drinking alcohol?
    P: They couldn't do that. That would be a lie. I don't even take aspirin and I can't stand any liquor.

51. I: Is there a possibility that they could have gotten any kind of a hint where they saw you drinking a glass of wine or where you bought diet pills?
    P: Nonsense. No way. Nobody would believe that about me. I don't touch anything.

Here you get into an ethical dilemma. Accepting a delusion as a patient's reality is one thing. Using it for diagnostic purposes is another. If it benefits the patient without any chance of harming him one might use his delusional thinking to obtain clinically useful information; otherwise you may want to discuss the problem with a medical ethicist.

Mental Status: The original section Q. 47–59 showed how easily the patient's suspicion can be aroused and how quickly she can turn against you. A patient who may appear disinterested in nearly any subject and show blunted affect through most parts of the interview often shows a strong affect if her delusion is challenged: the delusion is affect-laden.

Differential Diagnosis: DSM-III-R

1. Schizophrenia, paranoid type 295.3x vs. delusional (paranoid) disorder 297.10.

The patient's age of onset (about 34) is compatible with both schizophrenia, paranoid type and paranoid disorder. The onset of schizophrenic disorders falls usually into adolescence or early adulthood. In schizophrenic disorders, paranoid type however, the onset tends to be later in life (middle or late adult life) just as in paranoid disorder. Clear and orderly thinking is better preserved in paranoid disorder than in paranoid schizophrenia. The patient's delusions lack the bizarre flavor common in schizophrenic disorders; they are isolated and systematized rather than fragmented, multiple, and intrusive in all types of behavior as found in schizophrenic disorders. There is also no evidence of prominent hallucinations, incoherence, or loosening of associations. Therefore the diagnosis of paranoid schizophrenia is rejected in favor of paranoid disorder.

2. Major affective disorder with psychotic features 296.34 vs. delusional (paranoid) disorder 297.10.

Persecutory delusions are common in both disorders. The persecutory delusions of depressed patients usually contain an element of guilt. Previous failures or sins are named as the reason for the persecution. The above patient names her knowledge of computers as reason for her persecution which has more a grandiose than a depressive flavor. The depressions rarely persist for more than two years. The decisive difference between the two disorders however is the presence of affective symptoms in major affective disorder but not in paranoid disorder. The patient denies affective symptoms; therefore the diagnosis of affective disorder with delusions is not supported.

3. Paranoid personality disorder (301.00, Axis II) vs. delusional (paranoid) disorder 297.10.

Easily provoked suspiciousness is common for both paranoid disorder and paranoid personality disorder. Both disorders exist in the absence of an affective disorder. Persistent psychotic symptoms, however, such as delusions are not part of the paranoid personality disorder. Therefore this diagnosis is rejected.

4. Organic delusional disorder 292.11 vs. delusional (paranoid) disorder 297.10. To make the diagnosis of an organic delusional disorder requires the demonstration of a specific organic factor judged to be responsible for the development of the delusions. Further probing into the patient's history such as a search for evidence of ictal phenomena, conducting a physical examination such as demonstration of focal neurological signs, or gathering laboratory test results such as a brain scan

may provide proof of such factors. Since the patient was beyond age 30 when—according to her own account—her disorder started, such a search for an organic factor should be conducted. In this patient, further workup did not produce any evidence for an organic basis to her delusions. Therefore, by exclusion, the working diagnosis was delusional (paranoid) disorder.

Final Diagnosis: DSM-III-R delusional (paranoid) disorder, persecutory type 297.10.

Epilogue: The patient was placed on thioridazine 400 mg/day. After six weeks of treatment she was still convinced that computers were running her life, but she could hide this delusion well from other people. She talked about it only to her psychiatrist and social worker. She found a job as an executive secretary and functioned adequately, while being continued on neuroleptic medication.

5.   AVOIDANCE IN PHOBIA

Difficulties in interviewing patients with agoraphobia and social phobia arise from both an embarrassment about the silly fear and an avoidance of discussing this fear.

You can overcome this avoidance behavior with two tactics: 1. Chiseling away at it by asking short, specific questions, often closed-ended, when you find that open-ended questions encourage evasiveness. 2. Attempt to make the patient comfortable with supportive and accepting statements trying to reduce both his anxiety and avoidance.

Here is an example where short, closed-ended questions were used.

Brenda, a 23-year-old, white woman, was referred by a psychiatrist who had left the outpatient group practice. Her record was vague; paranoid feelings were mentioned, but the diagnosis was deferred. She had been treated with 50 mg Mellaril t.i.d. without a change in her complaints.

  1. I: You have seen Dr. V. for quite some time. He had given you Mellaril but it did not seem to help you?
     P: Yeah. Maybe I was a little calmer, but I don't think it made much difference.

  2. I: Please tell me, why did you come to a psychiatrist in the first place?
     P: I don't know. It is because of other people. (Patient looks downward.)

3. I: Other people?
   P: Yeah. (Long silence.)

4. I: What is it about other people?
   P: I don't know. Maybe it's my stepfather. (Patient again avoids eye contact.)

5. I: Your stepfather?
   P: Yes, I can't speak up when he's there.

6. I: Why can't you speak up?
   P: I'm all bottled up. I can't get a word out. (Patient looks away.)

7. I: You can't talk to him?
   P: I think he'll hurt me.

8. I: Has he ever done anything bad to you?
   P: No, he was always nice to me. I have no reason . . . He probably thinks I'm weird.

9. I: How long have you had this stepfather?
   P: Just the last two or three years.

10. I: Did you have trouble with other people before that?
    P: Yes.

11. I: What do you think they'll do?
    P: They'll do me in.

12. I: Do you in?
    P: Yes.

13. I: In what way?
    P: Just hurt me.

14. I: How does that make you feel?
    P: I don't know. I really don't want to talk about it. I just try to stay away from it. (Looks down again.)

15. I: Are they really out to get you?
    P: I don't know. I think I'm silly. But I can't help it. (Looks to the side.)

16. I: Have they ever tried to plot against you?
    P: Oh no, they don't plot against me. I'm not paranoid. I just have that . . .

17. I: That . . .?
    P: Fear. It's silly, but I really don't want to think about it.

Rapport: On the surface, rapport appears to be adequate. Brenda is neither hostile nor fearful but vague, which may indicate that she is concealing something.

Technique: The interviewer uses short, pointed questions which she answers in an equally short but vague way. Then, he echoes the patient's statements in Q. 3, 5, 6, 7, 12 to open her up, but to no avail. He probes with symptom-oriented, closed-ended questions (Q.15 and 16) whether persecutory feelings are responsible for her vagueness. Her answers reveal that unexplained fear but not persecutory feelings lead to her avoidance behavior. Looking at the recorded interview, it is obvious that the interviewer missed an earlier opportunity after A. 8 to assess an unfounded, silly fear which points to a phobic disorder. Instead of Q. 9 he could have asked:

"Your stepfather is nice, yet you are afraid of him and think that this is weird?"

Her answer could have very well excluded a persecutory delusional fear in favor of a phobic fear.

After A. 14, the interviewer could have confronted the patient with her tendency to be short and vague, or provoke her with the interpretation that she is concealing something. Such an intervention could have sped up the interview, leading directly to the discussion of phobic avoidance. But it would also have carried the risk of activating the patient's defenses.

Mental Status: Brenda is alert, giving goal-directed but short and vague answers without latency of response. There is no evidence of a formal thought disorder. The reasons for her vagueness are neither persecutory feelings nor the inability to express herself but tendencies to avoid her silly, phobic anxiety. Her statements show that she has full insight into the morbid nature of this anxiety.

Diagnosis: Brenda reports a silly, unfounded fear (Q. 8, 15) that she avoids discussing. Her full insight is typical of the anxiety disorders:

List No. 1: Included Disorders:
   social phobia
   agoraphobia
   agoraphobia with panic
   social phobia and panic
   panic disorder
   avoidant personality disorder.
List No. 2: Excluded Disorders:
   paranoid schizophrenia
   paranoid disorder
   paranoid personality.

The task now is to uncover the phobic stimulus, if any.

18. I: I want to understand what makes you suffer.
    P: I'm okay, when I'm by myself.

19. I: You mean, it's only there when you are with other people?
    P: Yes.

20. I: Are there any people in particular you are afraid of?
    P: I don't think so. It's just all the time. (Looks down.)

21. I: What about me?
    P: I'm afraid you'll laugh at me, and think that I am making a fool of myself.

22. I: With me?
    P: Yes.

23. I: Is that what you are afraid of?
    P: Yes.

24. I: And with everybody else?
    P: I'm just scared. I don't dare say anything.

25. I: Does it make any difference who is there?
    P: No.

Rapport: The interviewer expresses his empathy for her suffering (Q. 18) but she rebuffs it and points out that she is not suffering when alone (A. 18). After the interviewer has explored to what extent he himself is a phobic stimulus for her, rapport improves. She answers more specificly and maintains eye contact.

Technique: The interviewer screens with closed-ended questions for the objects of her phobia (Q. 19, 21). She reveals her fear: to be ridiculed by other people.

Mental Status: The patient conceals the obvious expression of anxiety, but has often avoided eye contact.

26. I: Or how many there are?
    P: It gets worse when more people are there. I feel lost and dizzy. My heart pounds. I get all sweaty.

27. I: How do you manage at work?
    P: Oh, I try to sit all by myself.

28. I: How about going to the cafeteria?
    P: I don't go. I bring food from home and eat at my desk.

29. I: You mean you can't go out to eat?
    P: No. I haven't been out for the last few years.

30. I: Do you ever go to the movies?
    P: No. I seldom go. When I go, I go late. I slip in when it's dark.

Technique: The interviewer presents a laundry list of phobic stimuli which Brenda answers clearly.

Diagnosis: A. 26 shows that she may experience panic attacks. Since she also avoids crowded places, she may qualify for the diagnosis of agoraphobia with panic attacks.

31. I: When did all this start?
    P: Oh, it started back when I was in school. I couldn't finish high school. After the summer vacation I was scared to go to school. I couldn't stand it. So I never did go through my senior year.

32. I: Why didn't you tell anybody?
    P: I was scared to. I think it's so silly, people will laugh at me and think I'm crazy.

Diagnosis: A. 31 reveals that the patient had suffered from separation anxiety disorder of unusually late onset, but a mild form may have been present before that time. The interviewer does not follow up on clarifying this point.

33. I: Did this ever affect your mood? Did you ever get depressed?
    P: I'm low most of the time.

34. I: Does this affect your sleep?
    P: I sleep mostly alright.

35. I: Does it affect your appetite?
    P: No, my appetite is fine.

Diagnosis: The interviewer excludes the presence of an affective disorder.

36. I: When you get scared, do you ever get really panicky so that you can't catch your breath?
    P: One time I did that. I was all upset. I couldn't breathe, I got all sweaty.

37. I: Did you feel your heart?
    P: It was pounding in my throat and my chest hurt. I thought I was going to die. It hit me all of a sudden on a Sunday morning, out of the blue.

38. I: How often did you have this?
    P: I've only had it once. But I feel scared an awful lot.

The interviewer now proceeds to a standard interview.

Diagnosis: The interviewer attempts to assess presence and frequency of panic attacks. There is only evidence of one clear-cut panic attack (A. 38) even though statements in A. 26 suggest that at least milder forms occur more often.

Rapport: Remains adequate.

DSM-III-R Diagnosis: Brenda reports symptoms of a *social phobia* (300.23). She expresses fear of other people and tries to avoid them (criterion A of social phobia). She also recognizes that this fear is excessive and unreasonable but still cannot overcome it (criterion F of social phobia). The presented interview section does not allow the interviewer to rule out avoidant personality disorder (301.82). If the patient avoids public social exposure and performance because she feels disapproval and embarrassment, has no or only one close friend besides first-degree relatives, and exaggerates the difficulties of some ordinary activity, she would qualify for this personality disorder. This aspect is however not explored further.

Agoraphobia without panic attacks (300.21) is also present. The patient avoids restaurants and movie theaters (criterion A), and is isolated and constricted in her life (criterion B). There is no evidence obtained that she avoids public places out of fear of having a panic attack. The patient does report one spontaneous panic attack but DSM-III-R requires four attacks in four weeks, or one attack, with fear of having another one, persisting for at least one month. The interviewer fails to assess whether she had that persisting fear after her first attack. Therefore, he cannot establish the diagnosis of panic disorder with agoraphobia.

There is no evidence for major depression, paranoid personality disorder, or schizophrenia. Obsessive compulsive disorder was not assessed in this part of the interview.

Follow-up: The diagnosis of social phobia and agoraphobia without history of panic was made. The patient was placed on phenelzine, an MAO inhibitor. After six weeks, the patient felt much better. She was less scared to talk to individual people, but still avoided crowds. She was able to identify her feelings clearly as unreasonable fears rather than as persecutory ideas. The interviewer developed a plan for deconditioning her agoraphobia. She agreed to visit crowded shopping centers, movie theatres, and crowded restaurants on a regular basis, with stays of more than one hour at a time.

6. DISBELIEF AND EMBARRASSMENT
IN PANIC DISORDER

Panic disorder shares some symptoms with generalized anxiety disorder: motor tension, autonomic hyperactivity, apprehensive expectation, and hypervigilance. In DSM-III-R, some symptoms of generalized anxiety are mentioned as associate features of panic disorder but they are not a necessary criterion. If anxiety symptoms affect daily functioning, patients accept diagnosis and treatment (even though they may claim that they are not really psychiatric patients).

In contrast, patients who suffer from panic attacks without generalized anxiety between attacks often believe they have suffered a heart attack and are convinced of the physical origin of their disorder. They have full insight into the morbid nature of the attacks, but they have difficulty in accepting them as a psychiatric disorder. This conviction may become the obstacle to rapport and therefore to diagnostic assessment.

Adjust your interview to the patient's beliefs:

1. Tell him that the attacks are metabolic in nature with a genetic component. Assure him that the attacks are not just in his head or an expression of a weak character.
2. Combine educational statements with symptom exploration. To win the battle for his confidence, show him that you are an expert on the disorder.
3. Intersperse supportive statements to relax him.
4. Tell him that his condition can be treated by medication.

"I'm glad you came to see me. It is good that we finally know what's going on. I think we can help you with your problem."

Christian is a 23-year-old, 245-pound, muscular, 6'4" male who had requested to see only the director of the outpatient clinic.

1. I: Hi, my name is Dr. O. I understand you requested to see me.
   P: Yes.

2. I: My secretary told me that you didn't want to see anybody but the chief of the clinic.
   P: Right.

3. I: Was there any particular reason why you wanted to see only me?
   P: Yes.

4. I: (Looks at the patient quietly and attentively.)
   P: Well, I thought you must know best.

5. I: Hmm.
   P: I wanted to be certain that I get the best opinion.

6 I: Hmm.
   P: I figured you must know best, because otherwise you would not be the head of the clinic.

7. I: It must be of concern to you to get the best opinion.
   P: That's right.

Rapport: Whenever a patient makes special requests explore them; they give important clues. Christian's request reveals both apprehension about misdiagnosis and difficulty in accepting his disorder as psychiatric.

Mental Status: Answers to Q. 4–7 reveal apprehension and possibly some distrust.

Diagnosis: Apprehension and distrust are compatible with:

all anxiety disorders
affective disorders with anxious or paranoid features
adjustment disorder with anxiety about a physical illness
obsessive compulsive personality disorder
dependent personality disorder.

Technique: The clue "I want to see the head of the clinic" is followed up by clarification and interpretation (Q. 7).

8. I: Tell me what made you come here in the first place.
   P: I did not want to come. My doctor sent me.

9. I: It does not sound like you really agree with your doctor.
   P: No, I don't.

10. I: May I ask who your doctor was?
    P: Dr. H.

11. I: The cardiologist?
    P: Yes.

12. I: Did he explain to you why he wanted you to see me?
    P: Not really . . . I guess he may have.

13. I: You don't really remember?
    P: No. It's not that. But I was so upset. I could not really listen when he talked to me.

14. I: Okay, maybe we can start at the beginning.
    P: I was so upset and angry. I felt like a nut. I could not listen. I don't remember a word. But he said something like that you are more familiar with my condition than him. And if I want to get rid of it I'd better see you. So, why not? And I have to get over it, because I want to make the team and can't just crack up.

15. I: What is it that upset you so much? You say you felt like a nut?
    P: Yeah, I thought Dr. H. thinks I'm nuts, that I imagine things and that it's all in my head. But I'm not a guy like that. I can knock the daylight out of those offensive linemen. I don't need to imagine things.

16. I: What Dr. H. told you must have really hurt your pride.
    P: That's darn right. I felt like Jerry Ford or something, getting too many hits on the head and then cracking up—all these jokes they made about Jerry Ford being slow and clumsy . . .

Rapport: It becomes obvious that Christian has a problem with insight. It is unclear whether he denies being sick, but it is clear that he rejects having a psychiatric disorder and therefore, he has no reason to see a psychiatrist. He has the common misconception that "psychiatric patients are nuts; they imagine things." Later, this misconception should be corrected to gain trust, cooperation, and compliance; however, presently the interviewer knows too little about the patient's condition to make such an educational effort. Since the patient is motivated enough to wait for a diagnosis, he gives sufficient information without having to be urged to accept his condition as psychiatric.

Mental Status: The patient is tense, talks a lot, and shows some mild flight of ideas in Q. 15 and 16.

Technique and Diagnosis: The interviewer attempts twice to take a history (Q. 8 and 14). He fails because the patient shows resistance to seeing a psychiatrist—he is too upset. The interviewer allows him therefore to ventilate his feelings about having to see a psychiatrist rather than pushing him to give historical information. He uses clarification and interpretation techniques (Q. 15, 16) which release the patient's tension.

17. I: Let me suggest again that we start at the beginning. What made you see Dr. H.?
    P: Okay, let's start there. It happened at spring training. It was the first training session and all of a sudden I felt that pain. I felt choked and sweaty. I trembled and my heart pounded like crazy. I thought that's it— I am having a heart attack. I felt I had to die. It was just awful.

18. I: Do you mean it came in the middle of a workout?
    P: No, that's the embarrassing thing, and it's so frightening. We hadn't even started yet. And I just zonked out.

19. I: What happened then?
    P: They gave me oxygen at the camp and then they rushed me to the hospital. There they started to draw blood and ran an EKG. And then the EKG did not show anything, but they said it's safer to put me in a cardiac intensive care unit because sometimes those changes show up later. They told me later that my blood was normal and that I did not have a heart attack.

Rapport: The patient has sufficient rapport to give a history of events.

Mental Status: The patient is colorful and dramatic in his description, with adequate recall of details indicating intact recent memory.

Diagnosis: The patient describes a panic attack. Panic attacks can occur during:

alcohol withdrawal
amphetamine and caffeine intoxication
major depression
schizophrenia
somatization disorder
panic disorder.

Besides alcoholism and depression, organic reasons for a panic attack have to be considered:

cardiological
paroxysmal atrial tachycardia
angina pectoris
mitral valve prolapse
endocrinological
hyperthyroidism
pheochromocytoma
parathyroid disease
hypoglycemia.

The history is obtained by asking a very specific direct question (Q. 17).

20. I: And then Dr. H. told you to see a psychiatrist?
    P: No, not really. He just said he would like to get a psychiatric consultation.

I: Okay?
P: I told him if he did that, I would sign out right then.

22. I: So that really hurt your pride?
    P: Just because they didn't find anything doesn't mean that I'm nuts and that it's all in my head and that I'm imagining things!

23. I: I agree with you. But did Dr. H. really say that you imagined it?
    P: No, but he thought so. Why else would he want me to see a psychiatrist?

24. I: So you think going to a psychiatrist means that one imagines things?
    P: Isn't that right?

25. I: Well, not really. So you refused to let a psychiatric consultant evaluate you and you didn't want to see a psychiatrist on the outside later on?
    P: Absolutely not!

Rapport: With Q. 20 the interviewer continues history taking, but introduces again the topic of psychiatric disorder. Q. 22 gives an interpretation, and Q. 23 and 25 assure Christian that psychiatric disorders are not imagined. Such statements emphasize that he has a "respectable" disorder. It allows the interviewer to split off the sick and build an alliance. It prepares the patient to accept a psychiatric diagnosis and to comply with treatment, if he will accept the interviewer as expert and authority.

26. I: What made you change your mind? You are seeing me now.
    P: Well . . . I had another spell. It came out of the blue just five days ago. I was just sitting there watching TV and it came.

27. I: So you decided then to call up here and see me?
    P: Well, my mother kind of pushed me to do it. But I thought if the X.X. (professional football team) found out that I'm loony, that would be the end of my career.

28. I: But I am glad that you came.
    P: (Stares at his hands.)

29. I: (Waiting.) Is there anything making you feel uncomfortable?
    P: Well, I guess I should tell you that I really did not call here right away. I was just thinking about it.

30. I: But you are here now.
    P: The darnest thing is . . . It was Monday night, no really Tuesday morning. I woke up early . . .

31. I: Yes?
    P: And I had another spell. I thought then I can't live like this. The hell with what they think in X.X., if they want to scrap me, okay. But I can't take

it. I can't go around having those spells and feeling like dying. I just can't. It was that morning that I called your clinic.

32. I: Why didn't you go to another cardiologist?
    P: Well, Dr. H. is the best man in town, they say. And it has happened to me before. That was when I still was in college. Way back then they could not find anything either. So I thought I would just give it a try.

33. I: I am glad that you are here. So when you had these three attacks, you were really scared?
    P: Yes, I really thought I would die.

34. I: And how is that now?
    P: Well, I still think it might have been a heart attack. Maybe? They just did not see it.

Rapport: A. 27 and 31 show Christian's embarrassment and how only the frequency of attacks made him finally come to see a psychiatrist without giving up his internal resistance to this step (Q. 34). The patient is given support (Q. 28, 33) to encourage him to cooperate further.

Diagnosis: A. 32 reveals that Christian may have had a longer-standing history of panic attacks than originally reported.

35. I: Tell me more about the attack in training camp.
    P: I just got drafted as a rookie. I was a ninth round draft choice for the X.X. I tried hard to make the team as a defensive end. And that's when it happened, when all of a sudden my heart started to pound, I felt choked, I could not breathe, fought for air, had horrible chest pain. Everything looked blurry, I was sweating and trembling all over. They all must have thought I had a real heart attack and now it's nothing. What will they say when they find out that I see a shrink? (Hides his face in his hands.)

36. I: Is that why you came a few hundred miles to Kansas City?
    P: No, my parents live here. When I got out of the hospital the coaches wanted me to take a break.

37. I: How long ago did this happen?
    P: About two weeks ago.

Diagnosis: A. 35 describes the main symptoms of a panic attack. The last three attacks occurred in the last two weeks (A. 37).

38. I: Before you had that attack, was there anything happening?
    P: Like what?

39. I: Do you have any other problems?
    P: I don't know what you mean.

40. I: Well, let me ask you a few things. Did your appetite change?
    P: No, I could always eat like a horse. Only when I'm tired and exhausted, I only want to drink then.

41. I: Drink?
    P: No, I don't mean liquor. Just water or soft drinks. I don't care much for alcohol.

42. I: And how was your sleep?
    P: Pretty good. Never had any problems. But the night before the tryout I may have tossed and turned. I just worried if I can make it.

43. I: Did you feel in any way down or depressed?
    P: No, I was really excited, because X.X. is a really good football team and if I could make it, that would just mean a lot to me.

44. I: Did you take any kind of drugs?
    P: No. There were some guys who took speed—you know what they say about football players. But I try to stay away from it. I tried some pot in college, but I even quit that.

45. I: And you don't drink liquor either?
    P: No, not really . . . I may have a couple of beers with the guys, but no hard stuff.

Diagnosis: This section works on list no. 2 excluded disorders as causes for panic attacks:

major depression
alcohol abuse
psychoactive substance use.

Technique: Open-ended questions (Q. 38, 39) do not yield a precipitating event. They do not work too well for this patient. Closed-ended questions produce believable answers and not merely "yes" responses.

46. I: Did anybody in your family have problems that made them see a psychiatrist?
    P: No.

47. I: Was there anybody in your family who was believed to have had a heart attack?
    P: Well, I don't know. I think my Dad mentioned something like that.

48. I: Do you know more about that?
    P: Well, see, when my Dad was younger, he had a drinking problem. I think he mentioned something about thinking he had a heart attack, but they didn't find anything.

49. I: I see.
    P: Does that have anything to do with me? I tell you I don't have a drinking problem.

50. I: But you have those spells.
    P: Well, I thought my Dad thought that those spells came from drinking too much.

51. I: What about your mother, did she have any drinking problems or spells?
    P: No.

52. I: Did she ever see a psychiatrist or psychologist?
    P: I don't think so, not that I know of.

53. I: Do you have any brothers or sisters?
    P: One older brother and two younger sisters, but they are all right. I am the only one.

54. I: I understand. I would like you to know that those spells often occur in more than one member of a family.
    P: You mean they are genetic?

55. I: We don't know for certain. But it is possible that you may have been born with such a condition. Strenuous exercise can bring it on. It has something to do with the buildup of lactic acid in the blood. And that happens often when you exercise very hard. There are several drugs that can help you. What you had is called a panic attack. They feel real because they are real.
    P: You say drugs can help it? You mean I have to take heart medication all my life?

56. I: Well, it's not exactly heart medication that you need. But a drug that is a muscle relaxant and an antianxiety drug, or another one that is a so-called antidepressant may help you. And there is indeed also one medication that one could call a heart medication. It is called propanolol or inderal. This may also be helpful for your condition. Would you say that you are an anxious person?
    P: Well, . . . when I was younger . . . my mother always said I was hyper or head strong. Yes, I remember now, she used to say: "You are always so apprehensive." Apprehensive, I think that is a pretty good word.

57. I: I think we can help you with both these things, your spells and your apprehensiveness. Now, let's go over some of the things that you may have experienced when you were a child and teenager.

Rapport: Q. 56 educates Christian about the nature of the disorder to make the condition more acceptable to him and to encourage him to comply with treatment. Somatic treatments are emphasized in Q. 57.

The patient is now willing to describe himself as "generally anxious." Full rapport is established. Christian accepts the interviewer as the appropriate expert and authority to treat his condition. The remainder of the interview follows the standard interview.

Technique: The interviewer informs the patient about panic disorder and combines his teaching with questions that confirm this diagnosis if answered positively. This strategy reduces apprehension and permits the patient to describe "embarrassing symptoms."

Diagnosis: The family history reveals possible alcoholism and panic attacks in the father. The description of general anxiety supports the diagnosis of panic disorder. A workup to exclude some of the above-mentioned medical conditions may complete the diagnostic process.

Christian reports the essential features of panic attacks: discrete episodes of dyspnea (I feel choked), palpitations (my heart pounded like crazy, chest pain) and discomfort (I felt pain), choking sensations, sweating, trembling, and the fear of dying. He describes seven out of thirteen symptoms for panic disorder; required are only four out of thirteen during at least one attack. Not mentioned were the other symptoms: dizziness, feelings of unreality, paresthesia, hot and cold flashes, faintness, nausea, fear of dying, and fear of going crazy. DSM-III-R calls for at least four panic attacks within a four-week period in situations other than physical exertion, (or for one or more attacks followed by a period of at least a month of persistent fear of having another attack). Our football player meets these criteria. He has a typical adolescent onset and a positive family history.

He does not meet diagnostic criteria for other mental disorders such as depression, schizophrenia, or hysteria, and there is no association with agoraphobia. The only associated feature the patient admits to is apprehensiveness.

DSM-III-R Diagnosis: 300.01 panic disorder.

7. PERSECUTORY FEELINGS IN MENTAL RETARDATION

To interview a patient with mental retardation is usually not difficult: the patient talks in simple sentences and uses concrete words. Once you suspect it, a few simple tests (see appendix B) help to confirm your impression. However, a mentally retarded or dull normal patient is more difficult to diagnose if he is keenly aware of his deficiency, and tries both to overcome and to hide it. He is extremely sensitive when he feels anybody alluding to his deficiency. He develops self-protective suspiciousness and hypersensitivity.

Such a patient is under chronic stress. Everyday situations test his limits. He seems to be in a perpetual "adjustment" situation of the "dull among the smart." To appear smarter than he is, he may pursue schooling fanatically, gather a broad vocabulary, and copy behaviors, tastes, and themes of conversation of people he considers smart. He hides his inability to think abstractly behind learned phrases. And he can fool the nonsuspecting. German and Swiss psychiatrists have applied the term *Verhältnisblödsinn* to such patients (Bleuler 1972). This word indicates that the patient's goals are out of proportion to his capabilities (intelligence).

Usually, such a patient comes to the attention of a psychiatrist when he develops symptoms such as dysphoria, anxiety, or suspiciousness. At times it is difficult to discern whether he has an independent generalized anxiety disorder, affective disorder, delusional paranoid disorder, or symptoms in reaction to being chronically overtaxed.

What are the characteristics of this type of patient? He is frequently the offspring of middle- or upper middle-class parents. He often has retarded intellectual development resulting from a birth injury or other unknown factors. These disturbances may not have affected all intellectual functions equally; they rarely impair ambition and the hunger for success.

In our outpatient clinic, psychiatric residents, social workers, and psychologists have misdiagnosed this condition. They have often entertained a diagnosis of affective disorder but were surprised that antidepressants worked less than satisfactorily. May is one of these patients. She was invited for a diagnostic conference in which five residents participated. Her treating resident psychiatrist described her as depressed and treatment-resistant to tricyclic and MAOI antidepressants.

May, a 30-year-old, boyish-looking, small, single, white woman, with sharp facial features, enters the conference room. Her straight brown hair is unevenly cropped; she is casually dressed in blue jeans and a beige jacket, giving the impression of a graduate student. She glares at the interviewer, who stands up from the conference table where he and five residents are sitting and walks toward her. The patient reaches out to shake hands.

1. I: My name is Dr. O. I'm the director of the outpatient clinic. Your name is May? Please sit down. Have you been told what this meeting is about?
   P: (Sits rigidly on the chair with shoulders back, head poised arrogantly, piercing the interviewer with her eyes.) Yeah, I know—you're gonna ask me a bunch of questions—and give me some advice!

2. I: (Moves his chair closer so that he can touch May's arm if assurance is needed.) Well, this is a weekly conference with the residents. Each time we invite one of our clinic patients so that we can see her progress. Today you are that patient. Does it bother you to speak in front of a group?
   P: (Answers quickly, looking only at the interviewer and not at the group.) Dr. O., I've been lookin' forward to this for two weeks.

3. I: Have you met any of these doctors before?
   P: (Looks around the room, examines everybody carefully, and points with her finger.) These two. I used to see another doctor, but I guess she isn't here anymore.

Rapport: At the beginning of the interview the patient's body language signals a conflict: She shakes hands and seeks eye contact, but expresses a reserved even hostile attitude in her posture. The interviewer therefore postpones diagnosing in order to improve *Rapport*. Since May avoids eye contact with the group, he invites her to look at the group members, thus including them in the interview situation.

Technique: The interviewer includes the group to reduce May's tension somewhat, and to make her talk spontaneously. He switches to concretely worded, short sentences to facilitate communication.

Mental Status: The concreteness and shortness of May's first answer may point to a difficulty with abstract thinking. The rapid and short second answer without eye contact to the group suggests anxiety as the most likely affect. May recalls the interviewer's name, indicating that she has good short-term memory, or that she had rehearsed his name prior to the interview to avoid failure. May recognizes her past resident physicians—obviously her recent memory is intact. She stays relaxed while facing a group of people which demonstrates that she has no extreme social avoidance.

Diagnosis: May interacts with the group—without avoidance behavior as seen in phobic patients—or guardedness as seen in patients with persecutory delusions—or joking interaction with individual group members as seen in patients with mania.

> *List No. 1: Included Disorders:*
> Mental retardation.
> *List No. 2: Excluded Disorders:*
> mania
> paranoid schizophrenia
> paranoid disorder
> phobic disorder
> paranoid personality disorder
> avoidant personality disorder.

Shift to Diagnosing

4. I: How long have you been coming to the clinic?
   P: For about a year.

5. I: What was your problem when you first came here?
   P: (Patient stiffens her back and seems to shoot out of her chair.) What d'ya mean, *Problem?* You think I got a *Problem?*

6. I: (Interviewer touches her arm and looks in her face for a second until the patient relaxes.) Maybe I should have said "reason" you first came to the clinic.
   P: (Appears dumbfounded, rolls her eyes sarcastically.) You're the doctor, you're s'posed to know what's wrong with me. (Pause.)

7. I: Can you tell me how I can help you?
   P: (Indignantly.) *I* didn't need help—my math teacher—*she* says I need help.

8. I: Your math teacher?
   P: (More jovially.) Yeah, we was playin' some tennis one day and she came up to me and she says: "May, you don't talk about things anymore"; I said to her: "I don't?" And she says, "You need to see somebody." And so here I am.

9. I: Did you agree with that? Did you also notice a change while in college?
   P: Well, yeah, because I started getting bad grades.

10. I: Was that a change from high school?
    P: Change? Of course it was a change! I made all A's and B's in high school.

11. I: Were you an honor student in high school?
    P: No.

12. I: What kind of grades did you have in high school English?
    P: English? I hated that rotten subject—I got a C out of the course—and I worked so hard for it.

13. I: What about math?
    P: (With increasing hostility.) What year?

14. I: Senior year.
    P: Well, I put in a lot of time but the teacher hated my guts and that's why I only got a C. (Looks down at her knees with an angry expression on her face.)

15. I: What about social studies?
    P: (With a hostile peek at the interviewer.) That's the worst course, most of the stories don't make any sense. I read lots of books for it. I hated that course worse than any of them. I got a D out of that course. (May bites her lower lip and breathes heavily.)

Shift to Rapport

16. I: I notice that you feel bothered by my questions.
    P: Darn right! Why do you have to pick on my weak spots? Can't you be nice for a change?

17. I: You are right. I should really ask you what courses you liked in high school?
    P: (Sighing with relief) I loved basketball and choir.

Rapport: May feels attacked by words such as her "problem" (Q. 5). The interviewer therefore substitutes "reason" for "problem" and touches her arm to calm her down but to no avail. She changes her attitude immediately when she can tell her story—showing that her irritation is not rooted in persecutory delusions (Q. 8). She resumes a hostile attitude, when she feels cornered by questions about her grades (Q. 11–15). The interviewer shifts therefore from diagnostic history taking back to rapport and confronts her with her emerging hostility (Q. 16). Only when he asks her about her strengths does she blossom.

Technique: Closed-ended, directive questions and deliberate probing into May's intellectual weaknesses provoke her anger and tension. Therefore, the interviewer shifts to open-ended questions, allowing May to choose the topic (Q. 17).

Mental Status: May interprets "problem" and "help" concretely as accusations. The rapid switch in her attitude from hostility to trust, when given the opportunity to tell her story, reveals that her hostile suspiciousness was not delusional but situational and self-protective in nature. These misinterpretations of words highlight her inability to abstract. Her concrete thinking surfaces again, when she does not summarize but repeats the complete dialogue with her math teacher—as a child would do—without going beyond the most literal meaning of the words (A. 8). May also accepts and follows naively her math teacher's advice. All indicate low intelligence.

Diagnosis: Her misinterpretation of words followed by hostility and her poor abstraction point to an organic mental disorder with persecutory ideas. Since these signs surface in a young person, they indicate borderline mental retardation. Since her persecutory ideas, or ideas of insecurity may reach back to her high school days, they point to an organic personality disorder.

The social withdrawal (as noticed by her math teacher) indicates either a superimposed adjustment reaction with depressed mood, or a depression.

> *List No. 1: Included Disorders:*
> organic mental disorder
> mental retardation
> organic personality disorder
> adjustment disorder with depressed mood
> unipolar affective disorder.
> *List No. 2: Excluded Disorders:*
> see above.

Shift Back to Diagnosis

18. I: How did you get along with the other students in high school?
    P: I was the most popular one.

19. I: What about teasing each other?
    P: (Proudly and emphatically.) Yeah, I did all the teasing.

20. I: Can you tell me a little bit about your friends?
    P: Well. (Pause.) I don't have many. Maybe one or two.

21. I: How did this happen?
    P: Because I hate people—they're rotten and they stab you in the back. I get all the bad breaks in life.

22. I: Could you tell me about some of your bad breaks?
    P: (Pleased.) Do you have all day? (Laughs.) Well, here's one of them. In college I was friends with the English prof and we were playin' tennis and he said I should take his class, so I did. At first, I was makin' A's and then B's, and somehow he gave me a D out of the course. I don't get it—he gave me a D on this last paper I wrote and then I gave it to a friend for her class—I knew it was cheatin' and all, but I felt sorry for her—well, she got an A out of the course and the teacher said it was the best paper he ever read! So, is that a bad break or what?

Shift to Rapport

23. I: Sounds like it. You must have felt really awful. She gets an A and a mention of the best paper, when you get a D for the same thing. I can understand your anger and disappointment.
    P: Yeah . . . Let me tell you another one! Once I had a girlfriend and I told her that I kinda liked this guy and before I knew it I found out she was sleepin' with him!

24. I: You told her your secret and she took advantage of it. That must have torn you up.
    P: You better believe it. I'm never gonna talk to that bitch again. I am through with her for life, Dr. O.

Shift to Mental Status

25. I: Do you feel there is a reason behind why you get all these bad breaks?
    P: Like what?

26. I: Is there anybody who has it in for you?
    P: What do you mean?

27. I: Like somebody who doesn't like you and plots against you.
    P: It looks like it, but I guess it's just bad luck.

Shift to Diagnosis

28. I: Any other bad breaks that you would like to tell me about?
    P: Yeah, I was workin' for the police department in the animal care department and what happened was that the officer there hated my guts, and finally he told me to go over to a house and pick up these dogs. So I went over there and picked 'em up. He called me in later and said: "May, what have you done? You went into a man's backyard and picked up his dogs!" But that is exactly what he told me to do and I told him so, but he just said, "Get the hell out of here—you're fired!"

29. I: Is there anything else you would like to tell me?

    P: I could sit here for twenty years and tell you about my bad breaks, be-cause I have them all the time. My car just blew up and I don't have any money. My parents hate me and my sisters are always putting me down. I felt so low, nothing turned me on anymore.

30. I: May, you got hit with so many bad breaks—did that ever affect your appetite at all?

    P: Yeah, some months back there were weeks where I didn't want to eat a thing.

31. I: Did you lose any weight?

    P: Must have, 'cause my jeans were baggy.

32. I: How was your sleep?

    P: I didn't. You wouldn't either, if you had so much on your mind.

33. I: So you must have really felt bad. Did you have any friends to talk to?

    P: No, shit, I didn't want to talk to anybody.

34. I: Did you have a boyfriend then?

    P: I had no interest in guys or sex, are you kidding? I had no fun with nothin'.

35. I: How is your sleep and appetite now?

    P: Oh, it's really much better since I take those pills for depression. Now I eat too much and oversleep. But I still don't care for other people.

Shift to Mental Status Examination

36. I: (Pause.) May, can I ask you some questions that will help us to assess the way you think?

    P: (Indignantly.) Dr. O., I am not here for my thinking. I'm here to get your help. Why are you trying to cut me down like everybody else?

Shift to Rapport

37. I: May, I don't want to cut you down. I think you can stand on your own. I just would like to ask you these questions to help you better.

    P: I don't want to do that right now.

38. I: Okay, May, that's fine. I would like you to know that I think you have a lot going for you. You speak up, you are quite motivated, and I think we can help you. Thank you for coming in.

Rapport: By referring to "all the bad breaks in life," the interviewer encourages May to complain and to reveal her suffering. When he shows empathy, she is no longer hostile, and continues to open up and elaborate on further frustrations. However, when the interviewer wants to test her intellectual functions, May resumes a hostile and defensive attitude. Instead of taking this examination as part of the interview, she misinterprets it as criticism. To finish on a positive note, the interviewer summarizes the patient's assets. She is grateful for the personal feedback and leaves the office head up and with a big smile (Q. 36–38).

Technique: The interviewer foregoes scrutinizing May's claim of being popular. He avoids breaking through her denial (which could endanger rapport). Instead, he focuses on her "bad breaks," and probes the borders between suspicious, delusional, and illogical thinking. The switch to open-ended questions allows May greater freedom to express herself.

Mental Status: The patient reports "bad breaks," a perception which is not due to persecutory delusional thinking or overvalued ideas (Q. 25–27), but to her inability to understand events around her as results of cause and effect.

May's monosyllabic, simplistic, and concrete word choice again underscores her limited intellectual capacity. Taking things literally impairs her judgment, e.g., she does no realize she could pick up only stray dogs and not dogs in someone's backyard. Her concrete thinking fosters misinterpretations and suspiciousness. They lead to anger and frustration.

Differential Diagnosis: 1. Depression in remission: May fulfills diagnostic criteria for major depression. A restricted affect and lack of emotional tone are still noticeable. The diagnosis of depression excludes—according to DSM-III-R—an alternate or additional diagnosis of adjustment reaction with depressed mood (Q. 30–35).

2. Borderline intelligence: Continually poor performance in high school and college, concrete thinking, and poor word choice support this diagnosis.

3. Organic personality disorder DSM-III-R 310.10: May made persecutory interpretations, and is defensive and hostile when she feels threatened. Denying any need for help, because she wants to appear competent and self-sufficient, limits her insight. Her paranoid tendencies may originate in an organic impairment and may, therefore, be diagnosed as an organic personality disorder. The diagnosis of a paranoid disorder cannot be made because delusions were not detected.

4. Psychosocial stressors: College exerted continual pressure to perform which she could not master.

Comment

This is an incomplete diagnostic interview. It did not address diagnoses such as: drug abuse, alcoholism, mania, anorexia nervosa, phobias, panic disorder, and paranoid schizophrenia. Furthermore, the course of present disorders, family, social, and medical history were not assessed. Feedback to the patient was not given by the interviewer, but was later provided by the resident.

Later, May's birth record was obtained. It supported the impression of an organic impairment. She was born prematurely (seven months), and needed prolonged care in an infant intensive care unit—a possible reason for her below average intelligence. A Wechsler Intelligence Test taken later confirmed the clinical impression. Of further diagnostic relevance would be:

1. premorbid history from outside sources
2. neuropsychological testing
3. assessment of so-called "soft neurological signs" which may be indicators for brain insult at birth.

This interview shows that without the index of suspicion of mild mental retardation, the lack of improvement could not be understood. May's mental status and the nature of her social difficulties revealed her impairment in thinking, problem solving, and judgment.

CHAPTER NINE

DISORDER-SPECIFIC INTERVIEWING: PERSONALITY DISORDERS

SUMMARY

Chapter 9 describes how to establish rapport, select your interviewing techniques, and modify your mental status examination to diagnose patients with personality disorder.

It is worse to be sick in soul than in body, for those afflicted in body only suffer, but those afflicted in soul both suffer and do ill.

Plutarch, Moralia:
Affections of soul and body, sec. 501 E. About 95 A.D.

Each of the thirteen personality disorders listed in DSM-III-R poses specific obstacles to interviewing. For instance, a patient with dependent personality disorder may endorse symptoms that, in fact, he has not experienced but feels compelled to admit to in order to please the interviewer. In contrast, a patient with antisocial personality disorder may lie about his past and deny problems to impress the interviewer.

It is the interviewer's task to spot such behavior and trace its origin. Such pursuit often leads right into the center of personality pathology. Since patients with a personality disorder have no or only limited insight into their disorder, and therefore cannot report their pathology in terms of symptoms, the observation of the patient's behavior during the interview becomes an important tool for the diagnosis of personality disorders.

To facilitate this process we have highlighted the pathological behavior of each of the thirteen personality disorders which most likely emerge during and interfere with the diagnostic interview.

1. EMOTIONAL WITHDRAWAL AND ODD BEHAVIOR—CLUSTER A

Three personality disorders are in cluster A: paranoid, schizoid, and schizotypal.

The mental status of a patient belonging to cluster A is characterized by emotional withdrawal, lack of warmth, and odd, or eccentric behavior. Throughout the interview he lacks spontaneity, appears cold and sometimes sarcastic, and seems even to hide his feelings from you. Regardless of your technique, and the type of question you ask, the patient has a tendency to answer with "yes" and "no." It is difficult to induce him to talk spontaneously and the interview does not flow. You never get the feeling that you are truly in touch with him and have rapport.

The interviewing process differs according to the type of personality disorder, but in all cases you will experience a lack of rapport. If you analyze the reason for this deficit, you will find the patient's coldness is the culprit. Make it the point of departure for your interview. Explore whether the patient showed these characteristics throughout his life, resulting in social isolation. After exclusion of the axis I disorders such as schizophrenia and delusional (paranoid) disorder, you have narrowed down your diagnostic options to a personality disorder.

Suspiciousness in Paranoid Personality Disorder

Rapport: Rapport with a patient who has paranoid personality disorder is hampered by his pervasive perception that everybody, absolutely everybody, will harm or exploit him. He screens all questions for hidden meaning, and conspiratorial content. He questions your trustworthiness; your friendliness, which he may assume is fake, a cleverly disguised attempt to take advantage of his weaknesses; your limit setting, assuming a strategy of revenge; your offer to help him, a Trojan horse. You cannot win because he has exposed you. He is nobody's fool because he is nobody's friend.

Genuine openness may persuade him to temporarily trust you with some of his problems. If you openly tell him how suspicious you find him, he may be impressed by your frankness, or he may interpret your statements as hostile, critical, or insulting. He may decide to cooperate with you, but may, at any moment, feel betrayed and disappointed, and launch out at you with a hostile counterattack.

Mental Status: The mental status of a patient with paranoid personality disorder is overshadowed by hypervigilance and suspiciousness. His attire may be meticulous so as not to give anybody reason for criticism, or show some neglect if he is depressed. He may then express that he is not interested in pleasing anybody. His speech is usually fluent and goal-directed. But the content of these goals is characteristic of his disorder: checking out your intentions, expressing that he looks through your maneuvers, and voicing his displeasure about your secret plans. His affect vacillates between anxiousness, and overt hostility. Memory and orientation are intact, but his judgment is impaired by his suspiciousness. He may acknowledge his suspiciousness but staunchly defend it as justified and not accept it as a part of a personality disorder.

Interviewing such a patient is delicate. As he expects all your questions to have a hidden, and threatening meaning, he will scrutinize them:

"Why do you ask that?"

But he resents being scrutinized himself. Smooth transitions are absolutely necessary. Any abruptness will be experienced as an unjustified switch in topic and may lead to anger, counterattack, or abrupt termination of the interview. He will confront you but not tolerate confrontation himself.

Diagnosis: The patient does not present any difficulty other than having to interview him with great caution in order not to trigger his suspiciousness and hostility. Since his hostility is so pervasive, it comes to the forefront early on. To establish a diagnosis of paranoid personality disorder exclude persecutory delusions and any type of hallucinations; this eliminates paranoid schizophrenia and paranoid disorder. Organic mental disorder, substance abuse, depression, and mixed states of manic depressive disorder may be associated with suspiciousness and ideas of reference, however this suspiciousness rarely remains on a nondelusional level. The latter is also time-limited, shows a circumscribed beginning, and association with other symptoms of a specific disorder.

If social withdrawal, aloofness, and coldness emerge during the interview, and if the patient expresses some odd and superstitious ideas, you will explore the differential diagnosis of the personality disorder of cluster A. Notice that the border between delusional (paranoid) disorder (axis I) and paranoid personality disorder (axis II) is fluid. While the patient with paranoid disorder sees his behavior as the best response to a danger he perceives as real, the patient with paranoid personality disorder, who has an awareness of his increased suspiciousness, usually tries to keep it to himself but finds reasons to justify it. Here is a more severe case:

I: Hi, would you like to come in?
P: What do you mean—like to come in?

I: Didn't you want to talk to me?
P: Who gave you that idea?

I: Well, you made an appointment, didn't you?

P: Are you holding this against me? Maybe I shouldn't have.

I: Since you are here, why don't you sit down.

P: You think you've got me already. Ok. Let's get on with it. I will sit down, but don't think that I will submit to your tricks. I have had some experience with psychiatrists. They are basically all the same. They trick and outmaneuver you—at least that's what they try to do, but not with me.

I: You don't seem to like or trust me.

P: Besides Nixon I have not found anyone I trust as little as a psychiatrist.

Withdrawal in Schizoid Personality Disorder

Rapport: Rapport with such a patient is hampered by his pervasive emotional withdrawal. There is no emotional response at the start of the interview, and none at the end. If you express empathy—it leaves him cold. He may talk about his depressive feelings, but you don't feel his suffering. Since emotional warmth is missing, you cannot judge whether the problems he talks about are central to him. You cannot appreciate whether he likes, trusts, and respects you, or resents you. It does not help when you ask him about it, because he does not know; and if he knows, it does not matter, because he does not care. He is indifferent. Rapport is a state where the patient is willing to reveal and discuss his symptoms, problems, and innermost feelings. Since the schizoid personality does not appear to have those feelings, you never get the impression of having rapport.

Mental Status: It is characterized by edgy body movements, lack of facial expression, and frozen and clumsy gestures. His speech is goal-oriented but lacks detailed elaboration. The tone of voice rarely ever changes, not even when he talks about the most intimate or traumatic events in his life. Neither the death of his mother, nor the loss of a friend seems to affect him. This lack of responsiveness underscores his main deficit: affective withdrawal.

The more intelligent patient with this personality disorder sometimes complains about his lack of interest and motivation. He may even name this state "depression," but he usually does not report associated sadness, guilt, or anguish.

A patient with schizoid personality disorder does not hallucinate or display delusional thinking; he may have some ideas of reference and a feeling that others don't care for him, but if they did, it would burden rather than please him. His memory is usually intact. He sees himself as less animated than others but does not consider this lack of interest a disturbance. His judgment concerning future plans is usually adequate; he rarely overestimates his potential unless he develops a schizophreniform disorder. Only if he/she is threatened with losing his job or spouse (male patients with schizoid personality disorder rarely marry) he may consult a therapist. Then he usually reports vegetative symptoms and depressed mood for which he seeks treatment.

Technique: You notice from the beginning that the patient only answers with "yes" and "no," or with very short, seemingly absentminded replies. You may misinterpret this poverty of words as sensitivity and become cautious not to hurt his feelings, but this would be an incorrect assumption. Any strategy seems to fail. No matter whether you invite him to talk about any topic of his choice, or try to push him with highly structured questions, the flow of information remains thin. You will detect that his restricted verbal and emotional expression is not due to self-protection but to mental and emotional emptiness. Therefore, you can start and end where you want—abruptly—nothing matters.

Diagnosis: Be aware that a patient with schizoid personality disorder usually comes to your attention when he develops a major psychiatric disorder (axis I) such as substance abuse, depression, or a schizophreniform disorder, or struggles with external stressors (axis IV).

The combination of a major psychiatric disorder with schizoid personality disorder is a source of confusion. A concomitant depression, for instance, may present in a younger person as a simple schizophrenia because of severe blunting of affect and severe social isolation. Fleeting hallucinations, due to substance abuse such as LSD, may make you consider incipient schizophrenia. The accuracy of your diagnosis will however be assured if you routinely include in your differential the combination of an axis I disorder with an axis II personality disorder.

Usually, it is not so much the chief complaint of the schizoid personality but the observed mental status that will tip you off. With your suspicion aroused, scrutinize the patient's social history. His life history is marred by loneliness, isolation, and desertion which seem to be more significant to you than to him.

The schizoid personality's behavior pattern and interactions seem to correspond to the symptomatology of patients with negative symptoms of schizophrenia: the same lack of initiative, blunted affect, poverty of gestures and verbal productions are seen. However, these patients are not hallucinating, they do not harbor delusions or show a formal thought disorder, and their reality testing is intact.

The following segment illustrates rapport and mental status with Mr. Forster, a patient with schizoid personality disorder.

I: Mr. Forster, can you tell me what kind of problems made you come to our clinic?
P: My work.

I: Would you tell me about the problems that you have at work?
P: No interest.

I: It must feel bad to work all day without being really interested.
P: Hmm.

I: What kind of work do you do? Tell me more about it!
P: Lab work.

I: What kind of laboratory do you work at?
P: Animal.

I: Please tell me what do you do in your lab?
P: Setting up experiments.

I: For how long have you had a problem with not being interested?
P: From the start.

I: How long have you been working at your present job in that laboratory?
P: Some years.

I: Has it always been that bad with your interest as it is now?
P: No.

I: When did this problem start?
P: Lately.

I: Can you give me a more accurate time frame?
P: Maybe spring of this year.

I: How have you been feeling lately?
P: Not so good.

I: I'm sorry to hear that you have not been feeling so good. What seems to give you the most trouble? Is it the type of work? Or other people at work? Can you give me some idea?
P: I'm feeling bad.

I: Can you pinpoint this?
P: Not really.

I: How are things at work? What is it about your work that makes it so uninteresting?
P: It's slow.

I: Are you getting your work done in time?
P: Barely.

I: Does anyone complain, push you, or threaten you?
P: No.

I: Or does anybody ask you to do more work?
P: There isn't that much to do.

No matter how hard you try, no matter how emphatic you are, whether you ask short, elaborate, structured, or unstructured questions, his responses are monotonous and short. He does not elaborate. Any affective tone is missing. To establish a differential list you will have to review a laundry list of symptoms using structured questions that permit yes and no answers. Such an interview will frustrate you but not the patient, who will return for the next appointment and will be as monotonous and uninspired as the first time around.

Irrationality in Schizotypal Personality Disorder

Rapport: When you try to establish rapport with a patient with schizotypal personality disorder, you will be amazed by his unusual formulations, surprising statements, and peculiar ideas. Rapport is hampered as long as the patient feels that you cannot appreciate his experiences.

Empathy for his feelings and thoughts can lure him out of his reserve. When you indicate that you don't reject him, and that you understand his perceptions and feelings, his confidence in you will grow and he will open up to you the sanctuary of his secret, autistic world. He will share with you new insights, personal references, sensitivities, and an individualized awareness that transcend reality. This responsiveness allows you to shape your rapport with the schizotypal patient which contrasts with the establishment of rapport with the schizoid patient, where none of your interventions makes a bit of difference.

Mental Status: The mental status shows several characteristic features.

The patient's attire may be somewhat peculiar; he may carry a talisman around his neck. He may use words with an unusual meaning, or in an unusual context. His sense of humor may strike you as bizarre, and his thoughts may be hard to follow. He will make an effort to communicate his thoughts and feelings to you provided he trusts you and believes you are worthwhile talking to.

The patient's thought content is indeed remarkable. It may show paranoid ideation, suspiciousness, ideas of reference, and magical thinking. He may claim to have access to a fourth dimension, to have out-of-body experiences, ESP, telepathy, and premonitions. The peculiarities in formulation and thought content give you the impression that the patient is odd, strange, eccentric, and superstitious. His affect changes with the thought content. He may appear aloof and cold when you involve him in topics of your choosing, but becomes lively and even intense in his affect when he talks about his telepathic experiences and his convictions.

His orientation, memory, and information processing is intact and his speech is coherent. However, his judgment is influenced by thoughts situated outside the realm of verifiable reality. He has partial insight; he knows that others consider him as odd, strange, and sometimes hard to understand. But he sees them as unable to look beyond a simplistic reality and not as critics of his poor reality testing.

Technique: The patient answers all types of questions if you have established rapport. You frequently have to ask him to specify his impressions and give you examples. In this clarification process you detect that he sees relationships among events and people that are not obvious. You can follow the direction of thinking without being fully able to appreciate its elements. Any empathic and interested approach to listening together with continuation techniques usually suffice to make the patient explain his experiences. In contrast, doubting questioning and expressions of rejection of his views, or confrontations with his reality cause the patient to recoil.

A bright patient with schizotypal personality disorder often desires to find out whether you have experiences similar to his. For him it is not enough that you are interested in his views; he hungers to communicate on the same wavelength. To handle this situation is more a question of *rapport* than a problem of how to formulate questions most effectively.

Diagnosis: The patient's oddities remind you of a schizophrenic patient with positive symptoms. Yet, when you hunt for delusions or hallucinations, you find none, neither in his mental status nor in his past history, even though his thinking is reminiscent of a thought disorder, with overvalued ideas and ideas of reference. Scrutiny of the patient's past will reveal that even as a teenager he was considered odd and strange. Such chronicity alerts you to the presence of a personality disorder of cluster A.

The lack of predominantly paranoid ideas differentiates the schizotypal from the paranoid personality disorder. Preoccupation with the occult and the supernatural differentiates it from the schizoid personality disorder.

The following interview with Kevin illustrates some of the characteristics of schizotypal personality disorder.

1. I: Where shall we begin?
   P: I may as well start with them, the character disorders.

2. I: Tell me about them!
   P: I think the people who give you the most trouble—that's who they are.

3. I: It sounds that some people bother you a lot.
   P: You see, it all depends. I hate the character disorders who are cruel and who hurt you. You can feel their aggressive thoughts, but I quit my job so they can't get at me anymore.

4. I: It must feel awful to be harassed by those people.
   P: I just have to stay away from them.

5. I: Did they try to harm or persecute you?
   P: It's their thoughtlessness that hurts you.

6. I: Have they ever tried to follow you, observe your house, tap your phone, bug your bedroom, or living room?
   P: No, but I'm surprised that you ask. Are you in tune with them?

Kevin uses formulations such as "who are cruel and who hurt *you*" rather than "who are cruel and who hurt *me*." Such formulations seem to intend to declare his experiences as generally true. This interpretation is supported by his direct question (A. 6): "Are you in tune with them?" The interviewer evades a direct answer and emphasizes that he wants to understand Kevin's feelings, but avoids the claim to share them.

7. I: I want to understand how they bother you, how they get to you.
   P: The way they look at you, the way they don't talk to you.

8. I: Have you ever heard them even when they were far away?
   P: No, not really.

9. I: Have you heard any voices ever?

   P: My own thoughts, I think them in words. I imagine how they would sound if I were to speak them out loud. There is the quality of sound in thoughts. Thoughts go beyond people. They interconnect and survive.

10. I: Do you have access to those interconnecting thoughts? Are you familiar with ESP?

    P: I can sense them, I can sense the hostile thoughts of the character disorders.

11. I: Tell me about these character disorders! Who are they?

    P: Those people who impose on your thoughts—you meet them everywhere. These thoughtless, callous mental morons.

12. I: Do you think they are like a fraternity? Sticking together and conspiring against you?

    P: No, they are not like a conspiracy—more here and there, you know, just like people you meet and don't like. I don't think they are organized. It's more like a mind game.

After he found the interviewer receptive, Kevin communicates freely about his perceptions. The interviewer's attitude toward Kevin's odd views is similar to the position taken toward hallucinations and delusions (see chapter 4): he pretends he is interviewing an astronaut who has visited a remote planet. What he reports was certainly his experience even though not immediately verifiable by the listener.

2. EXAGGERATED, DRAMATIC EMOTIONALITY— CLUSTER B

The four personality disorders in cluster B are the antisocial, borderline, histrionic, and narcissistic personality.

The mental status of a patient belonging to cluster B impresses you by erratic, exaggerated, dramatic, and nongenuine emotional display with colorful affect. Most of the time the patient is not aware of his affectation or inappropriateness. His speech is usually fluent but often vague and evasive. Frequently, he gets caught in contradictions. He intends to impress you by his behavior rather than by the revelation of his problems or suffering.

Superficially, this type of patient is easy to interview. Open-ended questions usually lead to lengthy, emotionally colorful answers decorated with similes and metaphors. You have to ask him to specify, to narrow down; you have to curb the flow and steer his direction. Usually he is not irritated by accentuated or abrupt transitions but is easily hurt and angered by interpretations.

However, because of his superficially exaggerated emotionality, and his desire to impress you, it is difficult to establish rapport during the interview. You do not feel he is leveling with you. He may threaten, complain, beg, flirt, or tease. It is difficult for you (and for him) to get in touch with his true feelings which seem hidden behind the emotional display.

The mental status, and the type of rapport alert you to a personality disorder of cluster B.

Lying in Antisocial Personality Disorder

Patients with antisocial personality (sociopaths) rarely consult a psychiatrist for behavior problems. Instead, they come in for alcoholic detoxification, to get a certificate as excuse from work, to obtain stimulants or sedative hypnotics (drugs with street value), or to avoid prison after committing a crime by claiming mental disorder.

Rapport: Rapport with such a patient is a problem. It is easy to talk to him as long as you play along, but he will criticize you and be angry when you resist his manipulations. It is difficult to make him focus on deficits such as his lack of emotional control and his unwillingness to act responsibly, or to consider the negative consequences of his behavior. This lack of sincerity and genuineness prevents rapport. If he perceives you as an authority figure he will protest against you clandestinely or even openly.

It has been said that the sociopath lacks a sense of suffering. This is only partly accurate. He is usually not remorseful about his lying, stealing, angry outbursts, or hurting others, but he can be made aware of the fact that nothing is going right for him and that he is ruining his life. You can establish rapport and review the patient's difficulties free of lies and distortions, when you show him empathy for the consequences of his behavior and his failures:

"I agree that you've had a fair share of trouble. Maybe we can find a way to prevent it in the future by finding out where things go wrong."

When he feels that the interviewer is an ally who does not scold, judge, or punish him, but supports his constructive goals and shows understanding for his inability to obey rules and regulations—he may occasionally start to form a therapeutic alliance and become cooperative, dependent, trustful, and willing to level with the therapist. Then it is temporarily possible to discuss as part of his disorder his need to impress, his inability to postpone gratification, his lack of temper control and dependability, and his tendency to lie, steal, and cheat. However, it is rare for the sociopath to sincerely attempt to change his behavior.

Mental Status: The sociopath usually tries to make a quick impression through his appearance and behavior. Some come close to the following stereotype: The male patient may try to look very masculine—sporting long hair, excessive facial hair, or an open shirt or V-neck revealing chest hair and jewelry. Other clues are tatoos, scars, leather belts with large buckles, keys on chains, visible knives or firearms, tight pants with an apparent penile bulge, and boots.

The female sociopath may try to appear seductive and feminine. Here is her stereotype: brash, heavy makeup, unusually long or very short hair, tightly fitting clothes, short skirts, skirts with long slits, or transparent blouses. Alternatively, she may wear a hippie outfit—neglectful and sloppy—showing contempt or lack of interest in social rules.

Motor behavior, speech, and mood of the sociopath reveal some common characteristics. The male sociopath shows an erect posture, a forceful walk, and a strong handshake with a pronounced emphasis on movements—depending on whether he wants to appear cool and relaxed, strong and masculine, or display an "I don't care attitude." The female may try to reveal her upper thighs, stretch out her breasts and swing her hips in a provocative fashion.

Speech may reveal stiltedness, boisterousness, or—in males—a certain hoarseness trying to appear smart and impressive with foul language or words he does not quite understand. His statements are rarely clear, detailed, and informative, but instead exaggerated, vague, and contradictory which suggests lying.

His mood may be irritable, depressed, or elated. He may portray a special emotional state such as modesty which you will soon recognize as being merely pretended to get you on his side and have his way with you. Usually, he shows a lack of emotional control when caught lying, or when asked to obey rules.

The insight of the sociopath may be limited. He may have a tendency to blame the environment for his failure. However, when you do have rapport with him, he may admit that he screwed up his life with self-destructive behavior.

Judgment is often poor as well. On a superficial basis he may be able to read social expectations accurately, but he is rarely able to accept expectations as justified and is therefore unable to comply with them. A sociopath also lacks remorse which allows him to use unethical shortcuts in the pursuit of his goals.

Technique: His outfit may be the starting point for a conversation directed to make the patient discuss inability to comply with social rules. Although the patient may seek help for his drinking, drug abuse, or depression, his mental status may serve as an opener.

The patient with antisocial personality likes attention. He uses bragging and lies to get attention. He glows in the limelight. His attention span is short, rewards are strived for without delay. You can make him talk if you encourage him to boast:

"You are quite a salesman" or
"What a con-artist you must be" or
"You seem to be able to put anything across to people" or
"Were you quite a fighter?"

Such comments will stimulate him to display his accomplishments. The sociopath's tendency to lie and cheat will distort his stories. If he talks freely, avoid a judgmental or accusatory tone so as not to lose his cooperation. Do not approve of his crimes. Accept his boasting but explore the negative consequences of his deeds at the same time.

If the patient is uncooperative, not willing to answer questions, or if he adopts a complaining or hostile posture, withdraw your attention, display indifference, and initiate the termination of the interview.

"You don't seem to be in the mood to discuss your problems now. Maybe we would hit it off better some other time."

Be vague about when "some other time" may be—several days down the road. This way the sociopathic patient's short attention span will come into play and he may quickly change his posture.

A similar tactic is to offer the assistance of someone lower in rank:

"Maybe you would like to talk to the medical student (or the aid)—he can tell me later what is troubling you."

If the patient is interviewed in front of staff, offer to release the staff so that you can talk to him alone. Usually, the loss of audience is painful for him, and he may quickly become cooperative.

If the patient with antisocial personality and an affective disorder becomes homicidal or suicidal, but unwilling to cooperate with the assessment or treatment plan, set limits, forcefully, and right away:

"I want you to write a letter to the hospital administration right now, so that I can start commitment procedures against you."

Diagnosis: The diagnostic process is simple when you suspect antisocial personality disorder. All it takes is establishing rapport and collecting a list of teenage and early adulthood infractions against social standards and laws with questions such as:

"Did you have disciplinary problems in school? In the service? Did you have problems with the law? At work?"

Here is an interview with Brewster, a 26-year-old, white male, who was brought to a V.A. Hospital by two friends. They had found him with a shotgun in his hand aimed at his mouth filled with water. He was pulling the trigger. Because the safety was on, the gun did not go off and they wrestled the weapon away from him.

1. I: I heard from the admitting resident what you were up to. You must have really meant business.
   P: You are damn right. They meant well, but I wish these assholes would have let me do it.

2. I: Why do you want to shoot yourself?
   P: My best friend got shot in one of the street fights that we had in L. He was just buried two days ago. I felt real bad.

3. I: You felt real bad?
   P: I let him down. I was a real ass. I betrayed him.

4. I: In what way did you betray him?
   P: I screwed his old lady. Can you imagine? My best friend . . . and I take his old lady to bed. He trusted me all the way. That's the jackass I am.

5. I: You are really down on yourself.
   P: You aren't kidding. Jesus, what a smart ass! (Cursing at the doctor.)

6. I: Okay, let's get on with it.
   P: Listen, doc, I'm tired of talking to you. You can shove it.

7. I: Okay. You can talk to the resident. I'll be back on Monday.
   P: Screw you.

8. I: Well, I can't help you if you don't talk to me.
   P: Listen, doc, I didn't want to be here in the first place. Just let me out of this damn joint.

9. I: No way. You tried to shoot yourself. We have to evaluate you.
   P: I want to sign out.

10. I: You can write a letter to the chief of staff requesting your release, but I can tell you what will happen.
    P: What's that?

11. I: We'll have to commit you. In the staff's opinion you are a danger to yourself. You may suffer from a depression and I agree with them. So, I'll see you on Monday. I hope you will feel better by then.
    P: Damn, doc, I don't want to sit here the whole weekend just waiting until you come back. Let's get it over with.

12. I: Okay.
    P: What do you want to know?

13. I: I really don't want to know anything.
    P: What kind of shit are you pulling on me?

14. I: I really want to understand how you get yourself in that mess. What made you so upset?
    P: Well, I messed up my whole fucking life. I just can't lick it. I can't get myself to do anything useful.

15. I: You're not working?
    P: Nope. Well, I'm service connected. I got a medical discharge. They told me I'm a schizophrenic.

16. I: How did this come about?
    P: I was on this ship. I was always on the shit list. They made me scrub the deck. I tripped, I fell down the steps, must have bumped my head. I passed out. After that I told them that I had these bursting headaches. I could not concentrate. They would not let me go. So I got drunk and ran my jeep into a light post. Then they sent me to a psychiatrist. I told him that I hear the voice of my dead grandfather and that he tells me to kill myself. That got me some action. The shrink said that I'm schizophrenic and that I have no business in the service. So I'm 26 years old and I already have a nice pension.

17. I: Can you live off it?
    P: I suppose I could. If I take an apartment in the ghetto, one of the $150 deals, and live off fast food.

18. I: How do you live?
    P: Do you have to know all that?

19. I: I don't have any feeling for what's really bugging you.
    P: Well, I live with a motorcycle gang. They're the only friends I've got.

20. I: You mean you stay with them all the time?
    P: Yeah. We're hanging around in a trailer park.

21. I: Really?
    P: That's all confidential, isn't it?

22. I: It's confidential.
    P: We go out and get our kicks.

23. I: How's that?
    P: We stalk shopping centers. We wait til everybody is gone and then we move in. We grab the manager—he is usually the last to leave. We make him turn over the cash. But first we let him beg. We let him go down on his knees and we pull a pistol on him. We play some Russian roulette with him—click—click. (Laughs.)

24. I: You seem like one of those tough guys.
    P: You better believe it. That's the only thing that gives me a kick, to see a guy piss in his pants and beg us. We tell him that if he plays his cards right, we may let him off. Then we let him pay for his life, take his cash, kick him in the ass and run off.

25. I: Aren't you afraid that you might get caught?
    P: Oh shit. We put a scare in him. We tell him if he opens his fucking mouth, some of us will be back. We tell him we know where he lives. We won't get just him. We will blow off his whole shitty family. He understands. The police are busy dishing out speeding tickets to car pooling mothers—they aint doing anything. They go where it's easy.

26. I: Is that how you always got your kicks?
    P: What do you mean?

27. I: What did you do in school?
    P: Well, my father was a colonel in the army and my mother was a rehabilitation officer (laughs). They kicked the shit out of me.

28. I: Did you get in any trouble at school?
    P: No. We lived on base. We moved around a lot.

29. I: Were you a good fighter in school?
    P: Well, I could take and give a good lick.

30. I: You could?
    P: Yes.

31. I: Did you ever do it?
    P: I kicked the assistant baseball coach and gave him one with my bat. He woke up in the hospital.

32. I: What did the school do?
    P: Not much. They suspended me, but my Dad got me back in. Then we moved to another base.

33. I: Ever had a problem like this again?
    P: One of the kids was a real smart alec. I straightened him out. I knocked his teeth out. That taught him something.

34. I: Did you get in trouble for that?
    P: His dad tried to start something, but my Dad put on his uniform and went over to his house. He told him to tell his son not to provoke people and that he had told me that I should take care of myself if somebody crosses me. So I did. The teachers wanted me out, but my Dad straightened them out.

35. I: How are you getting along with your Dad now?
    P: He doesn't want to have anything to do with me anymore. I got in some kind of trouble and I finally ran away. I enlisted with the marines. I lied about my birthday. They shipped me right over to Nam.

36. I: How did you get along in the service?
    P: I had a great time in Saigon. We had pot and speed and heroin—everything. And you would screw the hell out of those little girls. We got hold of some stuff from the Navy and sold it. No problem. We always had money. But coming back was the pits.

37. I: What did you try to do here?
    P: I tried to work as a trucker. I got in an argument. I tried to work as a scuba diver, but everything bores me.

38. I: And now?
    P: And now I've had it.

39. I: Did you really want to pull that trigger?
    P: I felt like it, but I put them on. I knew that the safety was on. But it put the scare in them.

40. I: So you really wanted them to get you here?
    P: I guess, I must have.

41. I: So you really wanted to do something about your problems?
    P: I guess.

42. I: I can see.
    P: I'm messing up my life. I can't go on like this. I have nothing to look forward to. I can't just live for the kicks. I have to grow up.

43. I: Does that mean you want to get more out of life?
    P: Yeah.

44. I: Let's talk about it. Will you level with me?
    P: We'll see.

45. I: Okay. Let's see. I want to know about the voices.
    P: Oh shit, I pulled one over on this clown.

46. I: You did?
    P: I know enough psychology to give young Freud his hour's worth. I made it up. I just wanted to get out of there. This shrink couldn't tell a shit.

47. I: Okay.
    P: What do you think is wrong with me?

48. I: Well, I think you don't care about rules, you don't care about lying, you don't care about cheating. You live on impulse. If you get angry you just get mad.

At the beginning, Brewster appears angry but cooperative. Showing him empathy seems to work. However, he starts to test the interviewer's ability to control the situation in A. 5. When the interviewer sets firm limits (Q. 7,9,10,11), Brewster cooperates again. The interviewer expresses interest in him and in the way he gets himself into a mess (Q. 14). The patient becomes willing to discuss his problems—at times even sincerely. He finally levels, gives up his boisterous display of anger, and tells his recent distress starting with A. 14.

Lability in Borderline Personality Disorder

Rapport: The patient with borderline personality disorder presents special resistance to rapport by the instability in his mood, goals, and in relating to the interviewer. He may show intense emotions, then unexpectedly switch his tone. He seems to trust and like you and tell you that you are the best doctor he has ever met. Then he will reverse his judgment when he feels lack of support and understanding.

You handle rapport with a patient with borderline personality by focusing in an empathic manner on his instability. You attempt to separate it as a pathological part that needs to be explored for the patient's benefit. However, since the lability in feelings, judgment, and goals also affects his relationship to you, it is difficult to maintain his instability as the focus of the interview. To neutralize the negative influence on rapport, you may have to come back to it many times. When you thus demonstrate that you recognize the instability, the patient may be more willing to open up to you, thus furthering rapport.

Technique: It is difficult to keep the patient on a subject. You have to direct him, encourage his pursuit of a topic with remarks of support, and curb his diversions. He may tell you about his goals and then renege on what he just told you. He may talk enthusiastically about a new relationship just to devalue it, moments later, when some unpleasant experience in this relationship comes up.

Confront him with his contradictions but express that you understand the nature of his ambivalent feelings—what appears good and right at one time may seem the opposite at another.

The patient with borderline personality disorder usually talks in a more genuine way if you ask open-ended questions and help him to stick with a subject by curbing, rather than trying to get precise answers with closed-ended, pointed questions.

Mental Status: The overriding feature in mental status is the intense but labile affect. It varies from euphoric to depressed, from appreciative to angry and critical. The affect shows a close relationship to both, the content of the patient's story and the way he experiences you, the interviewer. The labile affect is paralleled by the description of a labile mood which you can abstract from the patient's reports about life events.

The excessive intensity of affect and mood are impressive. Unlike the histrionic personality in which the affect appears more intensely expressed than felt, the patient with borderline personality genuinely experiences an intense affect and mood. The flair of phoniness is missing. Investigators have found that the borderline personality shows a strong relationship to manic-depressive disorder and may be a variant. Mood and affect in manic-depressive disorder again are intense by nature but not by the patient's intent.

The lability in emotions persists also in the patient's social attitude. Intense ambivalence to close friends leads to contradictory reports about their characteristics: they are either overidealized or devaluated.

Since a patient with borderline personality has no distance from his intense feelings, he has no insight into the source of his difficulties.

Diagnosis: The diagnostic process is fueled by the patient's report of a string of intense interpersonal conflicts, possibly suicidal or self-mutilating behavior, and by your mental status observations. All you have to do is collect the pieces that complete the set of DSM-III-R criteria. Unless you disrupt your interview by critical, rejecting remarks, you will have no problems with the diagnosis.

This is an interview with Janet, a 29-year-old, white female demonstrating this instability.

1. I: What brought you here today?
   P: They sent me up here from the ER. I had taken too much Parnate and too much cold medication. They gave me an infusion, because my blood pressure went so high.

2. I: What made you take so much medication?
   P: I had an argument with my boyfriend—I wanted to teach that bastard a lesson.

3. I: How would it teach him a lesson, if you end up in the emergency room?
   P: I really don't like your questions. They're really dumb, reminds me of my boyfriend.

4. I: So you must have felt really desperate.
   P: (Sarcastically.) Mustn't I? Why else would I take an overdose?

5. I: Can you tell me a little bit about what brought on that argument with your boyfriend?
   P: Oh, just his stupidity.

6. I: How is that?
   P: It really tears me to pieces. But he can be so nice at other times. We bought a house real cheap and fixed it up together to live there . . . (After a pause.) I really think I should call him. He probably wonders what's going on.

7. I: You just told me that you have these bad arguments with him and that you were ready to teach him a lesson.
   P: Maybe it's all my fault and I shouldn't have been so impulsive.

8. I: Are you impulsive often?
   P: He brings out the worst in me. But I still love him a lot.

9. I: It seems difficult for you to sort out these feelings.
   P: You hit it right on the spot. (Sarcastically.) You must really be a pretty good psychiatrist.

A suicidal gesture or suicide attempt in a young female suggests borderline personality to be included in the differential. This diagnostic impression is substantiated for Janet when the reason for her attempt is not depressed mood and delusional guilt but anger and revenge (A. 2).

Despite the evidence of a borderline personality diagnosis, the interviewer makes a mistake in technique in Q. 3. Rather than being supportive and understanding and telling her

"This fellow must have really hurt you that you were pushed so far to overdose,"

he asks a rational and critical question—and she lashes out in response. When he tries to correct his mistake (A. 4) by expressing his empathy, she remains sarcastic. She probably feels that he is not genuine.

When the interviewer restrains himself from supportive statements and focuses on the facts instead, she provides them freely. While she reconstructs her last argument with her boyfriend that led to the overdose, surprisingly, she changes her feelings about the event. The catharsis of her anger seemed to have freed her positive feelings about her boyfriend, and she shows a bout of guilt (A. 7). When the interviewer pursues her insight and makes an implicit interpretation that it seems difficult for her to sort out her feelings, she abandons the insight track and rejects his interpretation with sarcasm, demonstrating her defensiveness against facing a core symptom of her personality disorder.

Phoniness in Histrionic Personality Disorder

Histrionic personality disorder is more frequently diagnosed in females than in males.

Rapport: When you attempt to establish rapport, you deal with exaggerated emotionality and lack of depth. Together with frequent contradictions in her story she gives you the impression that she lacks sincerity; she appears "phony." It is a common response by novices to dislike and disrespect such a patient.

With a male interviewer the female histrionic patient likes to flirt, to impress him with stories of sexual adventures, and to display her physical attributes seductively. With female interviewers, she may initiate rivalry, or a power contest. Since the histrionic patient seems to be more interested in approval and admiration than in a professional relationship, rapport is severely hampered.

Mental Status: The mental status of a histrionic patient is dominated by a display of emotionality: vivid facial expressions, dramatic gestures, and a highly modulated voice. However, she can be interrupted and redirected to a different topic which she will take up in the same dramatic fashion. Her distractibility differs from mania, since there is no push of speech or flight of ideas (see glossary). The constant drama gives you the impression that she does not really experience any intense feelings. Her strong show of emotions is for your benefit, not a catharsis for her. In spite of excessive facial expressions and abundant gesturing she appears uninvolved in her story. The term *la belle indifférence* has been coined for this internal emotional distance.

Technique: You have to overcome the patient's vagueness and dramatic exaggerations to obtain specific information for a diagnosis. Unstructured, open-ended questions usually do not work, because the patient becomes sidetracked and gets lost in reproducing stories in which she was victimized. Therefore, settle on a main theme, like a marriage problem, a conflict at work, or a fight with her children, and keep her focused on this theme with curbing and specification. Get concrete examples. Even then you may not get a clear picture because the patient contradicts herself. Confrontation with her contradictions often results in anger and a loss of rapport. To get her to reflect on her behavior you have to express understanding and encouragement. Use phrases like

"You seem to be a sensitive person."
"You seem to feel that other people can't appreciate what you went through."

When the patient expresses that she feels understood by you, you may ask her

"How do you think your husband would report the same event?"

By comparing his and her perception you may help her to develop a better understanding of her conflicts and give her some insight. Such insight, however, is usually short-lived.

You can sometimes help her to develop insight into her behavior by asking emphatic questions. When you side with her, the patient may be encouraged to admit at times some of her deficiencies. As soon as she feels that your support, understanding, and empathy is slipping away, she will return to dramatization. A histrionic female has often experienced rejection which she does not understand. She tries to overcome it by exaggerating her pain and this tactic earns her contempt rather than empathy.

Another approach is to address the exaggerated dramatic behavior from the patient's point of view, such as:

"It seems to me that you have a hard time making people understand what you are going through. You tell them about your problems and they just don't seem to care. I think we should try to understand why this happens."

If pursued, the patient may complain about being rejected and ridiculed even by her family. She may admit that she wants to be loved, praised, and admired. Those admissions bring you closer to her true feelings and allow you to penetrate her strategy game.

The next step is to induce the patient to tell you the reasons why she is criticized. This may lead to a confession of her weaknesses. At this point, you have temporarily helped the patient to overcome her phoniness—at least for the moment.

Diagnosis: As for most personality disorders, it is the patient's mental status that will alert you. When you suspect a histrionic personality disorder, invite the patient to tell you how she is getting along with people close to her. Since the histrionic patient usually has conflicts, i.e., with parents, children, spouses, she will report lifelong conflicts with them. She often divides her relatives into "the good and the bad guys." Besides the exaggeration typical of the histrionic personality, you will also often encounter passive aggressive features and intense ambivalent feelings typical for the borderline personality disorder.

This is an interview with Jane, a middle-aged, white, married female who has chronic marital conflicts.

1. I: What kind of problems brought you here?
   P: Before we begin let me tell you something. I understand that you wanted me to be seen by some other doctor in the clinic, but I wanted the best. That's why I insisted on seeing you.

2. I: Thank you. But what makes you say I'm the best?
   P: Well, you are the director of the clinic, aren't you? And Dr. T. from Health Plus, who referred me here, said you specialize in sleep problems.

3. I: Tell me about your sleep problems.
   P: Oh, it's terrible. There are whole nights when I can't sleep at all. I toss and turn, and I get up in the morning without having closed my eyes for even a second.

4. I: This happens only some nights?
   P: It happens when I have these terrible, terrible fights with my husband. He just tears me to pieces. (Patient rolls her eyes dramatically upward.)

5. I: Does he or anybody else notice what you are going through?
   P: They don't have the foggiest idea. I can scream and yell and they still don't understand.

6. I: When you have these fights, is your mood affected?
   P: I get these devastating depressions and I have to cry the whole time.

7. I: What are these fights about?
   P: I'm not sure. Just anything. We have not had sex for the last four months. I can't understand how a man can be so cruel and hateful.

8. I: I have a hard time understanding what your fights with your husband are all about.
   P: He criticizes me and puts me down. He has left me more than thirty times in the last few years.

9. I: Maybe you can give me an example?
   P: Well, he comes back from his trips and rips me all apart.

10. I: So his criticism is the main part of your problems?
    P: I suffer so terribly much. A nice man like you probably cannot understand how a man can be as mean as my husband.

11. I: Maybe I should have a chance to talk to both of you.
    P: I'd rather not do that. He tells his side of the story in such a way that it fools everyone.

12. I: What do you think he would say?
    P: Just the same old thing, that I'm a bad housekeeper, that I haven't done anything, that I'm just sitting on my fanny while he has to do all the work . . . He'll just carry on like that.

13. I: So he talks about your shortcomings. Does he ever ask you how you feel and why you are having trouble getting things done?
    P: He has no understanding whatsoever. It's like he's made of wood and he looks so cold. I'm getting tired easily and when I rest and watch television, the time is gone and I can't get things done.

14. I: I see. Do you think then that he has a point?
    P: Are you taking his side? I thought I'm your patient, I'm the one who's suffering. I thought you understand that.

15. I: Okay. Let's start to talk about your problems and talk with him later.
    P: Well, when you talk to him you will not believe how nasty and mean he can be.

16. I: At this point do you see a future for your marriage?
    P: I still love him, I enjoy the closeness when we have sex.

17. I: Well, as you said, that has not happened for a long time.
    P: Oh, it was just last Friday. And some hours later he was tearing me apart.

18. I: I thought you had not been intimate with him for quite some time.
    P: Why do you use whatever I say against me? Can't you understand? I meant the time before last time.

Even though Jane talks freely, it is difficult to get precise information. At first, she does not describe the circumstances of the fights with her husband, nor does she agree to have him interviewed. She expresses her suffering in an exaggerated way, but she is reluctant to furnish the facts. She wants the interviewer to feel sorry for her; the mere fact that she suffers should be reason enough that the interviewer sides with her.

Her vagueness is temporarily overcome when the interviewer asks her to project what the husband would report about her. But when he tries to explore whether the husband's statements are to some extent justified, she protests. She prefers to indulge in suffering rather than to analyze her underlying problems.

When the interviewer explores whether she considers a divorce, her dependency needs surface. She has a hard time fending for herself. She starts to emphasize her husband's positive features. Thus, it appears that the patient is more interested in complaining about her problems than solving them.

Grandiosity in Narcissistic Personality Disorder

Throughout the interview, the narcissistic personality gives you the feeling that you are there to endorse his self-promoted importance. As long as you play along you will be idolized as a wonderful interviewer. However, if you support his grandiose self-perception, you will not help him to test his grandiosity against the grey reality of everyday life. Yet, helping the patient recognize his limits and the reality of the situation shatters his self-inflated ego.

To you the grandiosity is in glaring contrast with reality, but the patient has no insight to tell the difference between his healthy, critical self and his pathological tendencies. Alliance between you and the patient's healthy part is not possible. His lack of insight prevents rapport.

Here is an interview with Henry, a child psychologist at an eastern pediatric department:

1. I: Hello, Henry.
   P: Before you say anything, let me give you the background of my visit. I am here to discuss with you, as a smart and knowledgeable insider, some of the problems that I have dealing with incompetent diagnostic morons. One should call them medical technicians; they have no grasp of the essence of the problems they deal with. We have a long-standing conflict that is now coming to a head. Even after I published my book they doubt my expertise in the field. I have to make a decision whether I should quit this clinic that supports those morons or try to get them fired.

2. I: What does Dr. L. (the clinic director) think about it?
   P: I have been over that one with her several times. I have pushed her toward an ultimatum, I had her crying, but she is incapable of taking the necessary actions.

3. I: Who are the doctors that you have a conflict with?
   P: Several pediatricians at my clinic. They have no clinical savvy whatsoever. Their judgment with regard to the trustworthiness of molested children is just horrendously impaired.

4. I: How's that?
   P: As a forensic psychologist I have the experience that allows me to decide whether or not a child is lying. But all they are concerned about is the evidence: did the child have a conduct disorder, or did he abuse drugs? Intuition, recognition of defenses, and understanding of the family dynamics escape them completely.

5. I: Well, Henry, I'm not up on the field, maybe you can tell me on what kind of criteria you base a child's trustworthiness.
   P: That's so obvious. I'm surprised that you ask such a question. Haven't you read my book? I did send you a copy. Do you really expect me to teach you the basics here?

6. I: Well, since one of your discussions with your colleagues centers around trustworthiness of witnesses, I would like to know how you approach the question.
   P: Let me tell you what. I'll give you six criteria: experience, experience, experience, knowledge, understanding, and judgment. How does that strike you? I guess that does not sit well with your obsessiveness.

7. I: Come on, Henry. You can do better than that.
P: You have really lost your clinical touch since you have been away from clinical psychology and psychoanalysis. Medical School has gotten the best of you, I guess there is no sense in talking to you any longer!

8. I: Okay, Henry, I think I'm not helping you. It seems the pediatricians really do not grasp your contributions.
P: Now we're getting somewhere.

9. I: I'd like to know why you think they misunderstand you!
P: I told you! It's their intellectual flatfootedness!

10. I: Okay, if that's right, is there anything you could do to improve matters?
P: Listen, don't put it on me! Who do you think I am? You know I have dealt with all kinds of people who were not the smartest, but at least they had intuition, and esprit. You don't really expect me to get down to their level and worry about what pediatricians think!

11. I: Well, it depends on your goals.
P: What do you mean? I am not on trial here. You always point at me, thanks anyway—thanks, but no thanks!

12. I: Come on Henry, we have been friends, I want to help you to find out what's going wrong! Do you want to show them how ignorant they are, or do you want to get your diagnostic reasoning across?
P: Bull . . . I'm not enjoying this conversation. Let's forget it.

13. I: Well, Henry, you seem to feel insulted and misunderstood.
P: The hell, I do. They think because they are M.D.'s, they have one up on me. And you seem to be on their side too, just because they're M.D.'s like you. Maybe you did the right thing by going into medicine. Next time around I would do the same (his eyes fill with tears). You don't believe how much I have suffered for not being an M.D. By the way, do you know Rick D., the surgeon? We have the same little nursing student in the works. She really is a cute ass. Are you still giving talks?

14. I: A few of them. Why do you ask?
P: If you know anyone who needs a speaker, I would be willing . . . you can recommend me.

This interview shows how a narcissistic client tries to maintain his self-importance in light of an adverse reality. The interviewer's attempts to make Henry review his behavior are overrun. When the interviewer expresses empathy for his repercussions (due to his grandiose distortion), the patient collapses briefly but attempts to regain his posture by bragging about his amorous success.

As with other personality disorders, an empathic addressing of the narcissistic goal such as:

"You only feel worthwhile when you convince yourself and others that you are tops,"

or empathy for the consequences of the narcissistic behavior such as:

"I see you are hurting. Let's find out how you get hurt and how we can stop it,"

may only temporarily enable the patient to consider his narcissistic behavior as the cause of his problems. Usually, each insight is followed by grandiose repair of his shattered image.

3. ANXIOUS, RESISTIVE SUBMISSIVENESS— CLUSTER C

Four personality disorders fall into cluster C: the avoidant, the dependent, the obsessive compulsive, and the passive aggressive personality.

The mental status of a patient in cluster C is dominated by an anxious, tense, and dysphoric affect. He worries whether you accept him. His speech appears overcontrolled, and he weighs each word to avoid mistakes. Cluster C personality disorder patients have more insight into their behavior than clusters A and B—anxiety produces self-awareness and self-consciousness.

Rapport develops along a specific pattern. The patient watches you closely to find out what you think of him. If he finds you supportive, receptive, nurturing, and nondemanding, he strives to overcome his anxiety by paying reverence to your authority. He may flatter you, ask your advice, laud you as an expert, and tell you what he thinks you want to hear. He clings to you, and expects you to take charge. Rapport becomes lopsided.

Two of the personality disorders of cluster C are more difficult to interview: the passive aggressive and the obsessive compulsive personality. As the interview with these two types progresses, you may find it was only a token reverence that the patient paid you. After you respond with empathy and act protective of him, his internal resentment creeps up. Gestures and remarks slip out that indicate reluctance to cooperate. He may ask probing questions and let you know your inadequacies. He feels that you were not really worthwhile or powerful enough to justify his initial anxiety; he may resent his submissiveness and may shut you out. Special techniques will be discussed for the interview with the obsessive compulsive and the passive aggressive personality disorder patient.

Hypersensitivity in Avoidant Personality Disorder

Rapport: In a patient with avoidant personality disorder anxious guardedness and reticence can be approached with reassurance and empathy. Avoid confrontation that he may interpret as criticism. Instead, express empathic understanding for his suffering, which may encourage him to share his past tortures and his present anticipatory fears. If the patient feels that you understand his sensitivity and are protective of him, he will trust you and cooperate with you. The result is rapport. After he feels accepted and safe, the character of the interview may change dramatically. He may become explicitly detailed, may give you examples of social insults he has endured, and report to you the reliving and resuffering of his traumata.

Mental Status: The avoidant personality initially shows withdrawal which dominates his mental status. He is monosyllabic, vague, and circumstantial. Initially he may appear suspicious and paranoid, or anxious and phobic, but often void of clear-cut symptoms of DSM-III-R axis I disorders. After he feels comfortable with you and develops trust, he may reveal his sensitivity to being misunderstood and easily hurt by criticism or disapproval. He may then discuss his fear of rejection and inappropriate behavior.

Technique: After you have rapport, the patient is easy to interview. He feels relieved when he can describe his social fears of being criticized and rejected because he feels your empathy. He may experience these fears of being embarrassed as silly and express this. However, if you identify with this position, he may feel ridiculed and criticized and withdraw again.

Diagnosis: The patient's anxiousness and restricted affect at the beginning of the interview usually attract the interviewer's attention—an early clue. If he opens up, the diagnostic interview follows the standard phases (see chapter 7).

Donna, a 27-year-old, white, single female, had never been in treatment. When she entered the office, she sat down with her hands in her lap looking down. She refused to have coffee by shaking her head and mumbling "no." She appeared unusually tense. The interviewer decided—since small talk seemed to make her more uncomfortable—to ask for her chief complaint.

1. I: Maybe you can tell me what kind of problems bring you here . . . (Pause.) What would you like to talk about?
   P: (Silent, looking down at her hands with a tense expression on her face, then looks back at the interviewer.)

2. I: How do you think I can help you?
   P: I don't know.

3. I: Maybe you can tell me what's bothering you.
   P: (Looks down and shakes her head.) People, I guess.

4. I: (Silent, looking at her.)
   P: (Getting tenser and still looking down at her lap.)

5. I: (In a soft, soothing voice.) People? What is it about people?
   P: I can't really tell.

6. I: You seem to be scared of people.
   P: (Nods.)

7. I: What makes you scared of them?
   P: I don't know. I feel like they are closing in on me.

8. I: You feel they are out to harm you?
   P: No, not really out to harm me. They are so loud and pushy; they shut me up.

9. I: I understand. You feel that they can run over you any time; they close in on you and crush you . . . (Patient remains silent.) . . . Is this close to how you feel?
   P: Pretty close.

10. I: Is there anyone in particular?
    P: My father's brother. He comes in, pushes me aside, laughs at me. I hear it all the time; "Come on Donna, come off it, Donna, that's crazy, Donna, you're so impractical, Donna, damn, get your shit together, Donna, and put your foot down." (Patient shakes her whole body.) I can't stand it. I would like to hide in my room.

11. I: You must go through a lot.
    P: (Patient sighs.) Yeah . . . yeah, really. (For the first time the patient looks at the interviewer and establishes eye contact.)

12. I: How long has this bothered you?
    P: As far back as I can think. My past is full of hurts.

13. I: School must have been hell for you.
    P: Oh, it was. I remember when I had written a poem and the teacher made me read it to the class.

14. I: What happened?
    P: I did not want to do it. I was ashamed of having written a poem.

15. I: Did the teacher understand and help you out?
    P: She told me I could stay in my seat and read it there—it was awful.

16. I: What was awful?
    P: When I started to read, the kids in the front yelled: "Read louder, we can't hear you!" I started to swallow—finally, the teacher took the poem and read it. The whole class laughed. I swore that I would never write a poem again.

17. I: You have thin skin. Everything seems to get right through to you.
    P: I have no skin at all. I seem to be much too sensitive.

18. I: That makes it hard for you to speak up.
    P: I'll die before I open my mouth in front of a whole bunch of people again.

It takes the interviewer eight questions to piece together Donna's chief complaint. Rapport is established with Q. 9 and 11; Q. 9 expresses cognitive understanding and Q. 11 emotional empathy. In Q. 9 he summarizes what he has learned. He focuses then on the person whom she dreads the most. For the first time the patient gives a somewhat longer and emotionally laden account of a person whom she fears and hates at the same time. The interviewer expresses empathic understanding in Q. 11. The patient relaxes and the interviewer is now able to follow the standard interview and get her history (compare Q. 12–18).

Submissiveness in Dependent Personality Disorder

Rapport: It is easy to establish rapport with a patient with a dependent personality; after he loses his initial anxiety, he puts his trust in you. As long as you give pleasant advice, show empathy for his indecisiveness and failures, and are supportive, the interview flows easily. However, if you try to explore the background of the patient's submissiveness, he becomes uncomfortable and tries to persuade you not to be too harsh on him. If you pursue exploring his dependency, and if you do this from your own, rather than from the patient's point of view, he will show you how much he suffers. If you don't soothe the pain, the patient will change therapists to find a more sympathetic ear.

Mental Status: The mental status is colored by the associated disorders which bring him into therapy in the first place. The overriding features, however, are his dependency, submissiveness, anxiousness, and his need to please you. He tries to give you answers that he thinks you will like. His affect strikes you often as anxious and depressed with some obsessive features.

The thought content mirrors themes of low self-esteem, desertion, and anxiety of doing the wrong thing. The dependent personality is oriented and has good memory but fails to appreciate the degree of his lack of initiative, and its effect on his life. His judgment is hampered by his dependency.

Technique: Interviewing the dependant personality is easy. He cooperates and tries to meet your expectations. He answers questions to the point. He clarifies his answers on demand, so you can easily steer the direction of the interview. He tolerates accentuated and abrupt transitions, and allows you to probe very personal feelings. What he cannot tolerate is confrontation with and interpretations of his dependency.

Diagnosis: Several features of the interview tell you that you are dealing with a dependent personality. From the very beginning the patient elevates you to a position of authority.

His social history shows that he always seemed to share quarters with a person who took charge of his life. The combination of these features rather than any one alone will suggest to you that the patient has a dependent personality disorder. After you have included this diagnosis in your differential, two tasks remain: you have to show that first, the pattern of dependency is lifelong, and second, that his dependency can be separated from the symptoms of a disabling symptomatic psychiatric disorder, or from justifiable responses to such a disorder.

Susan, a white, divorced female in her late thirties has been attending a psychiatric outpatient clinic regularly for many years. During the first interview with a new psychiatrist she demonstrates some characteristic features of the dependent personality.

1. I: I'm taking over for Dr. V. I understand that you have been coming to this clinic for quite some time.
   P: Oh yes, at least the last fifteen years.

2. I: What seems to be the problem?
   P: (Pauses.) I don't know how to answer that question. Maybe you can tell me what's going on.

3. I: Hmm. Maybe you can help me by telling me what you've been struggling with lately.
   P: I really need your guidance. You can probably sort it all out. That's why I am coming here. I need your help and advice.

4. I: You have a hard time to get along?
   P: Yes, since my husband deserted and divorced me, people have been taking advantage of me, says Dr. V. I'd been better off if my husband hadn't divorced me. But he always said I cling to him too much. And so he left me, and I had done everything for him.

5. I: It seems you still miss him.
   P: I still see him once in a while. He's married again. They have three children. It gives me a pain in the chest when I see them and how happy they are, and I'm so miserable. Maybe you can help me.

6. I: Are you living alone now?
   P: No, I moved back in with my mother. She never liked my husband. Now I'm not dating at all. I don't even go out. I don't want to hurt my mother.

7. I: Have you ever thought of marrying again?
   P: My mother wouldn't like it. It would be like deserting her a second time. Sometimes I think it would be nice to find a man who would love me and would like to take care of me. Maybe an older man.

8. I: Why don't you want to find a man your own age?
   P: They are so demanding; they want you like a partner and not as a wife. I'm pretty traditional when it comes to marriage. I think the husband should be a gentleman and show you love and care for you.

9. I: Being a partner in a marriage seems to be tough for you.
   P: I think with real love men will be understanding. I feel that you understand.

10. I: It sounds to me that you have to find out how much you have to be on your own, how much responsibility to take.
    P: You sound like Dr. R. He did not seem to like me. He was not like Dr. V. who was always on my side.

11. I: I feel I have touched on something very painful for you.
    P: (Silent.)

12. I: I think it may be helpful for you if we can discuss it.
   P: My mother criticizes me all the time . . . but I don't make enough money to live by myself. (Her eyes fill with tears.) I'm really trapped. Please don't criticize me, I can't take it, I want you to help me.

Most long-term patients have a chronic disorder—one of the axis I disorders that is, such as schizophrenia; rapid cycling, nonresponding bipolar affective disorder; or nonresponsive chronic depression. If such a disorder is missing, yet the patient visits the clinic over many years, a personality disorder of cluster C is likely, especially dependent personality.

This may surprise the reader since by definition all personality disorders are chronic. However, not all result in long-term therapy as the cluster C disorders do. Therefore, a patient who is well-off and psychologically minded, with deep, nonresolving dependency needs, is a prime candidate for long-term psychotherapy. The interview with Susan bears it out.

From the beginning of the interview Susan attempts to put the interviewer in charge (A. 2,3). He does not confront her with this tendency but assesses her life circumstances instead. She describes a situation typical of the dependent personality.

In Q. 10 the interviewer attempts to address her ability/inability to rely on her resources. Susan misunderstands this exploration as an implicit criticism and responds with tears and a plea for not wanting to be criticized. This response shows that you should not confront the patient with her pathological dependency in the first interview. Instead, explore the patient's view of her dependency and then make her gradually aware of the consequences of her behavior. Chances are that, in spite of your interviewing skills, you will end up with an eternal patient rather than a responsible adult who faces and solves her problems.

Circumstantiality and Perfectionism in Obsessive Compulsive Personality Disorder

Rapport: The obsessive patient is blind to the situation because he is fixed on details. Therefore, in the interview you will be involved in an endless struggle about words, issues, and who is in charge without being able to develop an atmosphere of cooperation and understanding.

If you show empathy you will have a problem. He is proud that he doesn't have any feelings, that he is objective. Therefore, he is perturbed when you express empathy for his suffering and rejects it as irrelevant. Not his suffering but his problems are important; however, they are unsolvable. This struggle may prevent you from establishing the split between the healthy and the diseased part of his personality.

You may overcome this struggle by continuously trying to get and keep the patient in touch with his anger. This may work as long as he believes that you feel his anger is justified. But if you attempt to make the anger the object of the interview, he will defend or deny it. He will put forth more obstructive obsessive thinking, actively preventing a split between the healthy and the sick part of his personality. To form an alliance is difficult, and the interview often consists of aborted attempts, struggles, and frustrations.

Mental Status: The mental status of the patient with obsessive compulsive personality is overshadowed by one difficulty—making decisions. This shows in his ambivalence and the way he keeps you in limbo when answering questions. Should he open up to you, or would he be misunderstood? He may decide not to open up, but will wonder is that right? Should he spend his money on seeing you and then risk not getting a true reading of his problems? How can he get your best opinion if he holds back? Are you really the right person to talk to? Probably not. If he was sent to see you involuntarily, he probably would not have picked you, or would he have? He has to find out from you what's wrong. He should ask the questions, you should provide the answers. Who is in charge? Him? Or should you be in charge, since you are supposed to be the expert?

The obsessive compulsive patient perceives himself as being neutral, a quite distorted view. You sense a low-grade, chronic anger that can flare up into tenacious, persistent, bothersome questioning that cannot be satisfied by any answer. His anger will become overt when his obsessive expectations are not met, when he feels shortchanged in interviewing time, overcharged for his visit, or not rewarded with useful answers to his questions.

Technique: Your position as interviewer is precarious because his ambivalence is hard to overcome. He doubts your assurances. Your open-ended questions lead to confusion. He wants more circumscribed questions, but if you comply he interprets them as too narrow.

Diagnosis: The mental status gives the patient's diagnosis away; no secret here. The problem is to get the details of the associated disorders, if any. It appears that obsessive compulsive disorder itself, depression, phobic disorder, and sometimes delusional (paranoid) disorder are common concomitants if the patient presents at a clinic.

Here is a taste of obsessive compulsive personality found in Wynn, a 35-year-old scientist.

1. I: How can I help you?
   P: I'm concerned about a letter I wrote to my coauthor. She did not take it well at all.

2. I: What was the letter about?
   P: I don't know whether I should discuss this here. You may know her.

3. I: Are you concerned that something may leak out?
   P: Obviously . . . But maybe I can tell you if you can assure me of complete confidentiality.

4. I: How can I help you if you can't talk about it.
   P: Maybe the content of the letter is not the problem, but her reaction.

5. I: What is it about her reaction that concerns you?
   P: I'm just thinking that you can't really understand her reaction if you don't know about the letter.

6. I: Then let's look at the whole package.
   P: You are pushing me. Maybe I should think more about what I should tell you.

7. I: Alright.
   P: If I break off now, you couldn't really charge me for that short a visit, because it isn't me who can't guarantee confidentiality.

8. I: I'm sorry, this hour was reserved for you, I will charge you for my time.
   P: You really have a way with words. OK, if you charge me anyway, I may as well use the time. My coauthor agreed with one of the harshest critics who reviewed our paper. This really incensed me, because she's not really an expert in the area.

9. I: So you became angry.
   P: Not angry. I am very rarely distracted by my feelings. I consider them irrational. What I basically did is ask her to change the paper according to her criticism.

10. I: Could she do it if she is not an expert in the area?
    P: I cannot understand how someone can criticize work if they can't change it. Then she shouldn't have criticized it in the first place.

11. I: But wasn't her intention . . .

    P: I don't really care about intentions, I'm looking at facts. The facts are that she criticized the paper without being able to improve it. It's as simple as that.

12. I: But don't you miss the point, when you look at the facts without including the intentions?

    P: I don't think you have any appreciation for the facts. You are unable to see the facts. You have a hang-up on the emotional side. You are obviously biased.

13. I: My statements seem to make you angry.

    P: I'm not an emotional person. I just want to get the facts straight. But you won't let me do that.

Resentment in Passive Aggressive Personality Disorder

Rapport: Like the patient with dependent personality, the patient with passive aggressive personality establishes and maintains rapport as long as you agree with him and take his side. When you challenge his view, you trigger his anger. He is especially sensitive to demands put upon him; he resists them with tardiness, sulking, evasiveness, arguments, and occasionally open anger.

If you address his resentment toward demands, he becomes guarded, monosyllabic, and often hostile. If you fail to appreciate this sensitivity to demands, or even sympathize with the demanding person, you lose rapport. You regain it only if you return to the patient's point of view.

Technique: Slowly and carefully you should explore the patient's deep aversion to demands. The skillful interviewer expresses that he understands the patient's needs for leniency but points out at the same time that the unfulfilled expectations cause disappointment and resentment and poison all relationships. He knows if he temporarily sympathizes with the patient's resentment about demands, the patient may cooperate and allow him to explore the superimposed disorder (see below, under *Diagnosis*).

Mental Status: During the interview the patient may not show many abnormalities. His affect appears to be well adjusted and pleasant except when he starts to talk about situations where he was asked to perform. Then he shows signs of resentment, irritability, or anger. If you fail to identify these trigger situations, you may miss his underlying personality disorder.

Diagnosis: A patient with passive aggressive personality disorder rarely consults you for problems related to his disorder. His associated axis I disorders bring him to see you, such as alcoholism, affective disorder, or an anxiety disorder.

His story becomes transparent when he talks about social disappointments, interpersonal conflicts, and bad breaks. Typically, the patient does not openly oppose demands but accepts commitments and makes promises even when he knows he will not keep them. He says "yes" but acts "no." This characteristic leads to disappointments and rejection by colleagues, friends, and family members. And the patient complains bitterly about being rejected without understanding how he sets it off.

If you hit upon the "say yes/act no" attitude, explore whether it is limited to certain people, situations, or certain life periods when the patient was depressed. If this attitude tints all relationships lifelong, your patient has passive aggressive personality disorder.

Andy is a 34-year-old businessman with a family history of bipolar disorder, but without a psychiatric history of his own.

1. I: How can I help you?
   P: I just have to talk to somebody about the things that happened to me at work.

2. I: Ok, Andy.
   P: It will probably upset you as much as me.

3. I: You must have gone through some rough times.
   P: Have I ever . . . boy, if I could tell you. This friend of mine accepted a job down here and when I talked to him he asked me if I wouldn't like to join him.

4. I: So you did?
   P: Well, I did because I trusted him. So I went to work with him, and I thought we'd have a good time, because the guy seemed to be a lot of fun.

5. I: Was he?
   P: Let me tell you—the first thing he did was start with staff meetings in the morning—did I ever resent them. That was his sneaky way of forcing us to be on time.

6. I: Was there a problem with that?
   P: A problem? We were friends and he knew I had good ideas, but they don't necessarily come at 8 o'clock in the morning.

7. I: Well . . .

   P: When I came late, when I had car trouble, or when I had to run an errand, he didn't say anything, but I could feel that he didn't like it.

8. I: Was he ever late himself?

   P: Are you kidding? That guy is a workaholic. There he was in the morning, and he stayed late in the evening. If I'd known that he was such a slave driver, I would not have come here in the first place. But I got back at him when I had that accident. I don't know whether he believed me, but I brought the splinter from my foot with me back to work to show it.

9. I: Did your friend see it?

   P: I showed it to some colleagues when he was passing by in the hall.

10. I: Did he see it?

    P: You know what that bastard said? "If you don't believe Andy's story today, he'll bring a bigger splinter in tomorrow!" Boy, was I miffed.

11. I: So you expected him to treat you more as a friend than as an employee.

    P: That's exactly right. What's the use of working for a friend, if you have to slave along anyway?

12. I: So he should have given you some privileges and leeway.

    P: Isn't that obvious? You don't suppose that I should run like clockwork for that guy.

13. I: Well, you said he's at work at 8 o'clock.

    P: Listen, I think I made a mistake talking to you about it. You seem to be just like him. I want you to know there is more to life than work, work, work.

14. I: Let's go back, Andy, and explore some more of your feelings about your friend's demands.

    P: Listen, my friend, I have to explore nothing with you anymore. I'm here of my own free will. I resent your domineering attitude.

15. I: I'm sorry. I must have missed the point completely. I failed to see how your friend's pettiness has cost him your friendship and devotion.

    P: (Sarcastic.) What a sudden turn in your view.

16. I: (Ignoring the sarcasm.) You're right, I failed to see things from your vantage point. Your friend knew you before you went to work for him— he should have told you what to expect.

    P: That's right. I would never have worked for him if he'd told me that it's worse to work for a friend than for just any other employer.

The patient makes the underlying assumption that everybody who works for a friend can expect privileges such as being tardy, taking it easy, and extra time off. When the interviewer addresses these expectations indirectly (Q. 8), Andy avoids a response such as

"You are right, he sets a good example, why shouldn't I do the same?"

but instead criticizes the friend as a workaholic. Andy responds with anger when his friend humors him for missing work because of a splinter in his foot (A. 10).

When the interviewer confronts Andy with his expectation of receiving privileges, he becomes hostile. His response shows that he is more interested in mustering support for his position—if he indeed discusses his conflict—rather than facing his distorted expectation.

4. DESTRUCTIVENESS—CLUSTER OF PERSONALITY DISORDERS NEEDING FURTHER STUDY

DSM-III-R lists two personality disorders for which criteria have been developed but which have not been evaluated or accepted to the same extent as the personality disorders in clusters A, B, and C. These are: sadistic personality disorder and self-defeating personality disorder.

Demanding Cruelty in Sadistic Personality Disorder

DSM-III-R lists eight characteristics of the patient with sadistic personality disorder. The physical and mental cruelty and lack of empathy that such a patient shows for his victims will impress you each time you encounter one. He is quite capable of finding victims—usually he chooses somebody under his control, such as a child, wife, student, employee, or elderly person. If his rank does not assure him superiority, he will pick on somebody physically weaker.

He finds pleasure in dominating, torturing, and inflicting pain on his victim. Not only is he interested in the dominance and the ensuing increase in self-esteem, but in the pain that he can unnecessarily and deliberately cause.

Means that can enhance both dominance over and torture of others have a magic fascination for him. Therefore, he likes weapons, the martial arts, and professions that allow him to use them.

A patient with sadistic personality disorder does not seek treatment to have his sadism diffused. Sometimes, you may encounter sadistic features in patients who suffer from other problems such as persecutory delusions, alcoholism, or drug abuse, and you diagnose the sadistic personality disorder as a comorbid condition. Usually, however, you meet him through his victim.

When you interview such a patient, he may attempt to intimidate, bluff, and make you, too, suffer. He will use his techniques to impose his will upon you.

The following interview takes place between a psychiatrist and the husband (H) of a patient who demands his wife's release from the hospital. Mr. Richardsen is a pale, 5′8″, thin man with dark, slightly disheveled hair. He sits stiffly and straight up on a chair with his fists pressed against the armrests, white knuckles protruding. Out of narrowed eyes he stares piercingly at the interviewer without blinking.

1. I: Hi, Mr. Richardsen. I'm Dr. O., the attending physician here. Our nurse, Mrs. J., just called me and told me that you would like to talk to me.
   H: (Stands up, walks toward the interviewer and positions himself in front of him, with legs spread. With a low, pressed voice.) You got that right. I want to sign out Irene (his wife). She just took off from home and the next thing I know is that the social worker calls me and tells me that she has checked into this hospital here.

2. I: Hmm . . .
   H: And she tells me that Irene doesn't even want to talk to me.

3. I: (Frowns.) I don't understand . . . (with a puzzled look on his face) and you want to check her out?
   H: (With suppressed excitement in his voice.) You can't hold her here.

4. I: (Stretching out his right hand nearly touching Mr. R.'s chest.) Wait a moment . . . What did the social worker tell you?
   H: She told me that Irene has checked in here and that Irene wanted her to let me know that she's here, but that she doesn't want to talk to me.

5. I: Hmm . . .
   H: She didn't even want to come to the phone when I called back.

6. I: (Shrugging.) Well . . .
   H: (Protruding his chin.) Well . . . what?

7. I: (Shrugging some more and leaning slightly backwards.) Seems like your wife has made her wishes clear.

   H: (Steps forward half a foot.) I don't believe that. That's a bunch of crap. She wouldn't dare do that! It's the social worker who put her up to that. I know those bitches. They put their noses into everything.

8. I: (Raises his eyebrows.) You say your wife wouldn't dare? (Puzzled) I don't understand.

   H: (With emphasis.) She wouldn't! She knows better than that! We have a kind of old-fashioned marriage. She knows what I expect from her. But you liberals wouldn't understand that.

9. I: (With a very low voice.) Maybe you're right I don't understand.

   H: (Loud but less pressed.) In our marriage my wife is the wife and I'm the man. She wouldn't go against me.

10. I: (Leaning his head to the side with a thin slightly provoking smile.) What makes you so convinced?

    H: (With open anger in his voice.) Listen, I don't owe you any explanation . . . (condescending) but I'll tell you anyway.

11. I: (Turns his back to the patient, walks to a chair and sits down, stretching out his feet and looking the husband straight in the face but not saying anything.)

    H: When we got married my wife was quite immature. Whenever we had an argument she was on the phone to tell her mother. I put a stop to that shit.

12. I: (With mild interest.) How did you do that?

    H: (Walking toward the interviewer and standing in front of him) I guess you don't believe me. Let me tell you what. I'll give you an example.

13. I: (Interrupting.) Why don't you sit down?

    H: (Insecure, looking around the waiting room and finally taking a seat, but sitting stiffly and bent forward.) Okay, I told my wife not to call her mother anymore. The next thing I know she's writing her a letter. That was it for me.

14. I: What do you mean "That was it?"

    H: I grabbed that bitch by the neck and gave her a good shake and then . . .

15. I: And then what?

    H: And then I let her eat her words.

16. I: (Raises his eyebrows.) What do you mean?

    H: I let her read the letter to me aloud and I just looked at her. When she was through, I told her: "Eat it!" She looked at me and knew that I meant it. I had her tear up the letter in little pieces and eat it.

17 I: That is what you did? What did you expect to get out of that?
   H: Exactly what I got. She quit doing that crap. And now she has the rules down pat.

18. I: Hmm.
   H: Let me tell you a joke that my father used to tell. He was from Italy, the old country, you know.

19. I: Alright, go ahead if you have to. Why don't you sit down!
   P: (Mr. Richardsen takes a seat but sits just on its edge.) There was a newly wed guy and after a few months of marriage he met his friend and his friend asked him: "How's it going with your marriage?"

"Bad," the newly wed guy said. "My wife is doing as she pleases and I feel like a clown. She talks about me to her family and friends and makes fun of me."

The friend laughed and said: "You forgot to rip the cat apart."

When the newly wed guy said that he didn't get it, his friend said: "You see when I got married, I came home, grabbed the cat by its legs and ripped it apart. The cat was my bride's pet. She understood who's the master."

"Well," the newly wed guy said, "my wife has a cat too."

A few days later, the newly wed guy met his friend again. The friend was surprised because the newly wed guy had a black eye and wore a bandage around his neck.

"What happened?" he asked him.

"Well, I followed your advice. I came home, I grabbed the cat and killed it. My wife took a big wooden spoon, hit me in the face and took the kettle with boiling water and threw it at me."

The friend laughed and couldn't stop laughing. "You fool, now it's too late. You should have killed the cat during your wedding night."

I never forgot that story. It stuck with me. And I thought when I get married I make sure that I wear the pants. And I did.

20. I: So . . . that kind of kids' stuff impresses you?
   H: Okay, let's just stop beating around the bush. I will take my wife home, and I mean now.

21. I: But Mr. Richardson, I don't understand you. You just heard from the social worker that your wife doesn't even want to talk to you. Why do you think she wants to go home with you now?
   H: Listen, buddy, I tell you what. I want her to tell me that to my face, and then we will see.

22. I: Your wife doesn't want to see you. Mr. Richardson, you just heard that your wife doesn't want to talk to your face. Is that so hard to understand?

H: That's enough of that. (He jumps up from his chair.) I consider this a case of kidnapping. If my wife is not down here in two minutes, you will hear from my lawyers.

23. I: (Remains seated.) Mr. Richardson, that is just fine. If I can be of any help, here is the telephone.

H: Your kind really gets to me. I want to tell you something in confidence. I've been a hitman for the mafia. It doesn't mean a thing to me to blow anyone away.

24. I: Mr. Richardsen, I realize you are angry. There is no reason for threats. You can't tear apart any cat here. I would prefer you sit down and answer a few questions about your wife. I believe you have some concern for her, even though you have a hell of a way to express it.

H: (Stares at the interviewer; after a few seconds.) Ha . . . let's see what you can come up with.

25. I: That all depends how much you can tell me to make me understand what's going on between you and your wife. You already gave me a little taste of it.

H: Damned, that was exactly what I was afraid of.

26. I: I guess you're right. If you did not get mad about all this, nothing on earth would have gotten you here to talk to us. So since you're here, we may as well make use of it.

H: Holy cow . . . I don't believe this . . . but let's get on with it.

This encounter shows some of the key features of sadistic personality disorder as described above. The interviewer uses a set of strategies that seem to work for this man.

First, whenever Mr. Richardsen made a threat, the interviewer told him that he does not understand, to force him to spell out the threat. That gave Mr. Richardsen the message that he could not intimidate the interviewer "indirectly." That way, Mr. Richardsen was placed in a position comparable to a flasher who gets deflated when his intended victim asks him:

"Is that all you've got? Why do you show it off?"

Second, when the patient with sadistic personality disorder spells out his threats, the interviewer shows no emotion, especially not disgust, horror, or intimidation. Instead, he indicates his lack of understanding for the patient's fascination with violence. He shows him a neutral, unimpressed, "professional" side.

Third, the interviewer does not give way to the threat nor does he try to make a counterthreat. Instead, he confronts Mr. Richardsen with his aggression and tells him that nothing can be accomplished with it.

Fourth, he sidesteps the affront and focuses on a legitimate topic of conversation, namely the husband as the informant for the patient's psychiatric problems.

Sacrifice and Self-Destruction in Self-Defeating Personality Disorder

You encounter a patient with self-defeating personality disorder (formerly called masochistic personality disorder) under one of two sets of circumstances:

First, the patient has a major psychiatric disorder. At the beginning of the treatment you often notice some social problems that you think can be interpreted as resulting from the major psychiatric disorder. Typical problems are related to work, and to interpersonal conflicts in the family. Since the patient often suffers either from major depressive or an anxiety disorder, you see his problem as the consequence of his coping deficit or his guilt feelings. However, you notice during treatment that many of the social problems persist and that new problems surface that the patient had hidden from you previously. Thus, your view of the patient's disorder can change dramatically during treatment; increasingly, you notice the coping deficits due to his personality disorder.

Second, a patient consults you with symptoms that superficially fit criteria for adjustment disorder with depressed, or anxious mood, or mixed emotional features, or with withdrawal or disturbance of conduct. However, at closer examination you detect that similar adjustment reactions under similar circumstances have occurred before. You notice that his problems are less specific to stress than to a coping deficit. The patient seems to arrange some of the failures, reminding you of Freud's notion that some patients seem to have a compulsion to repeat their mistakes. Behind the adjustment problem the self-defeating personality disorder emerges.

Under both sets of circumstances the characteristics that the patient displays are the same. He sacrifices his own interests for others. He gives up his pleasure and his professional opportunities in favor of somebody else's. His sacrifice is often not solicited, and therefore a bother to others and not appreciated, which can cause rejection rather than appreciation. Typically, he misinterprets the reason for this rejection. He believes that he has not given enough, and thus increases contempt rather than ameliorating the situation. Dysphoric feelings and hopelessness result.

If you explore his needs and confront him with his denial of those needs, he will indicate that they are egotistical, and that it is repulsive to him to pursue those needs. He seems to consider it a sin to even talk about them. If you point out how his self-denial contributes to his misery, he may reject you as materialistic and nonunderstanding, and lose interest in you.

You will find this pattern more often in physically, sexually, or psychologically abused females, and in passive men who often serve loyally in underpaid, dependent positions.

This is an interview with Mary, a 38-year-old, white, separated female. She has been hospitalized for four weeks. She was treated with amitriptyline; all vegetative symptoms of her major depressive disorder had improved. She could concentrate better in recreational therapy; signs of psychomotor retardation were gone and she denied depressed mood; but she still stayed by herself in her room lying on her bed. When the interviewer enters her room, she is in bed. She has a thin smile on her lips. When he walks up to her, she sinks back into her bed. She looks several years older than her stated age.

1. I: (With a soft voice.) Mary, you have been with us here for a while; you sleep well now, you eat well, you seem to get around the hospital fine, but you look like you carry a big cross. You seem sad most of the time.
   P: Yes, I'm here in the hospital when I should be at home taking care of my kids (patient has eleven children).

2. I: Well, I'm concerned because you stay so much by yourself; that's why I thought you should stay a little while longer.
   P: But I really feel better.

3. I: That's what they say in the staff meetings, and also the recreational and the occupational therapist say that you're doing so much better.
   P: I am, at least for the last week or so.

4. I: (Surprised and slightly irritated.) Why didn't you tell me? I talked to you every day . . .
   P: I thought you would tell me when I'm ready.

5. I: (Puzzled.) Hmm, you said you felt overpowered by all your problems.
   P: (Sitting up.) Yeah, but I wasn't depressed anymore.

6. I: (With doubt.) But you isolated yourself and stayed in bed and . . . you're still back here in your room.
   P: Because I don't want to bother others with my problems, they have enough to worry about themselves, Really, I think I should be with my kids now.

7. I: Who takes care of them now?
   P: My sister and her husband. But that's not right. They shouldn't be doing that just for me. I'm really letting them down so much . . . (Tears well up in her eyes.)

8. I: Mary, you were pretty depressed. I think it's best for all of you that the family helps out.
   P: (Shakes her head.) No, I have to go back to work to make some money for food and the rent.

9. I: What about your husband?
   P: He left.

10. I: He left? . . . Why didn't you ever tell me about it?
    P: I was ashamed . . . but we are still married . . .

11. I: I'm sorry to hear he left . . . How long ago did he leave?
    P: Nearly a year now.

12. I: What happened?
    P: Well, I guess it became too much for him.

13. I: What do you mean?
    P: Well, when he came home there were always the children, always a lot of commotion, they were all over the place, I guess he just couldn't take it.

14. I: (Surprised.) Couldn't take it?
    P: You know, he had a lot of pressure at his job and he couldn't get along with his foreman anyway and then he came home and there was some more pressure.

15. I: But they are his kids, aren't they?
    P: Well—yeah, of course, we had a good marriage and it lasted for fifteen years; but then when I was pregnant with John, he just couldn't take it anymore.

16. I: Couldn't take it?
    P: He had the problem before; and once in a while when it got too much for him, he would just stay out.

17. I: Stay out?
    P: With a lady friend of his or just with the guys from work.

18. I: How did you handle that?
    P: Well, he told me there is no discipline with the kids, they are all over the place. He said it was my fault that I couldn't control them any better.

19. I: But what about him? Couldn't he help out?
    P: Well, he was at work and not around much.

20. I: And what about you?
    P: I worked too most of the time, because we couldn't pay the bills on one paycheck; but he didn't like it. He liked me to be home when he came back at night from his job.

21. I: Hmm.
    P: We argued a lot and there was a lot of fighting.

22. I: (Surprised.) Fighting? You never mentioned that before.
    P: I guess I felt guilty.

23. I: What were the fights about?
    P: Oh, about anything, but often about me working.

24. I: You working?
    P: Yeah . . . He said I rub it in . . . When we went bowling, I let everybody know that I had to work. It made him mad and he started fighting.

25. I: Physically?
    P: Physically and mentally. When he was drinking, he could get pretty upset.

26. I: He was drinking? That's news.
    P: Well, I'm sorry, I didn't know you and I didn't want to tattle on him.

27. I: Hmm.
    P: I must have angered him a lot.

28. I: Angered him?
    P: Yeah, he got pretty mad. I got him so angry one time that he hit me in the face and broke my nose.

29. I: Hmm.
    P: Another time he hit me in the eye and my retina came off. That's when I lost my job, because I couldn't see well enough any more to put the chips in the holes and do the soldering.

30. I: Mary, it sounds like you took a lot of abuse.
    P: But it was my fault, he told me. I brought it on.

31. I: What did your kids say when there was so much fighting?
    P: They got mad at him and then he got mad at me, because he said I put 'em up to it. So I tried to hide it from them because he's still their father and I don't want them to be caught between us.

32. I: Where is your husband now?
    P: He's around somewhere.

33. I: Does he not pay child support?
    P: He's supposed to, but he don't.

34. I: Don't you want to take him to court?
    P: No, he was my husband, and I don't believe in suing him. And I don't want to do it because of the kids . . . so I'm stuck.

35. I: Stuck? But he let you down . . . Can't you get any other kind of child support?
    P: If I apply for that, those agencies will go after him and I don't want that to happen.

36. I: But Mary, your husband ran away and let you hold the bag.
    P: I have to get through it. There is no need to talk about it. I just have to.

37. I: Do your older children help out?
    P: They really want to be with their high school friends, you know, go out with them and have a good time—I just have to get through with it by myself. I'm trapped, I just have to do it. There's no way out. I have to get through it.

38. I: Are you living alone with your children now?
    P: Well, kind of . . . There is a friend of mine who stays with me most of the time.

39. I: Oh, I see. Does he help out?
    P: Well, George has enough problems of his own. He's a veteran, he got injured in Vietnam, they had to amputate his foot, and he still has pain in the foot even though it's off. It really got to him mentally. He just got out of the state hospital; they said he had schizophrenia.

40. I: How do you feel about that?
    P: I feel bad about it because I'm Catholic and I think it's a sin. Because as a Catholic I'm not really divorced.

41. I: That's not what I meant. I mean how you feel about George . . .
    P: I feel sorry for him, because he's not able to work and he has only the VA pension.

42. I: So you took on an additional burden . . .
    P: I can't help him as much as I should because since I lost my job at the plant because of my bad vision, I have to work as a waitress and that doesn't pay enough to really help him out.

43. I: It appears to me that you have a hard time thinking about yourself and your own needs.
    P: I don't think one should just think about oneself. I can't just feel sorry for myself. And it wouldn't help anyway.

44. I: We should try to find out why you can't think about yourself . . .
    P: I'm not that kind of a person.

It is easy to get apparent rapport with the patient. And that is the first difficulty. She seems to open up, and is ready to talk about her failures in spite of all her efforts. That is where the interviewer can get trapped. It may escape him—as in Mary's case—that the patient carefully edits what she reports so that she appears as an innocent victim.

Another difficulty arises when you attempt to discuss her problems and make her recognize her behavior as self-defeating. If the interviewer focuses on the underlying self-sacrificing behavior, the patient feels criticized without being able to see its pathological nature.

Self-defeating personality disorder is one of the few conditions in which expression of empathy does not work because it devalues the patient's self-sacrifice as a symptom. The patient still suffers from the nagging feeling of not investing enough. If you suggest that she is overburdened you threaten her identity, which she cannot comprehend as pathological.

If you suggest to her that she denies her needs and foregoes assertiveness to gain love and protection through sacrifice, she will be appalled by your misunderstanding of her motives. Since the patient cannot be helped without gaining insight into her behavioral traits, her personality disorder defeats effective help.

EPILOGUE

Shall I tell you what knowledge is? It is to know both what one knows and what one does not know.

Confucius 551–479 B.C.

INTERVIEW BETWEEN THE AUTHORS (A) AND A HYPOTHETICAL READER (R)

1. R: Are we done now?
   A: Not really. We have only set the stage.

2. R: For what?
   A: For the *why*.

3. R: I don't understand.
   A: We have discussed how experienced mental health professionals interview for the *what*.

4. R: You mean *what* is disturbed in psychiatric disorders? *What* the symptoms are, and *what* the disorder?
   A: Yes. But we have not told you *why* it is disturbed.

5. R: Why not?
   A: Because it is not known.

6. R: Not known? What about the neuroreceptors, the overprotective mother, and the aloof father?
   A: You are right. We are experimenting with a gamut of approaches to find out.

7. R: Such as dexamethasone suppression test, CSF, TRH/TSH stimulation test, insulin/GH stimulation test, REM-latency test, MHPG, VMA, HIAA, blood or urine levels respectively, PET scanning, MRI, BEAMS . . .
   A: And family studies, epidemiological studies, psychoanalytical explorations of internal psychic mechanisms, psychic development, learning, and conditioning.

8. R: That's right—it all contributes to the *why*.

   A: To answer the *why* though, the *what* is necessary—a *what* unadulterated by theories and schools of thought—we mean a descriptive *what*.

9. R: And who shall have the last word?

   A: Since we preach empathy—you.

APPENDIX A

THINKING

TIGHTNESS OF ASSOCIATIONS

In the following, two types of disturbed association are described where the goal is totally or partially preserved: circumstantiality and tangentiality.

1. CIRCUMSTANTIALITY

Circumstantial speech has tightly linked associations which in the end reach their goal, but the thinking is sidetracked over a long circuitous route lined with irrelevant details, as in the following interview with Dorothy.

I: What brought you here?
P: (1) I have this feeling. (2) Let me explain this. (3) I remember when I was eight years old I had a dirty spot in my pants. (4) I may not have wiped myself properly. (5) I always had the feeling that I'm contaminating myself. (6) Wherever I put my stuff it becomes contaminated. (7) I have to avoid it. (8) It does not have to be actual dirt, just the thought that the dirt is there. (9) I would contaminate my clothes. (10) The contaminated clothes can contaminate me. (11) So when I look behind me I want to see if I am clean or if I have contaminated the chair. (12) That is why I look behind me to see if there are any signs of contamination. (13) I know it's silly. (14) Even when I'm not completely clean it will get through my clothes. (15) I have the feeling that I have to look behind me all the time. (16) This is what brought me here.

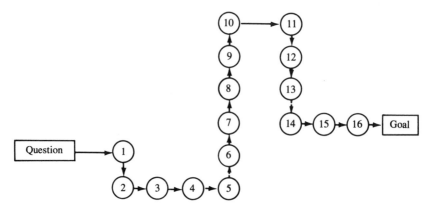

FIGURE A. 1
Speech pattern

The patient's speech can be diagramed in the following way: Each circled number represents a sentence or part of a sentence. A solid arrow reflects a tight, a broken arrow a loose connection between subsequent sentences. An arrow interrupted by two lines indicates no detectable association. The direction of the arrow is horizontal if the sentence contributes to reaching the goal; it is vertical when the sentence is irrelevant to the goal; and reverse when it leads away from the goal. Dorothy's answer would be sufficient if she had only answered with sentences 3–5, 11, 15, and 16 which lead to the goal. The additional sentences elaborate or repeat relatively unnecessary details. Dorothy shows perseveration in theme and circumstantiality which is typical for obsessive compulsive and organic mental disorder. Circumstantiality is also seen in mania where it presents as enrichment with many irrelevant free associations only loosely connected to the goal of the thought. Therefore, the minute details of the previous example do not fit manic circumstantiality.

2. TANGENTIALITY

Tangential thinking may show tight or loose associations. The patient's answers miss the goal, but land in close vicinity.

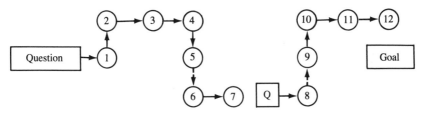

FIGURE A.2
Speech pattern

I: What brought you here?
P: (1) I have this feeling. (2) I have it all the time. (3) It's all the talk that's around me. (4) Can you imagine how it feels when it spreads? (5) It was first at my job. (6) Then in my neighborhood. (7) It seems it's now everywhere.

I: Does this talk bother you?
P: (8) It has to do with what others think. (9) It shows what they think. (10) It is like loud thinking. (11) You hear it everywhere and (12) you know they think again because they talk.

Goal-Orientedness and Sentence Association

The patient who thinks in a goal-oriented manner can give you a coherent history and answer questions to the point. In severe thought disorder the goal is lost and the associations are disturbed. Here are ten different types of disturbances:

(1) Perseveration

The patient repeats the same phrases and words, even if the subject is changed, or he sticks with the same theme:

I: What brought you here?
P: (1) I came for my manic problem. (2) You know, it has to do with my situation. (3) At home, my things disappear. (4) That is the situation, you know. (5) I believe my son-in-law has to do with it. (6) In my situation I don't know what to do. (7) That is the situation.

The patient repeats the term "situation" several times. The repeated word is called a stock phrase. Another example of perseveration: the patient is unable to shift from one topic to another.

I: What did you have for breakfast?
P: Cereals.

I: What did you have for lunch?
P: Cereals.

I: For dinner?
P: Cereals.

Perseveration is seen in depression, frontal lobe damage, and catatonic schizophrenia.

(2) Verbigeration or Palilalia

Catatonic and sometimes manic patients repeat words or phrases automatically, especially at the end of a sentence.

I: What problems brought you here?
P: My problems brought me here, problems brought me here, me here.

(3) Clang Association

Clang association is neither dictated by logic nor meaning, but by similarity of sounds.

I: What brought you here?
P: All the things said the swings. Whatever brings and tings and clings.

Some clang associations sound like rhyming, others appear forced as if the patient succumbs or is possessed to associate words by clang. It is seen in patients with chronic brain disease, with phonemic paraphasia, schizophrenia, and mania.

(4) Blocking and Derailment

In blocking, the stream of thought is suddenly interrupted; after a pause the patient may start with an entirely new thought, called derailment.

I: What brought you here?
P: I had this argument with my neighbors and they started to . . . (pause) Nobody should support the mayor.

The patient did not complete his first thought, but stopped midstream. In simple blocking, he may continue the original thought after a pause. If you ask what happened when the patient blocked, he will tell you that he suddenly lost his train of thought. This experience has been called thought omission. Blocking resembles petit mal seizures in children; however neither the EEG abnormality nor the blank stare typical for petit mal have been demonstrated in blocking.

(5) *Flight of Ideas*

Flight of ideas is non–goal-oriented speech due to distractibility. While the patient answers one question, he switches to a new train of thought, often triggered by a word in the previous sentence.

I: What brought you here?
P: (1) I got here by getting on my feet. (2) But I have hurt my feet while jogging. (3) Do you think jogging is good for me? (4) It may not help against heart infarct, aspirin may be better. (5) But I don't like to take drugs. (6) Drugs and crime go together.

First, the patient gives a concrete answer. Subsequently he never reaches his goal of explaining why he came, because he associates freely to important words in the preceding sentence.
In this diagram we chose the diagonal to indicate flight from the goal.

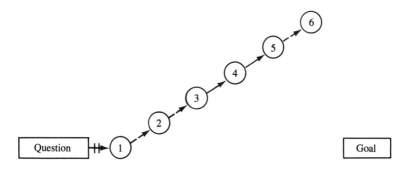

FIGURE A.3
Speech pattern

Here is another example:

I: What brought you here?
P: I was not brought here, but I walked, not with a car. I like new cars, especially foreign ones. Do you like the Mercedes? It is the best, but the gas consumption is high. You would have difficulties in Russia. There are not many gas stations over there. But it would help the economy. I knew it all along that the Russians put the cyanide in the Tylenol capsules.

In flight of ideas—typical in manic patients—you can identify the words that trigger the connections between subsequent sentences, but they don't arrive at a goal. Flight of ideas is usually associated with accelerated speech. You can follow the succession of ideas which is in contrast to schizophrenic speech where the content is cryptic.

We captured flight of ideas visually. This 19-year-old, female college student was asked to draw a watch. In rapid strokes she sketched the following picture in four stages.

I: Draw a watch

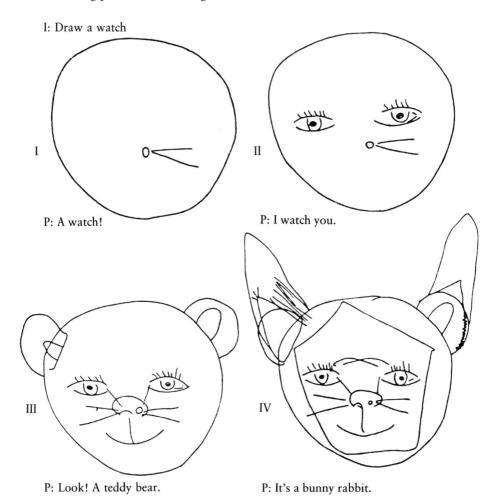

I

P: A watch!

II

P: I watch you.

III

P: Look! A teddy bear.

IV

P: It's a bunny rabbit.

FIGURE A.4
Draw a watch

(6) Non Sequitur

A non sequitur is a totally unrelated response to a question, on a concrete or abstract level:

I: What problem brought you here?
P: There is some evidence but it is not appropriate for my age.

You find this type of thought disorder in coarse brain disease and schizophrenia.

(7) Fragmentation

Patients with fragmented speech talk in phrases unrelated to each other. They show continuous non sequiturs in subsequent phases.

I: What brought you here?
P: I have been over . . . There is the street light . . . Can I go . . . No one will be . . . Let them all fly . . . Bye and hi.

Fragmentation is not specific for any psychiatric disorder. You may hear it from patients with mania, catatonia, schizophrenia, or coarse brain disease.

(8) Rambling

Patients who ramble use groups of sentences that are closely connected but followed by other groups without connection or goal.

I: What brought you here?
P: What a stupid question. Can't you see? But you look cute. Aren't you cute? Okay? Let me tell you, I don't want to repeat it, but I tell you here and now these damned bastards, why can't they leave me alone. I have not done anything. There is the cook. Comes and cooks again. Go away. Just leave me alone.

This type of speech is often seen in patients with acute organic mental disorder, such as alcohol intoxication. Watch for other signs of intoxication such as slurred speech, gait ataxia, and nystagmus.

(9) Driveling

Patients who drivel speak with preserved syntax and subsequent sentences appear linked, yet the speech cannot be understood.

I: What brought you here?

P: Okay. There was all of the others rounded by the broom, but nevertheless gathering the lomb. So what is the downward onvent creatibility? If nothing on those things never recreate a ribboned layer of all times.

In driveling you find no verbigeration and perseveration, but some neologisms. Neurologists have termed this type of speech jargon agrammatism. It can be observed in Wernicke's aphasia, but also in chronic schizophrenia.

(10) Word Salad

In some hospitalized chronic schizophrenics the meaningful connection between words is altogether disrupted. Whereas in fragmentation the loosening occurs between phrases and sentences, in word salad consecutive words are not linked by meaning; speech is incomprehensible.

I: What brought you here?

P: The, my, not, rode, for, new, cold, it, what, may, so.

Bleuler called this phenomenon "schizophasia." It resembles global aphasia (see chapter 4.4: Testing).

A thought disorder is not pathognomonic for schizophrenia as often assumed—not all schizophrenics exhibit thought disorder. On the other hand, patients with organic brain syndrome and affective disorder may also display thought disorder. Like most other symptoms and signs, evaluate formal thought disorder in the context of all other psychopathology, psychosocial functioning, and family history.

TESTING MENTAL STATUS FUNCTIONS

1. TEST RECENT MEMORY

Strub and Black's (1977) Paired Associates Test

Ask the patient to learn five to eight sets of unrelated paired words. After he has learned the pairs, wait ten minutes, then reexamine him by giving him the first word of each pair. The number of words he misses determines the degree of impairment. Here is how to give the test (Strub and Black 1977):

Tell the patient "I am going to read you a list of words, two at a time. Listen carefully because I will expect you to remember the words that go together. For example, if the words were big-little, I would expect you to say the word little after I said the word big." When the patient is clear as to the directions, continue as follows: "Now listen carefully to the words as I read them." Read the first presentation at the rate of one pair every two seconds. After reading the first presentation, test for recall by presenting the first recall list. Give the first word of a pair and allow five seconds for a response. If the patient gives a correct response, say, "That's right" and proceed with the next pair. If the patient gives an incorrect response, say, "No," provide the correct association, and proceed to the next pair. After the first recall has been completed, allow a 10 second interval and give the second presentation list, proceeding as before.

Test Items

Presentation Lists

First Presentation	Second Presentation
Weather-Bag	House-Income
High-Low	Weather-Bag
House-Income	Book-Page
Book-Page	High-Low

Recall Lists

First Recall	Second Recall
House-_____	High-_____
High-_____	House-_____
Weather-_____	Book-_____
Book-_____	Weather-_____

Scoring

The nonretarded patient is expected to recall the two "easy" paired associates (high-low, book-page) and at least one of the "hard" associates on the first recall trial, and to recall all paired associates on the second trial. Less adequate performance is indicative of impaired new learning ability. Some patients will be able to learn the paired words with strong natural associations, but are unable to learn the pairs without such associations. This discrepancy demonstrates a reliance upon semantic cues and inability to learn new material which cannot be associated with memories already in storage (Strub and Black 1977).

2. APHASIAS

Aphasic patients find it difficult to comprehend language or express themselves verbally. Deficiencies can be classified into two types: sensory (receptive) and motor (expressive). The aphasias also include reading and writing. The inability to read, called alexia, represents a sensory (receptive) aphasia, the inability to write, known as agraphia, represents a motor (expressive) aphasia.

Testing for sensory aphasia assesses whether the patient comprehends the meaning of words, phrases, or sentences of increasing complexity.

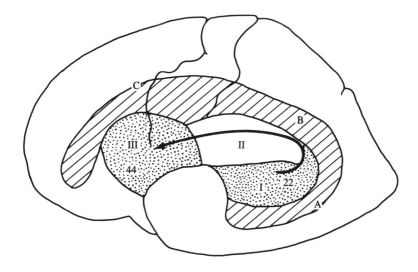

FIGURE B. 1

Location of cerebral lesion in different types of aphasias of the dominant hemisphere

Legend:

Roman numerals refer to the lesions seen in central aphasias:

I. Brodmann's area 22 in parietal lobe and posterior part of superior temporal lobe (Wernicke's receptive aphasia)

II. Brodmann's area 44 of prefrontal and frontal lobe of dominant hemisphere (Broca's expressive aphasia)

III. Connecting fibers between Wernicke's and Broca's speech areas (global aphasia).

Letters refer to lesions seen in pericentral aphasias:

A. Border zone posterior to area 44 (transcortical sensory aphasia)

B. Connecting fibers from occipital lobe to limbic system in the second and third temporal gyri (anomic aphasia).

C. Superior border zone to area 44 (transcortical motor aphasia).

Testing for expressive aphasia examines whether the patient can repeat words or name objects of increasing complexity. Testing for alexia investigates the ability of patients to read letters, words, and simple sentences. To screen for aphasia, start with a difficult task; if no deficiency is detected move to the next test. If you spot problems try simpler tasks to assess the severity of the disturbance.

Aphasias are further subdivided into four central and four pericentral types. The central types include Broca's expressive, Wernicke's receptive, conduction, and global aphasia. The pericentral types are transcortical sensory, anomic, transcortical motor, and isolation aphasia.

Central Aphasias

1. *Broca's Aphasia:* This is a result of a brain lesion of the prefrontal anterior speech area (Brodmann's area 44) (see figure B.1): the patient uses nouns and verbs without correct grammatical connection. Speech is nonfluent, dysarthric, and laborious, called telegram style language.

2. *Wernicke's Aphasia:* This results from lesions of Brodmann's area 22 (see figure B.1) in the parietal lobe and in the posterior portion of the superior temporal gyrus. The patient has difficulty in auditory comprehension of your question. His language is characterized by fluent, effortless, well-articulated speech devoid of nouns. He may have push of speech. Since the patient often has no insight into his speech problem and has sometimes no apparent hemiparesis, sensory loss, or altered level of consciousness, his language disturbance may be considered functional in origin and misinterpreted as psychotic language (manic or schizophrenic).

3. *Conduction Aphasia:* This is due to a lesion of the connecting fibers between Broca's and Wernicke's speech center. Repetition of words and sentences is severely disturbed. The patient's speech is fluent, but has pauses, because word finding is disturbed. Literal paraphasias are common. "I like to drive my tar."

4. *Global Aphasia:* The patient can neither express his thoughts nor comprehend other people's speech. Only some syllables are uttered. This severe speech disorder is seen in extensive lesions of the dominant hemisphere.

Pericentral Aphasias

Pericentral aphasias are due to lesions surrounding the central sensory and motor speech areas of Wernicke and Broca.

1. *Transcortical Sensory Aphasia:* The patient repeats well, his spontaneous speech is fluent, but he does not comprehend what he hears or repeats. His speech is paraphasic. The deficit is caused by a posterior borderzone lesion (see figure B.1, area A).

2. *Anomic Aphasia:* The patient speaks fluently, but with pauses to find words. He can repeat and comprehend well, but has difficulties in naming objects. He can neither name shown objects nor point to named objects. His word finding difficulties lead to paraphasias (figure B.1, area

B). The most severe anomias are found in lesions involving the second and third temporal gyri, which interrupt passways from the occipital lobe to the limbic system. Higher lesions in the parietal temporal area are associated with substantial alexia and agraphia.

3. *Transcortical Motor Aphasia:* The patient can repeat and comprehend well, but does not have fluent speech (figure B.1, area C).

4. *Isolation Aphasia:* The patient cannot name, or comprehend, and his speech is nonfluent. However, he can repeat and may have a tendency to repeat everything that is in hearing range, like a speech-trained parrot. This speech abnormality is called echolalia. The lesion involves the whole pericentral area (figure B.1, areas A, B, and C).

Testing of Aphasias

Rarely will the nonneurologist encounter an aphasia, but if he does, it is less important to identify the subtype than to recognize its neurological origin. When you encounter the rare case you can follow a simple sequence of tests to identify the type. Refer to table B.1 which gives the performance profile for the aphasias. Figure B.2 shows the decision tree. If you suspect an aphasic syndrome, test at least writing, repetition, fluency, and comprehension.

1. *Writing:* All tests for aphasia show some degree of *agraphia* (writing difficulties). Writing ability should be tested first (see table B.1), even though agraphia can occur without aphasia, as in the cases of agraphia with alexia or with the Gerstmann syndrome (see glossary). Agraphia cannot be established by asking the patient to write his name, because even in the presence of gross agraphia name writing may be preserved.

Screen for agraphia by giving the following instructions:

"Write down, in one sentence, what the main problem is that brought you here."

If the patient fails this test, continue with systematic assessment. Testing of writing ability starts with dictation of letters and numbers. Next, the patient should be asked to write down body parts or common objects. If he is successful with these tasks, he is asked to write a short sentence describing his family, the weather, or a picture on the wall. Agraphia should be diagnosed when basic language errors in spelling or substitution of letters, syllables, or words (paragraphias) not due to educational deficits are encountered.

TABLE B. 1
Performance Profile of Different Types of Aphasias

Aphasia Type	Writing	Repetition	Fluency	Comprehension	Naming	Reading Aloud and Comprehending it	Cerebral Lesion (Fig. B.1)
Central							
Wernicke	−	−	+	−	+ −	−/−	I
Conduction	−	−	+	+	+ −	−/− +	II
Broca	−	−	−	+	+ −	−/− +	III
Global	−	−	−	−	−	−/−	I + II + III
Pericentral							
Transcortical Sensory	−	+	+	−	−	−/−	A
Anomic	−	+	+	+	−	+/+ −	B
Transcortical Motor	−	+	−	+	−	−/+	C
Isolation	−	+	−	−	−	− +/−	A + B + C

Legend: + = intact
      − = disturbed
      − + = sometimes disturbed
Source: Modified after Ross, "Disorders of higher cortical functions."

2. *Repetition:* The repetition of spoken language is only disturbed in the central aphasias, in which the central speech areas that bank the Sylvian fissure are lesioned. The pericentral aphasias are caused by lesions surrounding the central speech areas and thus have good repetition. Repetition can be affected by impaired auditory functions, disturbed speech production, or by disconnection between the receptive and expressive language areas.

Test repetition by asking the patient to repeat words and sentences of increasing complexity. Ask the patient to repeat the material after you. Listen for errors in grammar, omissions, additions, paraphasias, and the inability to repeat the given material. For screening purposes, use the most difficult sentence (no. 10) first. If repetition is obviously disturbed, start with the easy tasks in order to establish a baseline for the extent of the disturbance.

1. Walk
2. School
3. Steamboat

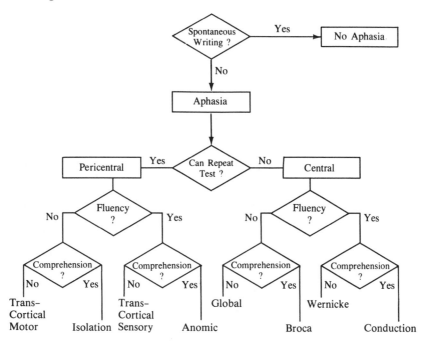

FIGURE B.2

Decision tree for eight different types of aphasias

4. Nursery
5. Mississippi River
6. The woman went to the store.
7. Everybody left the house at the same time.
8. Let's go out to the park to fly kites.
9. The tall fat maid cleaned the floors upstairs.
10. Every aspect of the problem needs more detailed discussion.

3. *Fluency:* This is observed in the patient's spontaneous speech during the interview. Nonfluent speech is sparse, laborious, agrammatic, and filled with pauses for word finding. Nonfluent speech consists predominantly of nouns (telegram style). Fluent speech may also be unintelligible (jargon aphasia) or otherwise empty of content, full of abnormal words (paraphasias) and neologisms (self-invented words or phrases).

There are two types of neologisms: the symbolic, repeatedly used neologism of the schizophrenic and the paraphasic neologism of the patient with a lesion in the speech center. Neologisms indicate either pathological creativeness or inability to find the correct word. Examples of the first are:

"The compterum that controls me and observes me."
And the newly invented random and nonsymbolic neologism of the aphasic:
"The onlyness is how wellabit can I not take."

In milder forms, aphasic language contains abnormal words (paraphasias) which affects mainly verbs and nouns; it is filled with articles, conjunctions, and interjections. There is often pressure of speech, distinguished from mania by the fact that manics have neither paraphasic nor aphasic problems. Lack of fluency points to a cerebral prefrontal lesion, fluency with paraphasia to a postcentral upper posterior temporal lobe or parietal marginal gyrus lesion.

4. *Comprehension:* This should be tested in a fashion that does not require much expression, so that expressive aphasia is not misread as a comprehension disability. Ask the patient to point to his eye, leg, and nose. If he is successful, ask for sequences of increasing length, such as "first point to your nose, then to your right eye, then to your left ear, then to your right knee." Patients with normal comprehension are usually able to point to four objects in sequence. A second method consists in giving six or more yes/no questions.

Does Monday come before Wednesday?
Does the year have thirteen months?
Is winter in Chicago warmer than summer?
Do you harvest potatoes in Iowa in December?
Is snow frozen water?
Do women wear athletic supporters?
Does the earth go around the sun?

All questions should be answered correctly.

5. *Naming and Word Finding:* Ask the patient to name the objects that you point to. Repeat approximately ten times. Use parts of the body, parts of a watch, and parts of clothing. Naming is usually more disturbed in the pericentral than in the central aphasias (see table B.1).

6. *Reading Aloud and Comprehension:* These skills are tested by having the patient read names of objects aloud and then ask him to point to them. A more difficult task is to have him read sentences aloud and then ask him yes/no questions about the content.

"Two boys played soccer against two other boys."

"Were the soccer players female?
Were there more than two soccer players?
Did they play soccer with a baseball bat?"

Usually, reading, comprehension, or both are disturbed in the aphasic patient.

Aphasias are infrequent. However, be prepared to interpret aphasic language as part of a neurological syndrome and not as a schizophrenic thought disorder. A misdiagnosis can be fatal. If the aphasia is due to a tumor or abscess in the brain, surgical intervention, instead of long-term treatment with phenothiazines, is needed. Also, you should be able to differentiate pseudodementia without aphasia in a depressed patient, from true dementia with aphasia in an Alzheimer patient.

Difference Between Neologism and Paraphasia

Neologisms are new words invented by the patient or ordinary words that the patient uses in a special way. The neologism thus has a fixed meaning. This term is usually applied to word formations produced by schizophrenics.

Paraphasia superficially resembles neologisms, since paraphasic patients use the wrong word, invent new words, or distort the phonetic structure of words. However, paraphasias do not have a fixed meaning in the language of the neurological patient.

Neurologists recognize different forms of paraphasia:

In *semantic* paraphasia, the correct word is substituted by another correct, but inappropriate word: "I wrote the letter with my grass. I like to drive around in my tent."

In *literal or phonomic* paraphasia, only one syllable or letter is substituted: "I wrote the letter with my len."

In *word approximation,* the correct word is substituted by an incorrect word, which has some relationship with the correct word: "I wrote the letter with my writing toy."

Neologisms are newly created words: "I wrote the letter with my zemps. On Sundays I like to wash my flom."

3. AGNOSIAS AND APRAXIAS

The parietal lobes of the cerebral cortex integrate sensory input; damage to these lobes causes deficits called *agnosias*. Agnosias are disorders of 'knowing,' the inability to recognize forms and the nature of objects, or sensations. There are several types of agnosia, such as the inability to

TABLE B.2

Agnosias and Associated Neuroanatomical Lesions

Agnosia	Test	Lesion	Associated Syndrome
RIGHT-LEFT	Pointing to right and left parts of own or examiner's body	Genetic or dominant parietotemporo-occipital region	
FINGER	Lift, name and point to individual fingers	Same as right-left	
GERSTMANN SYNDROME	Finger and right-left identification, writing and calculation	Dominant parietal lobe	
ACTUAL VISUAL	Name presented object or describe its use without picking it up	Bilateral visual association cortex, areas 18 and 19	
ASSOCIATIVE VISUAL	Name objects after they were selected and their use described	Left occipital lobe and posterior corpus callosum	Alexia
PROSOPAGNOSIA	Recognize familiar faces without hearing their voices	Bilateral occipito-temporal and right inferior temporo-occipital	
ASSOCIATIVE COLOR	Name different colors	Disconnection of visual and language area	Alexia with agraphia
ACUTE COLOR	Point to different colors	Bilateral inferior temporo-occipital	Prosopagnosia
GEOGRAPHIC	Find way in familiar environment; find cities on a map	Generalized right or left hemisphere	Right-left agnosia Spacial neglect

identify objects by touch, to read letters traced on the skin, or to recognize objects and pictures of faces. Agnosias may include disorientation in space, the improper designation of body parts, right-left disorientation, as well as sensory inattention, or denial of illness or defect.

Agnosias are tested by asking the patient to identify objects (e.g., a key, or coin) placed in their hand, or to read numbers written on the back of their forearm. Finger identification and right-left disorientation can be evaluated simultaneously by asking the patient, for example, to lift up the ring finger on the left hand. In summary, agnosia is the inability to conceptualize complex sensations.

Apraxias refer to the inability to execute purposeful actions and goal-oriented manipulations of objects. Apraxias are caused by damage to the premotor gyrus of the frontal cortex or the right parietal lobe. There are several types of apraxias, such as inability to carry out a movement, to determine what the movement should be, to organize the logical sequence of movements for acts such as dressing, or to construct simple forms or copy designs.

Apraxias are assessed by having the patient perform some customary act (e.g., light a match), imitate an imaginary action (e.g., thread a needle), or construct a simple form (e.g., build a triangle from three pencils).

4. TEST ABNORMAL INDUCED MOVEMENTS

Ambitendency: The patient alternates between opposing movements, like bending down to sit down, but raising up instead and repeating this several times, until he finally stands up for the rest of the interview.

Cooperation (Mitmachen): The patient is instructed to resist all movements. In spite of the instruction he can be pushed in all directions with a light touch of a finger. The opposite behavior is seen in *Opposition (Gegenhalten):* The patient, even though instructed to allow the examiner to move his limbs, resists movements with a force proportionate to the applied force.

Echopraxia: The patient imitates actions, such as hand clapping or snapping, or copies complete actions of you and other people. Echopraxia is seen in transcortical motor aphasias and catatonia, and is normal in early childhood.

TABLE B.3
Apraxias and Associated Neuroanatomical Lesions

Apraxia	Test	Lesion
I *Ideomotor*		
BUCCOFACIAL	Blow out a match, protrude tongue, drink through a straw.	Any lesion in the following circuit leads to apraxia: 1. Verbal comprehension in dominant Wernicke area to 2. kinesthetic memories in supra-marginal gyrus to 3. transmission to dominant premotor area for activation of motor memory; 4. transmission to pyramidal neurons of motor strip for execution of action.
LIMB	Salute, use tooth brush, hammer a nail, comb hair, snap fingers, kick a ball, crush a cigarette.	As above; isolated left limb agnosia is due to lesion of 5. pathway from dominant premotor to non-dominant premotor area via anterior corpus callosum or 6. from this premotor area to motor strip
WHOLE BODY	Stand like a boxer, swing a baseball bat, bow.	Pyramidal and extrapyramidal motor system
II *Ideational*	Complex tasks such as taking a tooth brush from a holder, opening toothpaste and putting toothpaste on a brush; or complete dressing in the morning.	Widespread bilateral cortex, especially both parietal lobes

Forced Grasping: The patient shakes hands whenever a hand is offered, even though he has been instructed not to do so.

Impairment of Switching: The patient continues to repeat the first task and cannot switch to a second one. Both types of perseveration occur in schizophrenics and demented patients; the former more in schizophrenia, the latter more in demented patients.

Magnet Reaction: You touch the patient's palm and withdraw your fingers slowly; the patient follows the examiner's fingers with his hand. Both forced grasping and magnet reaction can be seen in dementia and catatonia.

Negativism: An accentuation of opposition in which the patient resists all movements of his limbs by the examiner (passive movement) or tries to do the opposite of what he is signaled to do.

Perseveration: The patient repeats a movement over and over after a command such as "Open your mouth." In compulsive perseveration he repeats the movement until he is asked to do another task.

5. TEST AFFECT

An approach to measure a patient's ability to recognize and imitate affect has been proposed by Ross (1982). He recommends to ask a patient with right cortical lesions to say, with as much expression as possible, as if he were an actor, emotionally charged sentences. In our practice, we have used this approach with psychiatric patients and have asked them to enact the following phrases:

I'm angry.
I'm sad.
I'm scared.
I feel depressed.
I feel persecuted.
I'm disgusted.
I feel happy.
I feel worthless.
I feel guilty.
I feel insecure.

We propose to standardize the scoring in the following way. Rate each affect on a scale from 0 to 4. Give one point for each of the following four elements of affective expression: modulation in tone, change in rhythm of speech, facial expression, and body language. Patients who get an average rating of 1 or less per sentence are retested; they are asked to imitate the examiner. Read each sentence that was rated 1 or less to the patient and demonstrate change in tone of voice, rhythm of speech, facial expression, and body language, i.e., you attempt to express the sentence in a manner that would give you a rating of 4. Then have the patient repeat the test.

Guidelines for scoring each of the four elements is as follows.

Tone of Voice: Patient changes loudness, pitch of voice, and melody of the sentence. If positive give one point.

Rhythm of Speech: Patient changes rate of speech, length of vowels, and stress on syllables. Noticeable changes are rewarded with one point. There are no extra points for dramatic or excentuated changes.

Mimic: Patient makes facial changes around mouth, forehead, and eyes. If yes, reward with one point.

Body Language: A patient changes body position, stance, and gestures. If it clearly expresses intense emotion, reward with one point.

This test is not yet validated for different psychiatric and neurological patient populations. Only a few clinical impressions have been collected.

Patients with damage to the right frontal lobe and possibly disturbances of the limbic lobe have difficulty expressing their feelings (Ross 1982); their average rating is less than 10 for the ten sentences. Patients with conversion, somatization disorder, and mania may exceed a rating of 30. However, only a low rating is of clinical significance in measuring affect.

For psychiatric patients, statements that reflect some of their genuine feelings appear to be more diagnostic. For instance, anhedonic schizophrenics with flat affect become more lively when they express thought contents related to their delusions. Karl Leonhard called these patients "affect laden paraphrenics." They have a better recovery rate than his "systematic schizophrenics" (Leonhard 1979).

6. TEST SUGGESTIBILITY

1. *Falling Backwards:* Ask the patient to stand upright, keep both feet together, and close his eyes. Then ask him to imagine that he is standing on one end of a six-foot-long board facing the other end. Let him imagine that somebody is slowly lifting the other end in front of him . . . that he is losing his balance . . . that he starts to sway more and more

and is falling backward. Assure the patient that you will catch him if he falls. Repeat to him:

"If you can really imagine it, how the board is slowly lifted, you will fall backward. You can imagine it . . . imagine it . . . now you are falling over."

The test is positive when the patient sways markedly or falls back.

2. *Tired Eyelid Test:* Ask the patient to look up to your lifted index finger, a foot in front of and a foot up from his forehead, without lifting his head. Then ask him to imagine that his eyes are tired and the lids get heavy, . . . that they will slowly close, while he is still looking at your finger. The test is positive when the patient's eyelids slowly close, while the eyes are still focused on your finger.

3. *Hand-Sticking Test:* Ask the patient to fold his hands and clasp his fingers tightly. Then ask him to imagine that the fingers stick together. He is told that he cannot pull them apart, no matter how hard he tries. The test is positive when the patient cannot pull his hands apart.

4. *Circle Test:* A small object (like a ring) is fixed to a string in a pendulum fashion. The patient holds the pendulum between two fingers of his nonsupported arm and hand. Ask him to imagine that the pendulum starts to swing, first in a small circle and then in a larger radius. The test is positive when the object starts to swing in a circle.

It is important that you do not put your authority on the line by suggesting that the patient will have a certain sensation, or make a certain movement. Always make it clear to him that it is *his* task . . . "If you want to imagine that your arm feels heavy, you will start to feel the weight." That way a failure is *his* and not yours.

7. STUPOR

Stupor in a *panic* state may paralyze the patient with fear.

Stupor in *somatization disorder* without incontinence of urine may indicate an avoidance of an unpleasant situation.

Stupor in *bipolar affective disorder* is recognized in Europe especially in confusional and motility psychosis. It effects mainly the reactive and expressive movements and less the goal-oriented ones. Incontinence is rare. Pathologically induced movements are absent. A similar stupor can be seen with extreme psychomotor retardation in depression; patients with affective stupor still react with deepening of their depressive affect to emotional stimuli.

Catatonic stupor is associated with increase in muscle tone, catalepsy, stereotypies, "dead-pan" facial expression, and incontinence of urine.

The increase in muscle tone can lead to an odd facial expression, the so-called Schnauzkrampf where the mouth is protruded due to the increased tension of the oral muscles. When these patients lie down, their head is raised an inch above the pillow because their sternomastoid muscles contract. This has been termed the "psychological pillow." Patients interviewed after a catatonic stupor may describe the ordeal as a bad dream and report hallucinations and delusions. They usually admit that they could hear the ward personnel or visiting family members talking, and they remember how they were treated. One patient was asked why he did not answer any questions while catatonic. He replied, "because I was in a different dimension."

TABLE B.4

The G. H. Kent Intelligence Test
(Reprinted with permission from Williams and Wilkins, Copyright 1946, The Psychological Corp., New York, N.Y.)

Defective	0–18
Borderline	19–20
Dull Normal	21–23
Average	24–31
Bright Normal	32–33
Superior	34–35
Very Superior	36

	Credit	*Score*
1. What are houses made of? (any materials you can think of) 1 point for each item, up to 4.	1–4	___
2. What is sand used for? 4 points for manufacture of glass, 2 points for mixing with concrete, road building, or other constructive use, 1 point for playing or scrubbing. Credits not cumulative.	1, 2 or 4	___
3. If the flag floats to the south, from what direction is the wind? 3 points for north; no partial credits. It is permissible to say, "Which way is the wind coming from?"	3	___
4. Tell me the names of some fish. 1 point each, up to 4. If the subject stops with one, encourage him to go on.	1–4	___

5. At what time of the day is your shadow shortest? 3 points for noon. If correct response is suspected of being a guess, inquire why.   3 ____

6. Give the names of some large cities. 1 point for each, up to 4. When any state is named as a city, no credit for New York unless specified as New York City. No credit for hometown except when it is an outstanding city.   1–4 ____

7. Why does the moon look larger than the stars? Make it clear that the question refers to any particular star, and give assurance that the moon is actually smaller than any star. Encourage the subject to guess. 2 points for moon is lower down. 3 points for idea of nearer or closer. 4 points for generalized statement that nearer objects look larger than more distant objects.   2, 3 or 4 ____

8. What metal is attracted by a magnet? 4 points for iron, 2 for steel.   2 or 4 ____

9. If your shadow points to the northeast, where is the sun? 4 points for southwest, no partial credits.   4 ____

10. How many stripes in the U.S. flag? 2 points for thirteen. A subject who responds forty-eight may be permitted to correct his mistake. Explain, if necessary, that the white stripes are included as well as the red ones.   2 ____

TOTAL SCORE   ____

TABLE B.5
Mini-Mental State Examination
Reprinted with permission from *J. Psych. Res.* 1975, vol. 12, 189–98. Folstein, M. F., Folstein, S. E., and McHugh, P. R.: "Mini-Mental State." Pergamon Journals.

Maximum Score	*Item*	*Achieved Score*
(5)	What is the . . . (year) (season) (date) (day) (month)? Give *1 point* for each correct answer.	/____/
(5)	Where are we now? (county) (state) (city) (hospital) (floor) or (address) Give *1 point* for each correct answer.	/____/
(3)	Name three objects: *table, comb, tree.* One second to say each. Ask the patient to repeat them after you have said them. Give *1 point* for each correct answer on the *first* trial. Repeat the 3 words until the patient can say the three words. Number of trials: _____	/____/
(5)	Spell "world" backward. Give *1 point* for each correct letter in *dlrow.*	/____/
(3)	What are those three words I said to you? Do not give clues. Give *1 point* for each correct word.	/____/
(2)	Show the patient a pencil and watch and ask the patient to name them. Give *1 point* for each correct word.	/____/
(1)	Please say what I say: "No if's, and's, or but's." Give *1 point* if no error.	/____/
(3)	A 3-stage command: "Please listen. Take this paper (point) in your right hand; fold it in half and put it on the floor." Do not repeat. Give *1 point* for each correct act.	/____/
(1)	Show the patient the card with the sentence: *Close your eyes.* Ask the patient to read it and do what it said. Give *1 point* if the patient closes his eyes.	/____/
(1)	Say: Please write a sentence here (give the patient a pencil and piece of paper). Any sentence will do. Give *1 point* if a complete meaningful sentence is written.	/____/
(1)	Show the patient the card with a figure. Ask him to copy it. Give *1 point* if the drawing resembles the figure. Ignore small tremulous lines.	/____/
(30)	TOTAL SCORE	/____/____/

PERSONALITY DISORDER CRITERIA

Table C.1 lists thirty-six criteria which represent maladjustive behavior patterns (rows) characteristic for thirteen personality disorders (columns) of DMS-III-R. For the first nine patterns the opposites (listed in parentheses) are also used. Plus ($+$) and minus ($-$) signs in table C.1 indicate whether a particular pattern ($+$) or its opposite respectively ($-$) is a criterion for a given personality disorder. A blank indicates that under usual circumstances this pattern is not present, at least not in a domineering form.

Notice that the first nine patterns characterize personality disorders of all three clusters. These patterns are useful to decide whether a patient has a personality disorder or not. Patterns 10 to 14 are shared by personality disorders belonging to cluster A. Patterns 15 to 26 are specific for personality disorders in cluster B, and 27–33 for cluster C. Patterns 34–36 apply to the sadistic and self-defeating personality disorders.

The thirty-six criteria in table C.1 allow you to arrive at a personality profile. If this profile is consistent with one particular personality disorder, assign that diagnosis. It is left to your discretion to decide whether the presence of an unexpected pattern invalidates a single personality disorder diagnosis in favor of more than one.

For instance, ideas of reference (criterion 11), if present in a schizoid personality, do not invalidate this diagnosis, even though ideas of reference are not typical for a schizoid personality.

TABLE C.1
DSM-III-R Criteria for Thirteen Personality Disorders

DSM-III-R Criteria	Cluster A			Cluster B				Cluster C					
	SCD	PRD	SCT	HST	NRC	BDL	ANS	DPN	AVD	OC	PA	SA	SD
1. Isolated (attention seeking)	+	+	+	−	−	−	−	−	+				
2. Emotionally cold (exaggerated)	+	+	+	−	+	−	+			+			
3. Hypersensitive (indifferent) to criticism, praise	−		+						+			+	−
4. Self-centered (submissive)				+	+		+	−		+			
5. Grandiose (low self-esteem)					+			−	−				
6. Dependent				+				+					
7. Exploiting (altruistic)	−	−			+		+						
8. Pleasure-seeking (ignoring it)			−		+		+						
9. Feels entitled (undeserving)										−			
10. Suspicious		+	+										
11. Ideas of reference		+	+										
12. Magical thinking			+										
13. Illusions			+										
14. Odd speech			+										
15. Suicidal gestures				+		+	+						
16. Labile affect				+		+	+						
17. Impulsive				+		+	+						
18. Temper tantrums				+		+							
19. Nongenuine					+								
20. Fantasy of success													
21. Unstable relations						+							
22. Disturbed identity						+							

23. Empty, bored
24. Law-breaking
25. Lying
26. Stealing
27. Acceptance-craving
28. Preoccupied with details
29. Indecisive
30. Workaholic
31. Defiant
32. Procrastinating
33. Stubborn
34. Causes pain
35. Feels unappreciated
36. Pessimistic

Legend:

SCD = Schizoid
PRD = Paranoid
SCT = Schizotypal
HST = Histrionic
NRC = Narcissistic
BDL = Borderline
ANS = Antisocial
DPN = Dependent
AVD = Avoidant
OC = Obsessive Compulsive
PA = Passive Aggressive
SA = Sadistic
SD = Self-Defeating
+ = present
− = opposite criterion (given in parentheses) present

If the profile satisfies criteria for two or more personality disorders, make those diagnoses. If the profile fulfills some criteria of one or several personality disorders without satisfying all criteria of any one single personality disorder, make the diagnosis of personality disorder not otherwise specified (NOS).

Here is an example.

A patient complains that his boss is overdemanding and has no understanding for his job-related problems. He claims that he can only cope by skipping a day of work here and there to get enough rest, or by pretending that he has not received certain memos, or by promising work that he knows he cannot complete. This defiant behavior points to a passive aggressive personality disorder; but you may not have enough information to decide whether it is complimented by a generalized tendency to procrastinate and by stubbornness (criteria 32 and 33). Pursuit of these patterns will establish a profile qualifying for the diagnosis.

GLOSSARY

In principle, this glossary defines only those terms in the text that are not found in the DSM-III-R glossary. Where this glossary expands on a DSM-III-R definition it invites you to compare the two.

abreaction: Release of discharge of emotional tension by recalling or acting out a painful experience which had been repressed (see *catharsis*).

acalculia: Inability to do arithmetic operations, seen in parietal lobe lesions; acalculia is a type of aphasia.

activity level: The ability to make decisions, to initiate and complete actions, and feel satisfied. A variety of brain areas participate in this complex mastery: the reticular activating system contributes alertness; the limbic system regulates emotional tone and motivation; the dominant hemisphere provides various parts of memory and language functions; the frontal lobe directs control functions.

adjustment disorder: Consider an adjustment disorder when the chief complaint describes a *stressor* linked to a maladjusted response. An adjustment disorder has a clear-cut onset; it is caused by an identifiable, convincing stressor. It is short-lasting and self-limiting with complete recovery after the stressor ceases, i.e., pre- and postmorbid states are identical. Therefore, a diagnosis of "recurrent adjustment disorder" is a misnomer.

agraphia: A type of aphasia; inability to communicate in writing, usually attributed to cerebral disorders.

akathisia: A condition marked by motor restlessness, ranging from anxiety to inability to lie or sit quietly or to sleep, as seen in toxic reactions to neuroleptics. It is associated with pacing, foot tapping, and walking on the spot. *Tardive dyskinesia* is a neuroleptic-induced, so far mostly irreversible movement disorder. It presents with mouth smacking, rotating tongue movements, and flapping finger movements, and can progressively involve the trunk and limbs.

amnesia:

amnestic states: Occur as a result of toxic insults to the brain. They are either temporary or chronic states of anterograde amnesia.

anterograde amnesia: Refers to forgetting of events that follow a brain insult. The patient cannot store permanently new memory traces. He cannot learn new material; he is unable to recall what you have discussed with him a few minutes ago. If you repeat the same joke several times during the interview, the patient will repeatedly laugh at the punchline.

chronic, Alzheimer type: Depends on the degree of cortical involvement; patients suffer first recent and immediate memory loss; later they lose their remote memory. Relatives usually do not understand memory disturbances. They may quote as "good memory" the recollection of events in the patient's childhood.

chronic, Korsakoff type: Occurs when recent memory is disturbed, but immediate and remote memory are intact. Korsakoff patients may be able to lay down new memory traces, but are unable to retrieve them spontaneously. They can, however, recognize some of the material that they were exposed to.

impaired retrieval: Occurs in normal forgetting and in retrograde amnesia.

psychogenic: The patient claims inability to recall certain events or claims complete loss of memory. In spite of his claimed disability, he finds his way around, is able to learn new material and take care of himself. Inconsistencies in his memory failure can often be detected. Hypnosis and sodium amytal interview may lead to recovery. This type of memory disturbance is a pseudo-neurological symptom that occurs in somatization and conversion disorder and in multiple personality. Psychogenic amnesia has to be distinguished from simulation.

retrograde: The patient has forgotten events prior to a brain insult. Psychiatrists encounter that state for instance in patients treated with electroconvulsive therapy.

simulated: The sociopath or the patient with factitious disorder may simulate amnesia to win compensation. This patient knows that he is simulating. He is usually suspicious and hostile when he feels that you as interviewer make attempts to retrieve the lost memory. Hypnosis and sodium amytal are not helpful in this situation.

anniversary reaction: Symptoms or disturbed behavior that occur on an anniversary of a significant experience in the patient's life (often a loss).

aphasia: Impairment of the ability to communicate through speech, writing, or signs, due to dysfunction of brain centers. It is considered global when both sensory and motor functions are involved.

apraxia: 1. Inability to perform purposeful movements without sensory or motor impairment or 2. Inability to properly use objects.

attention: This is the ability to focus on one subject or activity. It requires the interaction of the ascending reticular activating system which regulates alertness, the frontal lobes which regulate voluntary focusing, and the limbic system which adds emotional value to the focus of attention.

body type (Kretschmer 1925; Sheldon and Stevens 1942):
    dysplastic: Generally obese with abundance of fat tissue on the torso and the limbs.
    ectomorphic: Body type characterized by the predominance of the structures developed from the ectodermal layer of the embryo: slender, thin, with relatively long limbs—thought to be associated with schizophrenia.
    endomorphic: Body type developed from the endodermal layers, pyknic type—thought to be associated with manic-depressive disorder.
    mesomorphic: Type of body build in which tissues derived from the mesoderm, athletic type, predominate.
    pyknic: Fat body with protrusion of the abdomen.

catalepsy: A condition seen in psychotic patients who show generalized diminished responsiveness usually associated with a trancelike state and a prolonged maintenance of postures (see *waxy flexibility*).

catharsis: A technique of freeing the mind by having a person recall a traumatic event or experience. This technique was used by Freud initially in his psychotherapy. Catharsis is the method used to bring about *abreaction*.

coma: Loss of consciousness and responsiveness to outside stimuli.

concentration: This is the ability to maintain attention to outside stimuli as well as to mental operations such as puzzle solving and calculations. The ascending reticular activating system which regulates alertness, the frontal lobe which regulates voluntary focusing, and the limbic system which adds emotional value participate in this function.

congruency: Refers to the relationship between the content of hallucinations or delusions and the patient's prevailing mood. For example, if the mood is depressed, voices that belittle the patient, accuse or scold him are congruent with his mood; so are delusions of chronic illness, destruction, unforgivable sin, and eternal guilt. In contrast, command hallucinations or ideas of thought insertion, of being controlled by outside forces, or of living by somebody else's will do not reflect a depressive mood—they are mood incongruent.

Related to congruency of mood is the phase relationship between presence of hallucinations or delusions and abnormal mood. If hallucinations and delusions only occur when the mood is clearly disturbed, then they are in phase; otherwise, they are out of phase. This phase relationship applies only to patients with a clear-cut episodic mood disturbance.

consciousness: A state of subjective awareness and appropriate responsiveness to external stimuli. It is controlled by the ascending activating system which originates in the reticular formation of the brain stem and extends to the cortex via the diffuse or nonspecific thalamic projection system. A lack of alertness points to involvement of subcortical centers. Isolated cortical damage does not lead to loss of alertness. (For details, see Strub and Black 1977).

delusion: (Compare DSM-III-R glossary.) A fixed false belief firmly held despite obvious contradictive evidence. This belief is not ordinarily shared by others. Empirical evidence or logical arguments cannot change the patient's conviction. These ideas do not withstand reality testing. Fixed false ideas are also called apophanous phenomena, a term introduced by Conrad.

　congruency: Refers to the relationship between the content of a delusion and the patient's prevailing mood (see *congruency*).

　primary delusions (apophany): Experiences not deducted from other events. They take three forms: delusional mood, delusional perception, and sudden delusional (autochthonous) ideas. Delusional mood refers to the patient's feeling that he is in danger, or persecuted, or that something is brewing at work, that people are talking about him and avoid talking to him.

Delusional perception is based on a real perception to which the patient assigns a new meaning: A patient gets up during group therapy and explains that suddenly he understands communication among people. He explains that he saw a girl at a party putting her hands on her waist, spreading her index and middle finger thus forming an inversed letter V. This meant that she wanted to make love to him. He also explained other signs: touching an earlobe means she does not want to get involved. He explained that suddenly he understands this language and can respond to it.

The primary delusional (autochthonous) idea refers to the sudden occurrence of a fully formed delusion. A patient claimed that he was looking at his fingernails and detected white spots in them. All of a sudden he understood that he was supposed to enter the race for mayor and that he should choose his sister-in-law for advisor.

Distinguish a delusional idea from delusional misinterpretations in which the perception may have a logical place within the delusional system. For instance, a patient talks to her ex-husband on the phone and hears a cracking noise in the line. She concludes that he must be making a recording to prove that she is an unfit mother.

secondary delusions arise from other morbid experiences; for instance, from disturbed mood or hallucinations: a patient hallucinated that she hears the voices of her family over a long distance. They tell her that she looks like an ape. She concludes that her family wants her to be an animal, so her husband can be free and can control her. In this example, the origin of the delusion is a hallucination which is elaborated and extended by the delusion.

denial: A defense mechanism where the patient refuses to acknowledge the presence or existence of some external reality that is apparent to others.

dysgeusia: Impairment or perversion of the sense of taste. Patients with depression often report that meat has a strawlike, repugnant taste.

dyslexia: A condition in a person with normal vision and normal intelligence who is unable to interpret written language.

ego-dystonic: Denotes any thought content or impulse that the person experiences as not his own and not under his voluntary control and repugnant to or inconsistent with his conception of himself (its opposite is ego-syntonic).

ego-syntonic: Denotes ideas or impulses that are acceptable to and compatible with the ego. The person experiences them as his own and under his control.

euphoria: Morbid or abnormal sense of physical and emotional well-being.

euthymia: Joyfulness or mental tranquility.

excitement: A paroxysmal increase in motor activity. It may occur in the same disorders that are associated with stupor, namely catatonia, paranoid schizophrenia, and affective disorder.

>   **manic excitement:** The patient displays hostile or euphoric affect; shows flight of ideas and increase of goal-oriented and expressive movements.

>   **paranoid excitement:** Patients with paranoid schizophrenia who experience an increase in intensity of phonemes (hallucinations of conversing voices) may react with excitement.

>   **psychogenic excitement:** Sometimes seen in sociopathic patients who may become wildly aggressive when stressed, trapped, or embarrassed. Sometimes this behavior is expressed by destruction or self-mutilation. It has often an attention-seeking quality.

folie à deux: Occurrence of a similar behavioral disturbance in two closely associated persons occurring at the same time.

fright: Extreme sudden fear.

Gerstmann syndrome: Joseph Gerstmann (1888–1969), American neurologist, described a symptom complex: it consists of finger agnosia, right-left disorientation, aculculia, and agraphia. Additional features may be present: constructive apraxia, word finding difficulties, disturbed ability to read, impaired color perception, absence of optokinetic nystagmus, and disturbance of equilibrium.

Gjessing's periodic catatonia: Gjessing has shown in systematically controlled investigations that motor functions, ideation, and perception in periodic catatonia are closely correlated with changing levels of positive or negative nitrogen balance. Stuperous or excited catatonic states change periodically in these patients but can be arrested by continuous administration of thyroxine (Gjessing 1947, 1953a, 1953b; Gjessing and Gjessing 1961).

hallucination: (Compare DSM-III-R glossary.) A sensory perception without an exterior stimulus occurring during wakefulness. A hallucination is different from a dream which also contains perceptions without exterior stimuli but occurs during sleep. Hallucinations can affect all senses. There are auditory, visual, olfactory, gustatory, haptic (tactile), and vestibular hallucinations. Even hallucinations of pain may occur. The most common type of hallucination in a psychiatric population is auditory, followed by visual and haptic hallucinations. Hallucinations may occur in a subjective rather than in an objective space, such as voices may be heard in one's mind rather than outside the head. This is seen in both, schizophrenia and affective disorder.

auditory: Such hallucinations are also called phonemes. Patients with functional psychosis report three types of phonemes: 1. voices that give the patient orders (command hallucinations) which he may follow or resist; 2. voices which comment on, criticize, or praise the patient's actions and repeat his thoughts; 3. thoughts that become audible (the technical term is a German word, *Gedankenlautwerden,* which can best be translated as *thought echo.* These three types of phonemes, listed by Kurt Schneider (1959) as so-called first-rank symptoms, were thought to be pathognomonic for schizophrenia. However, the specificity of these hallucinations has not been verified by clinical studies—manic patients also experience first-rank symptoms.

complexity: Hallucinations vary from simple to complex. An example for simple hallucinations are noises, light flashes, sudden unpleasant smells or tastes (elementary hallucinations); they often occur in organic mental disorders, less often in schizophrenia; they may precede seizures, especially temporal lobe seizures, and migraine headache attacks (classic). Hallucinations can be *complex* and *organized,* such as music, intelligible voices and conversations, or dramatic scenes.

congruency of hallucinations: see *congruency.*

dysmegalopsia: The objects in visual hallucinations may occupy more space and appear larger *(macropsia)* or smaller *(micropsia)* than in reality. Both experiences are called dysmegalopsia.

functional: Some patients, especially chronic schizophrenics, hear voices only when some other noise is present like the fan of an air conditioner or a running car engine. They hear both, the noise and the voices which are not distorted, but clearly separated from the background noise. They are not illusions.

gustatory: Hallucinations of taste are often reported by schizophrenics with persecutory delusions whose food tastes drugged to them as if somebody slipped something into it (see *dysgeusia*).

haptic: Perceptions of touch. They are more common in organic mental disorders. An example is the sensation that insects are crawling over the patient's skin as reported in delirium tremens due to alcohol and sedative withdrawal. This sensation may occur isolated from a visual perception and is then called formication.

hypnagogic: Visual and auditory hallucinations that are associated with sleep onset REM periods. Dreamlike phenomena occur prior to sleep. These experiences are reported by patients with narcolepsy.

hypnopompic: Occurs at the end of sleep (see *hypnagogic*). They are associated with REM sleep but persist after cessation of dream sleep.

mood congruency: See *congruency*.

olfactory: Hallucinations of smell can precede seizures, especially temporal lobe seizures; they are described as elementary hallucinations of short duration, usually of unpleasant quality, like burned rubber and they may not always be followed by a full seizure. Patients with persecutory delusions suffering from either schizophrenia or organic mental disorder may report a strange smell such as of gas penetrating the house. Some patients report that they emit a foul smelling body odor originating from their sexual organs. This may occur as a monosymptomatic hallucination. These monosymptomatic, chronic, olfactory hallucinations are often resistant to treatment with phenothiazines, tricyclics, sedatives, MAO inhibitors, carbamazepine, phenytoin, ECT, and combinations thereof. Some may respond to neuroleptics which are also calcium channel blockers.

pain: Schizophrenics report hallucinations of pain, such as some force tearing flesh off their bones. They also report the sensation that an animal such as a snake is eating them alive from inside their bodies. Distinguish this hallucination from a delusion. The sensation of actual pain is absent in the latter.

space and time distribution: Hallucinations may occur outside the usual sensory space. A patient may see a person exactly behind him where he normally could not see him, or the patient can hear two people conversing over hundreds of miles (without telephones). These hallucinations have been called extracampine.

vestibular: Visual images affected by vestibular stimulation, often seen in alcoholic hallucinations. "Under vestibular irritation, these images show changes such as occur when the subject is submitted to passive rotating movements" (Campbell 1981).

visual: These hallucinations may occur isolated or combined with auditory ones. They are more frequently encountered in acute organic mental disorder in combination with clouding of consciousness. A special form is the vision of small crawling animals (insects, mice, or rats), either seen on the floor, or on the patient's skin. This perception seems to be common in delirium due to withdrawal from sedative hypnotics or alcohol.

impulsive actions: Goal-directed behaviors with an abnormal goal due to a deficit of insight and/or judgment.

insight: Refers to the patient's knowledge that the symptoms of his disorder are abnormal and morbid; for instance, a patient has insight when he realizes that his hallucinations or delusions are incompatible with reality and therefore a product of an illness. He has no insight when he assigns reality to them and claims, for instance, that only he has the ability to perceive them because of his special powers.

irritability: Hypersensitivity and hyperreactivity to outside stimuli.

mannerism: A peculiar modification or exaggeration in movements, speech, writing, or dressing.

memory: The ability to recall images of past events, experiences, facts, and impressions. It is usually subdivided into:
    immediate or short-term memory: Recall of events from the last few seconds.
    recent: Recall of events from the last few months and days up to the last few minutes.
    remote: Recall of impressions from childhood and years ago.
    These three types of memory correspond to different brain functions needed to reproduce them: the language cortex is essential for immediate recall, limbic structures for recent memory, and the association cortex for remote memory.

mental status: Cross-sectional aspect of psychological and higher cortical functioning, as opposed to the patient's history which reflects the longitudinal view of his psychiatric problems. The time frame of the mental status examination is the duration of the interview, whereas that of the psychiatric history is the patient's life. The history reflects the subjective experiences reported by the patient, the mental status includes the objective signs and behaviors observed by the interviewer who sees and hears pathology and witnesses the patient in action. The patient's history reflects the recurrent and stable features of mental functioning, the mental status the ever-changing here and now. Often, interviewers include phenomena such as hallucinations and delusions in their mental status examination, even if they do not occur during the interview but during the last 24 hours.

mood: The feeling of pleasure or displeasure by which a person experiences himself, the outside world, and his reactions to both. Mood has to be distinguished from affect. Whereas affect is the external manifestation of emotion observable by the interviewer, mood is the subjectively experienced background emotion that is not written on face and body but that has to be asked for.

reactivity: Refers to mood changes due to external events. The term applies to a depressed mood that normalizes as a result of favorable experiences.

movements:

athetotic: Slow, coarse, and wormlike writhing, involuntary movements of the extremities; they are more pronounced in the distal than in the proximal part of a limb.

choreic or choreatic: Rapid, abrupt jerking, involuntary movements which resemble parts of expressive and reactive movements.

expressive: They project the patient's emotions in facial expressions, gestures, and posture.

goal-oriented: Necessary to accomplish all physical tasks and purposeful actions.

myoclonic: Sudden muscular contractions restricted to one area of the body.

reactive: They occur in response to unexpected tactile, visual, or auditory stimuli. The responder startles and flinches, and automatically turns his head toward the stimulus.

spontaneous: They include nose and hand rubbing, ear lobe pulling, mouth covering, throat clearing, blinking, swallowing, foot tapping, pacing, nail biting, finger picking, grimacing, and stereotyped movements.

stereotyped: They are carried out in a uniform way. They may resemble goal-oriented or expressive movements; for instance, grimacing is a stereotyped movement of the facial muscles.

multiple personality: According to DSM-III-R, "the essential feature . . . is the existence within the person of two or more distinct personalities or personality states."

mutism: Absence of speech.

akinetic mutism: The patient is mute and immobile but his eyes follow people around and can be diverted by sound. A painful stimulus sometimes evokes a reflex or weak movements but no manifestation of pain or emotion. Akinetic mutism is presumably due to incomplete interruption of the reticular activating system.

myoclonus: See movements.

omega sign: Eyebrows drawn together with medial ends raised obliquely producing vertical and horizontal furrows on the mid-forehead.

orientation: Refers to the patient's ability to identify himself (orientation to person), to know where he is (county, state, city, address, hospital, room number—orientation to place), and to know the time (year, day of month, time of day—orientation to time).

paraphasia or paraphrasia: Disorder characterized by incoherent speech.

perplexity: A sign observed most commonly in organic mental disorders. The patient shows disturbance in grasping a situation, in association, in memory, attention, and will.

phonemes: See *hallucinations, auditory.*

posture: Maintenance of muscle tone against gravity.
    catalepsy: The patient maintains an abnormal posture for minutes or hours. To diagnose waxy flexibility or catalepsy the patient has to be instructed to resume a resting position after his limbs have been passively moved, but he fails to do so.
    posturing: The patient holds his body in a strange position.
    waxy flexibility: The patient offers some plastic resistance to movements imposed by the examiner, and maintains the final posture for some time.

pseudohallucinations: The term has several meanings. Hallucinations may be perceived in a subjective rather than in an objective space: "It is a voice in my mind," rather than "I hear the voice like I hear your voice." The patient may deny that his perception has the same quality as a real perception. He may feel that he has control over it, can make it appear and disappear, or he has insight and can identify it as a hallucination.

pseudoseizure: A clinical event which superficially resembles an epileptic attack but lacks essential epileptic components, such as electroencephalic changes, or has a feature incompatible with epilepsy, such as being induced or stopped by a simple command or a hypnotic suggestion. Such patients often claim they can hear and see what is going on in their environment but they cannot respond.

simulation: Pretense of having a disease, or a symptom.

speech: The mechanical forming of words by the muscular apparatus of the mouth, tongue, diaphragm, and vocal cords, and by the central directing and organizing functions of the speech centers in the dominant hemisphere of the brain.
    concept of words: The way words are used, correctly if they are used in the conventional manner and with the right level of abstraction.

flow: The continuity of verbal production.

mumbled: Hesitant speech with low intensity, poor articulation, and unnatural pauses and slowing (Huntington's chorea).

paraphasic: Speech in which the patient substitutes the correct word with a wrong word. This wrong word may be invented; for example, "I write a letter with my cryston" (neologistic paraphasia). The wrong word may be correct semantically but not logically; for example, "I write a letter with my car" (semantic paraphasia). The wrong word may show the substitution of only one otherwise correct letter; for example, "I write a letter with my nen" (literal paraphasia).

pressure of speech: The patient has the urge to continue talking; he cannot be interrupted.

push of speech: No pauses exist among words and sentences. Words are incomplete and flow into each other and a great deal is said in a short period of time. The patient can be interrupted.

retarded: Slow, with many pauses.

scanning: Vowels and sounding consonants *(m,n)* are stretched. Speech is slow with sliding cadence (multiple sclerosis).

staccato: The opposite of scanning speech—consists of words that are clipped and abruptly presented (psychomotor epilepsy).

stressor: A stressor is a stimulus that taxes the patient's ability to respond. Be aware of the circularity: a stressor is what causes an intense reaction; an intense reaction identifies a stressor. DSM-III-R defines both type of stressor and levels of severity. It lists eleven areas in which psychosocial stressors can occur (see DSM-III-R).

Holmes and Rahe (1967; Gundersen and Rahe 1974) have provided lists of psychosocial stressors ranked by their severity. DSM-III-R lists seven levels, unfortunately defined by examples and not by general principles.

DSM-III-R classifies stressors also as acute (lasting less than six months), or chronic (lasting more than six months), justified by the fact that children develop adjustment reactions to chronic, but rarely to acute events.

A stressor may be related to a psychiatric disorder in six different ways: as (1) time marker, (2) magnifier, (3) consequence, (4) pathological thought content, (5) trigger, or (6) cause of a dysfunction.

(1) Stressor as time marker
The patient considers a life event as the "cause" of his disorder, but reveals that the event merely occurred at the same time, often after the onset of the disorder.

(2) Stressor as magnifier

The stressor is part of the patient's routine life but suddenly he is unable to deal with it. The stressor reveals and magnifies the patient's dysfunction. For instance, a patient who could previously take over the responsibilities of a vacationing colleague, cannot do so when depressed. He may blame the increased workload as the cause of his depression, rather than the depression as a cause for his inability to cope.

(3) Stressor as consequence

Divorce or job loss reported as the precipitating event of a mental disorder are in fact its result. Analysis of the sequence of events reveals, for instance, that the disorder preceded the event. The irritability, social withdrawal, and decreased sex drive associated with depression did result in marital discord, or divorce rather than the divorce resulting in depression.

(4) Stressor as pathological thought content

During a depressive episode some patients who experience guilt feelings screen their past for reasons to feel bad. Sometimes these reasons are quite delusional in character. For instance:

"When I was five years old, I stole a stamp. Now people found out and I have to suffer the consequences. That makes me depressed."

Others may talk about recent bad news that pulls them down. Recognize these reasons as a secondary filling, i.e., the fitting of a content to the pessimistic outlook typical for depression.

(5) Stressor as trigger

A stressor may be a trigger of a psychiatric disorder if the patient has a predisposition for the psychiatric disorder. Females may report the onset of a depressive episode after childbirth or during the onset of menopause. However, the literature is controversial with respect to such a trigger function of a stressor.

(6) Stressor as cause

According to DSM-III-R, two types of disorders are caused by stressors: Posttraumatic stress disorder and adjustment disorder. Posttraumatic stress disorder requires extraordinary stressors like earthquakes, floods, war, rape, or atrocities. An adjustment disorder may be caused by a more common stressor such as physical illness, job loss, or loss of support. If you encounter such a stressor, examine the patient's response. For symptoms and signs of both disorders, see DSM-III-R.

It is unknown what makes these stressors pathogenic for some people but not for others. It is also not clear what makes them more noxious at one but not at another time. Before you accept a stressor as sufficient cause of an adjustment disorder, exclude alternate possiblities.

stupor: 1. Level of alertness: The patient appears unconscious and responds to pain only with some defensive movements or utterances. This is usually due to interruption of the impulses from the reticular activating system of the pons and midbrain to the cortex.

2. Special psychiatric condition: psychogenic stupor occurs as a fright reaction. The patient appears motionless and mute, but is alert without incontinence of urine or feces. Hypnosis or sodium amytal will interrupt this state.

3. In stupor with an organic basis, such as akinetic mutism, space occupying lesions of the third ventricle, the thalamus, or the midbrain can be found. These patients appear alert, react slightly to pain, but are unable to talk or follow commands. Patients usually have complete amnesia for this state if they recover. Some stuporous states are associated with repeated bursts of discharges in the EEG similar to grand mal seizures, or spike and wave charges. In Gjessing's periodic catatonia, slow waves in the EEG have been described.

catatonic stupor: The patient is mute, has increased muscle tension especially in the anterior neck muscles, masseters, and the muscles around the mouth, giving rise to the so-called snout spasm. The patient does not respond to painful stimuli or anesthesia, is incontinent of urine and may show catalepsy. The patient is usually alert. Sodium amytal injections may break the muteness, as does ECT.

depressive stupor: The patient may appear confused, perplexed, and bewildered. There is usually no obstruction, opposition, catalepsy, or increase in muscle tension. The patient is alert, but appears depressed. There is no incontinence of urine or feces; response to emotional stimuli is present. Most stuporous patients should have an EEG and lumbar puncture to rule out organic causes.

suggestibility: A condition in which a person responds readily to suggestions or opinions of others to the point of uncritical acceptance.

tic: Paroxysmal involuntary twitching of small muscle groups; tics may resemble a defensive reflex or an expressive movement.

thinking:
abstract thinking: The ability to use symbols such as "dog" and to generalize to a class of symbols such as "a dog is a four-legged barking animal."

concrete thinking: The inability to abstract.

thought blocking: Sudden involuntary cessation in the train of thought.

torpor: Abnormal inactivity, dormancy, numbness, apathy.

transference: The unconscious shifting of an affect and behavior pattern from one person to another; especially the transfer of the patient's emotion originally directed toward parental figures to the therapist as a result of unconscious identification.

tremor: Rapid alternation of contraction of antagonistic muscle groups of the eyelids, tongue, lips, head, upper trunk, extremities, and hands. Tremors can be classified by their frequency, amplitude, regularity, and relationship to volitional movements. The latter criterion is customarily used in most descriptions: Static or resting tremor occurs when a limb is in repose. It shows 3–7 beats per second and is suppressed temporarily with voluntary movements. Therefore it does not interfere much with voluntary motor acts such as writing.

> action tremor: Occurs when the limb is voluntarily maintained in a certain position. It disappears when the limb is relaxed. Normal people have very fine action tremor. It is 6 cps in children, and 10 cps in adults.
>
> hepatic flapping tremor: A special form of an action tremor. It is best demonstrated when the patient's hands are held in front of the body and sharply dorsiflexed, with the fingers maximally spread apart. Periodically, the hands will fall due to gravity. Voluntary attempts to bring them back into position leads to bursts of rapid arrhythmic flexion and extension movements (aristixis).
>
> intention tremor: A tremor that occurs with movements. It often increases near the end of the completion of the movement. If a patient is asked to touch the examiner's finger, the patient's finger may oscillate more and more the closer it comes to the goal.

undoing: One of the defense mechanisms consisting of a symbolic action that negates certain thoughts or acts.

Verhältnisblödsinn: Discordance between ambition and comprehension, between desire and capabilities. Many patients with Verhältnisblödsinn continuously start new businesses, persuade others with false arguments to invest money into their ventures, and then lose financial control, fail everywhere, and involve others in their downfall. Some patients obtain large grants or scholarships to presumably develop artistic talents that they don't have. The intelligence of patients with Verhältnisblödsinn suffices for a modest social level; however, such patients maneuver themselves into positions that they can't fill. Many of these patients have confused thinking (translated from Bleuler 1972, p. 585).

vigilance: The ability to sustain attention to an outward stimulus over some arbitrary time period.

waxy flexibility: Often seen in *catalepsy* (see above) permitting the limbs to be molded into positions in which they persist.

REFERENCES

Adler, A. 1964. *Problems of neurosis*. New York: Harper & Row.

Akiskal, H. S., and Webb, W. L., eds. 1978. *Psychiatric diagnosis: Exploration of biological predictors*. SP Medical and Scientific Books. New York and London: Spectrum.

American Psychiatric Association. 1968. *Diagnostic and statistical manual of mental disorders*, 2d ed. (DSM-II). Washington, D.C.: American Psychiatric Association.

American Psychiatric Association. 1981. *Diagnostic and statistical manual of mental disorders*, 3d ed. (DSM-III). Washington, D.C.: American Psychiatric Association.

American Psychiatric Association. 1985. Draft, DSM-III-R in development. Work group to revise DSM-III. Washington, D.C.: American Psychiatric Association, 10-5-85.

American Psychiatric Association. 1987. *Diagnostic and statistical manual of mental disorders*, 3d ed., revised (DSM-III-R). Washington, D.C.: American Psychiatric Association.

Anderson, S. C. 1968. Effects of confrontation by high- and low-functioning therapists. *J. of Counseling Psychology* 15:411–16.

Baker, A. B., and Joynt, R. J., eds. 1985. *Clinical neurology*, vol. 1, 2, revised ed. Philadelphia: Harper & Row.

Barrett, J., Hurst, M. W., and Discala, C. et al. 1978. Prevalence of depression over a 12-month period in a nonpatient population. *Arch. Gen. Psychiat.* 35:741–44.

Berne, E. 1964. *Games people play*. New York: Grove Press.

———. 1961. *Transactional analysis in psychotherapy*. New York: Grove Press.

Bierman, R. 1969. Dimensions of interpersonal facilitation in psychotherapy and child development. *Psychological Bulletin* 72:338–52.

Bleuler, E. 1972. *Lehrbuch der Psychiatrie*. Zwölfte Auflage neubearbeitet von M. Bleuler. Berlin: Springer Verlag.

Cameron, N. 1964. Experimental analysis of schizophrenic thinking. In *Language and thought in schizophrenia,* ed. J. S. Kasanin, pp. 50–64. New York: W. W. Norton.

————. 1963. *Personality development and psychopathology: A dynamic approach.* Boston: Houghton Mifflin.

Cameron-Bandler, L. 1978. *They lived happily ever after.* Cupertino, Calif.: Meta Publications.

Campbell, R. J. 1981. *Psychiatric dictionary,* 5th ed. New York: Oxford University Press.

Chapman, J., and McGhie, A. 1964. Echopraxia in schizophrenia. *Brit. J. Psychiat.* 110:365.

Confucius. 1955. *The sayings of Confucius.* Translated by J. R. Ware. New York: New American Library, Mentor Books.

Cox, A., Hopkinson, K., and Rutter, M. 1981. Psychiatric interviewing techniques II. Naturalistic study: eliciting factual information. *Brit. J. Psychiat.* 138:283–91.

Critchley, M. 1953. *The parietal lobes.* New York: Hafner Press.

DeBetz, B., and Sunnen, G. 1985. *A primer of clinical hypnosis.* Littleton, Mass.: PSG Publishing.

Dubois, P. 1913. *The psychological origin of mental disorders.* New York: Funk and Wagnalls.

Ekman, P. 1983. Autonomic nervous system activity distinguishes among emotions. *Science* Sep. 16. 221 (4616): 1208–10.

Erikson, E. 1969. *Identity: Youth and crisis.* New York: W. W. Norton.

Fenichel, O. 1945. *The psychoanalytic theory of neurosis.* New York: W. W. Norton.

Fish, F. 1967. *Clinical psychopathology.* Bristol: John Wright.

Folstein, M. F., Folstein, S. E., and McHugh, P. R. 1975. Mini-mental state. *J. Psych. Res.* 12:189–98.

Foulds, G. A. 1976. *The hierarchical nature of personal illness.* New York: Academic Press.

Freedman, A. M., Kaplan, H. E., and Sadock, B. J. 1975. *Comprehensive textbook of psychiatry,* vols. 1, 2, 2d ed. Baltimore: Williams and Wilkins.

Freud, A. 1946. *The ego and the mechanisms of defense.* Translated by C. Baines. New York: International Universities Press.

Freud, S. 1952–1955. *Gesammelte Werke chronologisch geordnet,* Bd. 1–17. London: Imago Publishing.

Frosch, J. P., ed. 1983. *Current perspectives on personality disorders.* Washington, D.C.: American Psychiatric Press.

Gauron, E. F., and Dickinson, J. K. 1966. Diagnostic decision making in psychiatry: I. Information usage. *Arch. Gen. Psychiat.* 14:225–32.

————. 1966. Diagnostic decision making in psychiatry: II. Diagnostic styles. *Arch. Gen. Psychiat.* 14:233–37.

Gedo, M. M. 1980. *Picasso: Art as autobiography.* Chicago: University of Chicago Press.

Gjessing, R. 1947. Biological investigations in endogenous psychoses. *Acta Scand.* 47 (Suppl.):93.

———. 1953a. Beiträge zur Somatologie der periodischen Katatonie. Mitteilung VII. *Arch. Psychiatr. Nervenkr.* 191:247.

———. 1953b. Beiträge zur Somatologie der periodischen Katatonie. Mitteilung VIII. *Arch. Psychiatr. Nervenkr.* 191:297.

Gjessing, R., and Gjessing, L. 1961. Some main trends in the clinical aspects of periodic catatonia. *Acta Scand.* 37:1.

Goldstein, K. 1964. Methodological approach to the study of schizophrenic thought disorder. In *Language and thought in schizophrenia,* ed. J. S. Kasanin. New York: W. W. Norton.

Goodwin, D. W., and Guze, S. B. 1984. *Psychiatric diagnosis,* 3d ed. Oxford: Oxford University Press.

Goodwin, D. W., Othmer, E., Halikas, J., and Freemon, F. R. 1970. Loss of short-term memory: Predictor of the alcoholic "black-out." *Nature* 227:201–2.

Griesinger, W. 1882. Mental pathology and therapeutics. Translated by C. Lockhart Robertson and J. Rutherford. New York: William Wood and Co.

Gunderson, J. G. 1984. *Borderline personality disorder.* Washington, D.C.: American Psychiatric Press.

Gunderson, E. K., and Rahe, R. H., eds. 1974. *Life stress and illness.* Springfield, Ill. Charles C. Thomas.

Hall, R. C. W., ed. 1980. *Psychiatric presentations of medical illness.* New York and London: Spectrum.

Heller, K., Davis, J., and Myers, R. A. 1966. The effects of interviewer style in a standardized interview. *J. of Consulting Psychology* 30:501–8.

Helzer, J. E., Clayton, P. J., Pambakian, R., Reich, T., Woodruff, R. A., and Reveley, M. A. 1977. Reliability of psychiatric diagnosis: II. The test/retest reliability of diagnostic classification. *Arch. Gen. Psychiatr.* 34:136–41.

Hersen, M., and Turner, S. M. 1985. *Diagnostic interviewing.* New York and London: Plenum Press.

Hinsie, L. E. 1937. *Concepts and problems of psychotherapy.* New York: Columbia University Press.

Holmes, T. H., and Rahe, R. H. 1967. The social readustment rating scale. *J. Psychosom. Res.* 11:213–18.

Hopkinson, K., Cox, A., and Rutter, M. 1981. Psychiatric interviewing techniques III. Naturalistic study: eliciting feelings. *Brit. J. Psychiat.* 138:406–15.

Horney, K. 1939. *New ways in psychoanalysis.* New York: W. W. Norton.

Horowitz, M., Marmar, C., Krupnick, J., Wilner, N., Kaltreider, N., and Wallerstein, R. 1984. *Personality styles and brief psychotherapy.* New York: Basic Books.

Isaacson, R. L. 1982. *The limbic system,* 2d ed. New York and London: Plenum Press.

Izard, C. 1977. *Human emotions.* New York: Plenum Press.

————. 1979. Emotions in personality and psychopathology. New York: Plenum Press.

Izard, C. E., Ekman, P., Levenson, R. W., and Friesen, W. V. 1983. Autonomic nervous system activity distinguishes among emotions. *Science.* 221:1208–1210.

Jaspers, K. 1962. *Allgemeine Psychopathologie,* 7th ed. Translated by J. Hoening and M. W. Hamilton. Manchester and New York: Manchester University Press. (Originally published 1959.)

————. 1963. *General psychopathology.* Chicago: University of Chicago Press.

Jung, C. G. 1971. *Psychological types.* Princeton: Princeton University Press.

Kaplan, H. E., and Sadock, B. J. 1985. *Comprehensive textbook of psychiatry,* 4th ed. Baltimore: Williams and Wilkins.

Kasanin, J. S., ed. 1964. *Language and thought in schizophrenia.* New York: W. W. Norton.

Kent, G. H. 1946. *E-G-Y scales, 1946.* New York: Williams and Wilkins, The Psychological Corporation.

Klein, M. 1952. The origins of transference. *Int. J. Psychoanal.* 33:433.

Kleist, K. 1928. Über zykloide, paranoide und epileptoide Psychosen und über die Frage der Degenerationspsychosen (On cycloid, paranoid and epileptic psychoses and on the question of degenerative psychoses). *Schweiz. Arch. Neurol. Psychiat.* 23:3–37.

Koenigsberg, H. W., Kaplan, R. D., Gilmore, M. M., and Cooper, A. M. 1985. The relationship between syndrome and personality disorder in DSM-III: Experience with 2,462 patients. *Am. J. Psychiat.* 142:2, Feb.: 207–12.

Kraepelin, E. 1968. *Lectures on clinical psychiatry,* revised ed. Edited by T. Johnstone. New York: Hafner Publ. Co.

Kretschmer, E. 1925. *Physique and character: An investigation of the nature of constitution and the theory of temperament.* Translated from the second revised and enlarged edition by W. J. H. Sprott. New York: Harcourt, Brace.

Leon, R. L. 1982. *Psychiatric interviewing: A primer.* New York: Elsevier/North Holland.

Leonhard, K. 1979. *The classification of endogenous psychoses,* 5th ed. Edited by E. Robins, translated by R. Berman. Irvington, N.Y.: Halstead Press, Div. of John Wiley.

Lion, J. R. 1981. *Personality disorders: Diagnosis and management (revised for DSM-III),* 2d ed. Baltimore: William and Wilkins.

Ludwig, A. M. 1985. *Principles of clinical psychiatry,* revised and expanded 2d ed. New York: The Free Press.

Ludwig, A. M., and Othmer, E. 1977. The medical basis of psychiatry. *Am. J. Psychiat.* 134:1087–92.

Luria, A. R. 1966. *Higher cortical function in man.* New York: Basic Books.

MacKinnon, R. A., and Michels, R. 1971. *The psychiatric interview in clinical practice.* Philadelphia: W. B. Saunders.

MacKinnon, R. A., and Yudofsky, S. C. 1986. *The psychiatric evaluation in clinical practice.* Philadelphia: J. B. Lippincott.

Mahrer, A. R., ed. 1970. *New approaches to personality classification.* New York and London: Columbia University Press.

Marquis, K. H., Marshall, J., and Oskamp, S. 1972. Testimony validity as a function of question form, atmosphere, and item difficulty. *J. of Applied Social Psychology* 2:167–86.

Masserman, J. H. 1955. *Practice of dynamic psychiatry.* Philadelphia: W. B. Saunders.

Mellor, C. S. 1970. First rank symptoms of schizophrenia. *Brit. J. Psychiat.* 117:15–23.

Mendel, D. B. 1964. On therapist-watching. *Psychiatry* 27:59–68.

Menninger, K. A. 1958. *A theory of psychoanalytical technique.* New York: Basic Books.

Meyer, A. 1957. *Psychobiology: A science of man.* Springfield, Ill.: Charles C. Thomas.

Millon, T. 1981. *Disorders of personality. DSM III: axis II.* New York: John Wiley.

Millon, T., and Klerman, G. L., eds. 1986. *Contemporary directions in psychopathology: Toward the DSM-IV.* New York, London: The Guildford Press.

Morris, D. 1987. *Bodywatching: A field guide to the human species.* London: Grafton.

Othmer, E., and Desouza, C. 1985. A rapid screening test for somatization disorder (hysteria). *Am. J. Psychiat.* 142:1146–49.

Othmer, E., Penick, E. C., and Powell, B. J. 1981. *The psychiatric diagnostic interview: Manual.* Los Angeles: Western Psychological Services. Copyright © 1981 by E. Othmer, E. C. Penick, and B. J. Powell. Excerpted and reprinted in this volume by permission of the publisher, Western Psychological Services, 12031 Wilshire Boulevard, Los Angeles, CA 90025.

Othmer, E., Penick, E. C., Powell, B. J., Read, M., and Othmer, S. C. 1988. *The psychiatric diagnostic interview.* Revision by E. C. Penick. Los Angeles: Western Psychological Services. Copyright © 1988 by E. Othmer, E. C. Penick, and B. J. Powell. Excerpted and reprinted in this volume by permission of the publisher, Western Psychological Services, 12031 Wilshire Boulevard, Los Angeles, CA 90025.

Payne, R. W., and Hewlett, J. H. G. 1960. Thought disorder in psychotic patients. In *Experiments in personality. Vol. 2, Psychodiagnostics and psychodynamics,* ed. H. J. Eysenck. New York: The Humanities Press.

Pope, B., and Siegman, A. W. 1965. Interviewer specificity and topical focus in relation to interviewer productivity. *J. of Verbal Learning and Verbal Behavior* 4:188–92.

Powell, B. J., Penick, E. C., Othmer, E., Bingham, S. F., and Rice, A. 1982. Prevalence of additional psychiatric syndromes among male alcoholics. *J. Clin. Psych.* 43:404–7.

Rado, S. 1956 and 1962. *Psychoanalysis of behavior,* vols. 1, 2. New York: Grune & Stratton.

Rank, O. 1952. *Will therapy and truth and reality.* New York: Alfred A. Knopf.

Reich, W. 1949. *Character analysis*. New York: Farrar, Strauss & Young.

Reitan, R. M., and Wolfson, D. 1985. *The Halstead-Reitan neuropsychological test battery: Theory and clinical interpretation*. Tucson, Ariz.: Neuropsychology Press.

Robins, E. 1981. The final months: A study of the lives of 134 persons who committed suicide. New York: Oxford University Press.

Rogers, C. R. 1951. *Client-centered therapy*. Boston: Houghton Mifflin.

Rose, F. C., and Bynum, W. F., eds. 1982. *Historical aspects of the neuro sciences: Festschrift for McDonald Critchley*. New York: Raven Press.

Ross, E. D. 1980. Disorders of higher cortical functions: Diagnosis and treatment. In vol. 5 of the *Science and Practice of Clinical Medicine: Neurology* eds. R. N. Rosenberg and J. M. Dietschy, pp. 589–602. New York: Grune & Stratton.

————. 1982. The divided self: Contrary to conventional wisdom, not all language is commanded by the brain's left side. *The Sciences* 22, 2:8–12.

Rutter, M., and Cox, A. 1981. Psychiatric interviewing techniques: I. Methods and measures. *Brit. J. Psychiat.* 138:273–82.

Rutter, M., Cox A., Egert, S., Holbrook, D., and Everitt, B. 1981. Psychiatric interviewing techniques IV. Experimental study: four contrasting styles. *Brit. J. Psychiat.* 138:456–65.

Saghir, M. T. 1971. A comparison of some aspects of structured and unstructured psychiatric interviews. *Am. J. Psychiat.* 128:180–84.

Sandifer, M. G., Jr. 1972. Psychiatric diagnosis: Cross-national research findings. *Proc. Royal Soc. Med.* 65:1–4.

Sandifer, M. G., Jr., Hordern, A., and Green, L. M. 1970. The psychiatric interview: The impact of the first three minutes. *Am. J. Psychiat.* 126:968–73.

Schneider, K. 1959. *Clinical psychopathology*. Translated by M. W. Hamilton. New York: Grune & Stratton.

Sheldon, W. H., and Stevens, S. S. 1942. The varieties of temperament: A psychology of constitutional differences. New York: Harper.

Siegman, A. W., and Pope, B., eds. 1972. *Studies in dyadic communication*. New York: Pergamon.

Strub, R. L., and Black, F. W. 1977. *The mental status examination in neurology*. Philadelphia: F. A. Davis. Excerpted and reprinted in this volume by permission of the publisher.

Sullivan, H. S. 1954. *The psychiatric interview*. New York: W. W. Norton.

Taylor, M. A. 1981. *The neuropsychiatric mental status examination*. SP Medical and Scientific Books. New York: Spectrum.

Taylor, M. A., and Abrams, R. 1973. The phenomenology of mania: A new look at some old patients. *Arch. Gen. Psychiat.* 29:520–22.

Truax, C. B., and Mitchell, K. M. 1971. Research on certain therapist interpersonal skills in relation to process and outcome. In *Handbook of psychotherapy and behavior change,* eds. A. E. Bojin and S. L. Garfield. New York: John Wiley.

Vaillant, G. E. 1986. *Empirical studies of ego mechanisms of defense.* Washington, D.C.: American Psychiatric Press.

Vaillant, G. E., and Perry, C. J. 1985. Personality disorders. In *Comprehensive textbook of psychiatry,* 4th ed., eds. H. I. Kaplan and B. J. Sadock, pp. 958–86. Baltimore, London: Williams and Wilkins.

Wechsler adult intelligence scale, revised (WAIS-R) manual. 1981. New York: The Psychological Corporation, Harcourt, Brace, Jovanovich.

Weinberg, H., and Hire, W. A. 1972. *Abnormal personalities: A book of case readings.* New York: MSS Information Corporation.

Wender, P. H., Kety, S. S., and Rosenthal, D. et al. 1986. Psychiatric disorders in the biological and adoptive families of adopted individuals with affective disorders. *Arch. Gen. Psychiat.* 43:923–29.

Wilson, I. C. 1967. Rapid Approximate Intelligence Test. *Am J. Psychiat.* 123:1289–90.

Winokur, G., and Crowe, R. R. 1975. Personality disorders. In *Comprehensive textbook of psychiatry-II,* vol. 2, 2d ed., eds. A. M. Freedman, H. I. Kaplan, and B. J. Sadock, pp. 1279–97. Baltimore: Williams and Wilkins.

Wolberg, L. R. 1967. *The techniques of psychotherapy,* 2d ed. New York: Grune & Stratton.

Zimmerman, M., Pfohl, B., Stangl, D., and Coryell, W. 1985. The validity of DSM-III axis IV (severity of psychosocial stressors). *Am. J. Psychiat.* 142:12, Dec.: 1437–41.

Zuckerman, M. 1978. Sensation seeking. In *Dimensions of personality,* eds. H. London and J. Exner. New York: John Wiley.

Zung, W. W. K. 1972. How normal is depression? *Psychosomatics* 13:174–78.

INDEX